D0073768

VOICE DISORDERS AND THEIR MANAGEMENT

VOICE DISORDERS AND THEIR MANAGEMENT

Edited by MARGARET FAWCUS

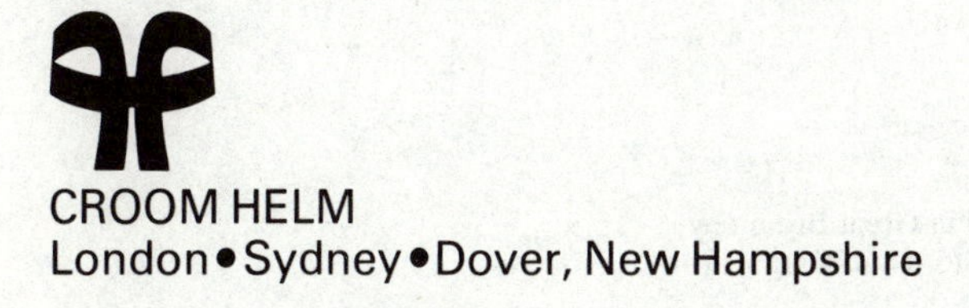

CROOM HELM
London • Sydney • Dover, New Hampshire

Croom Helm Ltd, Provident House, Burrell Row,
Beckenham, Kent BR3 1AT
Croom Helm Australia Pty Ltd, Suite 4, 6th Floor,
64–76 Kippax Street, Surry Hills, NSW 2010, Australia

British Library Cataloguing in Publication Data

Voice disorders and their management.
1. Voice disorders
I. Fawcus, Margaret
616.2′2 RF510

ISBN 0–7099–1070–3

Croom Helm, 51 Washington Street, Dover,
New Hampshire 03820, USA.

Library of Congress Cataloging in Publication Data
Main entry under title:

Voice disorders and their management.

Includes index.
1. Voice disorders. I. Fawcus, Margaret.
(DNLM: 1. Voice disorders—therapy. WV 500 V889)
RF510.V66 1986 616.85′5 85-31330
ISBN 0-7099-1070-3 (pbk.)

Printed and bound in Great Britain by
Biddles Ltd, Guildford and King's Lynn

CONTENTS

LIST OF CONTRIBUTORS

Judith Challoner, BA, LCST, Speech Therapy Department, West Middlesex University Hospital, Twickenham Road, Isleworth, Middlesex TW7 6AF: and The Gender Identity Clinic, Charing Cross Hospital.
David D. Clarke, MA (Cantab), MA (Oxon), DPhil, AB, PsS, Senior Research Officer, Department of Experimental Psychology, University of Oxford, South Parks Road, Oxford OX1 3UD.
Sara Collins, LCST, Senior Speech Therapist, ENT Department, The Radcliffe Infirmary, Woodstock Road, Oxford OX2 6HE.
Kay Coombes, Dip CST, MCST, Senior Lecturer in Speech Pathology and Therapeutics, Central School of Speech and Drama, Embassy Theatre, 64 Eton Avenue, London NW3 3HY.
Eryl Evans, LCST Senior Speech Therapist, Speech Therapy Department, Singleton Hospital, Swansea SA2 8QA.
Bob Fawcus, BSc, FCST, Director of Postgraduate Studies, Centre for Clinical Communication Studies, The City University, 214 St John Street, London EC1V 0HB.
Margaret Fawcus, MSc, FCST, Director of Undergraduate Studies, Centre for Clinical Communication Studies, The City University, 214 St John Street, London EC1V 0HB.
Margaret Freeman, LCST, School of Speech Therapy, Department of Science, City of Birmingham Polytechnic, Franchise Street, Perry Barr, Birmingham B42 2US.
Margaret Gordon, DTST, Area Speech Therapist, Greater Glasgow Health Board; Speech Therapist, Victoria Infirmary, Langside, Glasgow G42 9TY.
Thomas M. Harris, MA, FRCS, Laryngologist, ENT Department, The Radcliffe Infirmary, Woodstock Road, Oxford OX2 6HE.
Elaine Hodkinson, LCST, Director of Speech Therapy, Central School of Speech and Drama, Embassy Theatre, 64 Eton Avenue, London NW3 3HY.
Andrew Johns, MA, FRCS, Consultant ENT Surgeon, The Kent Aural and Ophthalmic Hospital , Maidstone, Kent.
Sheila Scott, BSc, MCST, Senior Speech Therapist, Drumchapel Hospital, Glasgow G15 6PX.

Malcolm Stockley, MA, MEd, Dip Ed, Dip CST, MCST, FRSH, FCP, LCST, Senior Lecturer, Central School of Speech and Drama, Embassy Theatre, 64 Eton Avenue, London NW3 3HY.
Margaret L. Stoicheff, PhD, Professor and Acting Chairman, Graduate Department of Speech Pathology, University of Toronto, Toronto, Ontario, Canada.
Sheila Wirz, MEd, LCST, Senior Lecturer, National Hospitals College of Speech Sciences, 59 Portland Place, London W1N 3AJ.
Brian Williams, MB, ChB, FRCP, Consultant in Administrative Charge, Division of Geriatric Medicine, Gartnavel General Hospital, 1053 Great Western Road, Glasgow G12 0YN.

INTRODUCTION

> The great functional vulnerability of the vocal organs may, at least in part, derive from a paradoxical situation, for we use for the delicate task of self expression a set of structures that originally was not created for this purpose. The sphincteric origin of the larynx and the pharynx makes them more suitable for closure, for shutting off, than for emission.
>
> Brodnitz (1959)

Voice disorders, seen against the broad landscape of communication problems, are unique in a number of ways: in the first place, the management of vocal dysfunction has been something of a grey area where voice training and speech therapy meet in a mutual interest in voice production. This was demonstrated in a recent voice symposium at the Royal Society of Medicine where both singing teachers and speech therapists were in the audience. It must be remembered that the majority of early therapists came from a background of speech and drama training and practice and these beginnings have obviously been influential in the techniques employed in remedial voice work.

Secondly, it has been an area somewhat bedevilled by a reliance on subjective judgements, both in describing the pathological voice and in attempting to evaluate the treatment. This has been true in spite of the feedback on the laryngeal condition provided by direct and indirect laryngoscopy. The therapist could hardly be blamed for this state of affairs, since until recently there has been little available in the way of a more objective approach to voice evaluation. The chapters in this book by Eryl Evans and Margaret Gordon illustrate the assessment procedures available in a specialist voice clinic compared to the rather more limited technological hardware available in the majority of general hospitals. The picture is gradually changing, but may be expected to change very slowly in the current economic climate.

While the emergence of more sophisticated and objective assessment procedures represents one of the most significant advances in voice management, the competent and experienced therapist may have to work quite effectively on a modest budget.

imaginative and interesting approaches to voice therapy and, perhaps most important of all, personality characteristics and non-verbal behaviours which enable her to establish a comfortable and reassuring environment. Collins and Harris have discussed the vital factor of patient satisfaction in evaluating treatment efficacy.

The idea for this book arose some years ago, and was born of an increasing concern that intervention strategies in dysphonia often seemed to have very little to do with the cause of the voice problem or the presenting symptoms of the dysphonic patient. Indeed some clinical practice appeared largely irrelevant to the patient's real needs. Increasing experience has done little to change this viewpoint, and has acted as a spur in producing this volume. Whether the exercise will prove a worthwhile one for the reader will depend on the answers to the following questions:

> Does the book meet the needs of those who are seeking to increase their own expertise in the management of voice disorders?
> Will it lead the clinician to question the rationale behind some of the more traditional approaches to voice therapy?

More than any other area of speech therapy, therapeutic techniques in the management of dysphonia have their roots in a speech and drama model of training. We should develop what is relevant and worthwhile in that model, but remember that much of the expertise gained in working with the normal voice in order to obtain high standards of artistic achievement (as in acting or singing) is largely inappropriate to voice use in less demanding everyday circumstances. This point will be discussed more fully in the chapter on hyperfunctional voice use.

It is hoped that this book will meet a very real need in student training, since it is seldom possible to give that depth of clinical experience which is needed to produce a confident and competent therapist. Many qualified therapists, except those working in association with interested ENT surgeons, may have relatively few voice referrals and therefore limited opportunities to develop a tried and trusted repertoire of therapeutic techniques. This book will give them the opportunity to share the knowledge, ideas and understanding of therapists who have had the experience of working more intensively with both the prevalent and more rare causes of voice disorders.

In editing this volume, certain rather arbitrary decisions had to be made in omitting important areas of voice production — background information on the physiology of the larynx and disorders of resonance, for example. It would not have been possible to do justice to the latter, a rapidly expanding area of expertise, in the space available. There is no chapter on the voice of senescence, although the problems of the ageing voice are discussed in Chapter 12. Very few elderly people are sufficiently concerned or handicapped by the gradual changes in their voice to seek professional help, probably regarding the process as a normal rather than pathological one. It was, however, felt that a book on voice would be incomplete without a chapter on the acquisition of voice in the laryngectomised patient. The post-radiotherapy voice is also considered by Stoicheff, since this is an area which is assuming greater importance as radiotherapy is becoming an increasingly refined and successful form of treatment in laryngeal carcinoma.

We would like to place on record the help we have received in many forms from our colleagues and friends. Many of us have stretched the tolerance of long-suffering families, whose only reward is to know it is all over! Finally, we are inevitably indebted to the patients, who have undoubtedly taught us more than any textbook.

Margaret Fawcus

1 THE CAUSES AND CLASSIFICATION OF VOICE DISORDERS

Margaret Fawcus

Introduction

The chapter titles of this book indicate the wide range of causes of voice disorder. Basically, there are three conditions in which phonation can be affected:

(1) The vocal folds may show structural abnormalities;
(2) The folds may appear normal at rest but may demonstrate a disturbance of movement patterns;
(3) There may be no apparent organic impairment in terms of either structure or function.

These three conditions will now be considered in rather more detail:

(1) The larynx is vulnerable to physical stress which can result in the build-up of tissue reactions (vocal nodules, contact ulcers or non-specific laryngitis). Physical vulnerability, upper respiratory tract infection and personality factors, as well as the demands of the situation, may all combine to produce a voice disorder. Where the vocal folds fail to present smooth vibrating edges, capable of full adduction along their total length, we may expect a voice characterised by air waste and a quality which may variously be described as 'rough', 'hoarse' or 'husky'.

As indicated, such changes in the smooth appearance of the vocal folds may be a direct result of inappropriate voice use. In other cases, there may be changes caused by physical trauma, such as intratracheal intubation during general anaesthesia, haematoma or granuloma, by infection, or by benign or malignant new growths (or the tissue changes which precede them). These are initially the province of the surgeon, although speech therapy may be needed in some cases following appropriate medical or surgical treatment.

Excessive alcohol consumption, smoking, chemical irritants, certain drugs and hormone imbalance may also lead to tissue changes in the larynx. In many cases these factors occur in combination to have an adverse effect on voice quality.

(2) The structure of the vocal folds may be normal but the movement of the cords may be affected. Disturbed vocal function may be part of the dysarthrophonic syndrome (Peacher, 1949) where there is a disease process of the central nervous system, affecting both articulation and phonation. The dysarthrias associated with cerebellar, extrapyramidal, lower motor neurone and bilateral cortical lesions have associated voice problems involving all aspects of voice production (see Scott and Williams, Chapter 7 of this volume).

At a peripheral level, there may be interference with the nerve supply to one or both vocal folds. The most common of these is a unilateral recurrent laryngeal nerve lesion (see Stockley, Chapter 8 of this volume).

(3) Voice disorders can exist in the apparent absence of any physical cause, although this may reflect the present state of the investigation procedures rather than the true state of affairs. In some of these cases, more refined techniques, such as laryngeal microscopy, may reveal previously unidentified physical signs. This shift of emphasis from a psychogenic to a physical cause is demonstrated very clearly in the case of spastic dysphonia (see Stoicheff, Chapter 15 of this volume).

Generally speaking, however, wherever there are no apparent signs, the dysphonia is labelled as 'functional', 'psychogenic' or even 'hysterical'. Freeman (Chapter 11 of this volume) has indicated the complexities of the situation and the need for a careful evaluation of the variables involved. Despite the increasing sophistication in our approach to these functional voice disorders, one can still receive a referral which states: 'This lady has a tensor weakness of the larynx with no evidence of local lesion. I have explained that this is an emotional problem. . . .'

There are two other areas where the client has a normal voice mechanism but the voice is perceived as abnormal: in cases of significant hearing loss and in transsexualism. Increasing interest has developed in recent years in the indirect but often very marked effects of profound hearing loss for the frequencies of voice production (see Wirz, Chapter 14 of this volume). The speaker has a *potential* for normal voice production which is never realised due to his severely impaired auditory feedback mechanism and, in the case of acquired profound hearing loss, the continuous auditory monitoring that enables us to maintain consistent and appropriate intensity, pitch and intonation patterns.

In the case of the transsexual (see Challoner, Chapter 13 of this volume), we may indeed challenge the concept of a voice *disorder*, since the vocal pitch (the only aspect of voice with which the transsexual is normally concerned) may be entirely in keeping with the physical constraints of the laryngeal structure. There is, however, a mismatch between the modal range and the desired gender which the transsexual wishes to convey.

We must now consider what we mean by a voice disorder, and examine the ways in which interested speech therapists, laryngologists and phoniatrists have attempted to classify the aphonias and dysphonias.

'A voice disorder exists,' says Aronson (1980) 'when quality, pitch, loudness or flexibility differs from the voice of others of similar age, sex, and cultural group.' It is on variants of these four perceived parameters of voice production that the listener judges the normality or otherwise of the voice he hears. Aronson considers that these judgements are made in relation to the listener's expectations regarding sex and age within a given cultural group. We must also consider the listener's individual preferences and biases, and his level of awareness of how voices sound and the differences between them. There is a continuum extending from the voice that is clear and audible to one which is unmistakably dysphonic.

Different listeners, asked to make a judgement about a speaker's voice, will not always place that voice at the same point on the continuum. For one listener, a voice may be acceptably 'normal', while for another judge the same voice may be noted as frankly abnormal. Wynter (1974) has emphasised the subjectivity of listeners' judgements which has given rise to a confusing variety of terms to describe voices quality. 'Typically they are based on subjective auditory judgements rather than on objective observations of vocal function' (Reed, 1980).

It is inevitable that problems occur in devising a satisfactory classification of voice disorders, because they so often represent the culmination of a number of predisposing, precipitating and maintaining factors. Perkins (1971) has commented that we are 'mired in a terminological swamp, with terms whose lineage is physiological, anatomical, acoustical and psychological'. While most writers are agreed that there is a need to strive for a greater objectivity, we must remember that descriptive labels may be important and meaningful to the voice user himself. As Thurman (1977) observes, the client's own terms may be inaccurate and difficult to define, but they may have more relationship to what he is doing vocally than the usual professional terms: 'The clinician should pick up the terms the client uses and attempt to identify the problem as the client sees it and to relate it to normal voice production.'

Dysphonia, Aronson (1980) reminds us, is a disorder of communication and has 'personal, social and economic significance'. In judging the normality of voice he poses the following questions:

(1) Is the voice adequate to carry language intelligibly to the listener?
(2) Are its acoustic properties aesthetically acceptable?
(3) Does it satisfy its owner's occupational and social requirements?

The answers to these questions provide an effective way of judging, in the first place, whether the patient actually has a voice problem, and secondly, in helping us to evaluate the efficacy of our remedial procedures.

There is, however, one further dimension of voice disorders which has received scant attention in the literature: how does the voice *feel* to the patient? The degree of discomfort experienced is a vital and sensitive barometer of the condition of the larynx and the state of voice use. However normal the voice may sound to the therapist, or to anyone else for that matter, if it does not feel comfortable to the patient then we have failed in our task of vocal remediation. *Absence* of physical awareness of the voice is the target to be achieved.

Before considering some of the ways in which voice has been classified, we must remember that labels may be applied at a number of different levels. Brackett (1971) has discussed this problem in a very comprehensive contribution on the parameters of voice quality. Much will depend on who is applying the label: the patient describing his problem; the laryngologist reporting on the appearance or movement of the vocal folds; the therapist noting the perceived symptoms; or the physicist measuring certain acoustic phenomena of voice production. In other words, are we making some sort of classification on the acoustic, anatomical, physiological or psychological correlates of voice disorder? As Brackett says, 'the nature of the disorder remains the same, although different labels may have been used in its descriptions'.

Classification Based on Acoustic Phenomena

Wilson (1979) has observed that voice problems are 'traditionally' classified under the *aspect* of voice affected (quality, loudness and pitch problems). While this is a useful and apparently simple form of classification, we are immediately faced with the fact that in the majority of dysphonic patients all aspects of voice production are affected.

As Van Riper and Irwin (1958) observe, 'seldom does the abnormal variation exist along one dimension of voice alone'. Classically, the dysphonic voice is weak in intensity, restricted in pitch and 'hoarse' or 'husky' in quality. While we may encounter conditions where a single feature of voice is affected, such as the level of intensity in the early stages of Parkinson's disease, these cases are relatively uncommon. Furthermore, such a classification does not tell us all we need to know about the causes underlying the disturbed acoustic features. There are, of course, exceptions: the overloud voice in an elderly person may suggest a fairly marked degree of presbycusis, and persistent monotony may be associated with depression. Such exceptions are scarcely sufficient to justify the use of a classification system which is more appropriate as an assessment tool.

The majority of voice cases present as 'weak', 'hoarse' or 'husky' (or whatever we may choose to apply in place of these terms) and demonstrate a disorder along all parameters. It is also important to consider those cases who are referred with a voice that appears essentially normal, but where the problem may be one of vocal fatigue and discomfort, with as yet little effect on the way the voice *sounds*.

When we examine the many terms which are used to describe voice quality there are three which occur most frequently: harsh, hoarse and breathy. While they represent an essentially subjective judgement of voice, there does appear to be surprising agreement in their use.

The term 'breathy' implies that there is a degree of air waste during phonation. Moore (1971) described the breathy voice as a combination of vocal fold sound and whisper noise produced by turbulent air. 'The quality of the breathy voice,' he says, 'varies over a wide range that is determined by the ratio of breath noise to phonatory sound.' Air waste occurs when there is incomplete adduction of the vocal folds, which may have an organic cause (bowing of the cords or vocal nodules), or may be an habitual pattern of voice in the absence of organic changes.

The harsh voice, by contrast, implies that the vocal folds are adducting normally, but that the speaker is employing excessive tension. An alternative synonym for harsh is strident, again a term which occurs frequently in the literature. Van Riper and Irwin (1958) state categorically that the essential feature of the harsh voice is tension. They quote a study by Brackett (1971) in which inflammation of the vocal folds was achieved experimentally by the deliberate use of harsh voice. They say that the intensity of the harsh voice appears louder than normal, but consider that this may result from the effect on resonance of tension in the oral and pharyngeal cavities. It is commonly characterised by a hard glottal attack. Brackett (1971) has described this as hypervalvular phonation '. . . the vocal folds strike each other vigorously at the beginning of the closed phase and separate violently when the opening phase is initiated'. In addition, 'the vocal folds offer increased resistance to air flow with subsequent increase in subglottal air pressure'. The harsh voice has been described as generally lower in pitch than normal. Bowler's (1964) study found a mean fundamental frequency of 94 Hz for harsh voices compared to 127 Hz for normal adult male voices.

Depending on the physical vulnerability of the vocal folds, such habitual vocal misuse may eventually lead to tissue changes of chronic laryngitis, vocal nodules or contact ulcers. The therapist hearing a voice which has this harsh, strident quality is alert to the risk of vocal abuse, particularly if the patient complains of vocal discomfort after voice use, or periods of vocal weakness and pitch breaks.

The majority of dysphonic voices, however, present as 'hoarse' and this is the label most often encountered. Wilson (1979) states that 'hoarseness in its simplest definition is a combination of harshness and breathiness, with the harsh element predominating in some hoarse voices and the breathy element in others'. In addition to the turbulence created by air waste, there is also an aperiodicity of fundamental frequency. Van Riper and Irwin

(1958) describe an experiment in which a husky (breathy) and a harsh voice were blended in simultaneous recording of the same sentence. Eight of the ten judges listening to the resultant recording described the voice as hoarse. The tension present in hoarse phonation may represent the patient's physical effort to compensate for a weak, breathy voice. In some cases this tension may represent a long-term pattern of vocal behaviour (hyperfunction) which resulted in a weak (hypofunctional) voice (Brodnitz, 1959). On the other hand, tension may have been of more recent origin — for example, occurring after an attack of acute laryngitis, where the patient was trying to make himself heard. Boone (1977) wrote of these 'temporary laryngeal changes which cause compensatory vocal behaviours that persist and become the individual's particular *set* for subsequent vocal behaviour'.

As we have already said, one important constraint of a classification based on perceptual factors is the limited information it offers about the condition of the larynx in terms of muscle movement and tissue change, and the causes of the voice disorder. Clearly, we have to look elsewhere for a more satisfactory classification, leaving the areas of pitch, intensity, intonation and quality to be the focus of careful assessment and evaluation.

The Functional Versus Organic Dichotomy

The classical approach to classification is the broad one of a functional versus organic dichotomy, but as Van Riper and Irwin (1958) comment, 'both organic and functional factors are often present and it is difficult or impossible to weigh their influence properly'. Aronson (1980), who gives a comprehensive survey of organic voice disorders, describes the cause as organic 'if it is caused by structural (anatomic) or physiologic disease, either a disease in the larynx itself or remote systemic illnesses which impair laryngeal structure or function'. Brackett (1971), in discussing some of the theoretical difficulties involved in using such a classification, makes three important points: in the first place, a speech structure may be used in a variety of ways and therefore we may use the normal voice mechanism to produce a number of different acoustic effects; secondly, the way in which a structure is used may have an effect on that structure — it is well documented that hyperfunctional voice use leads to vocal nodules, inflammation and oedema; thirdly, certain structural anomalies, such as laryngeal web, will place constraints on voice use. 'Present understanding,' says Brackett, 'does not permit a clear differentiation between the two terms functional and organic since both the condition and the use of the structure are determinants in the assessment of the disorder.'

The condition of vocal nodules is a very clear example of the oversimplification which the organic/functional dichotomy represents. The essential element in the development of nodules is the manner in which the patient is using his voice. Van Riper and Irwin (1958) provide a graphic picture of the 'repeated impact of highly tensed vocal cords hitting each other under conditions of excessive strain' which eventually leads to a tissue reaction in the epithelium of the larynx. It is these organic changes, in the form of small, bilateral, localised fibrous growths, that prevent full adduction of the free edges of the vocal folds, and result in a voice characterised by air waste, and, in most cases, by the hoarse quality that indicates the excessive effort the patient is making to overcome the vocal weakness. The organic problem is indeed having its effect on the voice, but initially it was the way in which the vocal mechanism was used which created the organic condition. This same patient may experience considerable anxiety about his dysphonic voice and its effect on his career or social activities. This can lead to still further localised or generalised tension. He may try to compensate for his weak voice by making greater vocal efforts, which inevitably lead to a worsening of the organic condition. This illustrates the complex interaction between functional and organic factors, and underlines the essential limitations involved in using this form of classification. As Wilson (1979) says, 'the continuum' (between organic and functional) 'is a two-way path because a pathology can result in a poorly functioning mechanism, or a poorly functioning mechanism can result in organic changes or an organic condition'.

This brings us to a more careful consideration of the term functional. Brackett (1971) says that functional applies to the physiology or use of the structures in attaining particular objectives. Aronson (1980) takes a very different view in claiming that functional is a synonym for psychogenic, and that psychogenic voice disorders are caused by psychoneuroses, personality disorders and faulty habits of voice use. The voice is abnormal 'despite normal anatomy and physiology'. Wilson (1979) uses 'functional' as an umbrella term to include both vocal misuse and emotional disturbances.

In using the word 'functional' in clinical practice, it is clearly important that we define our meaning. For many speech pathologists, the term implies a psychogenic voice disorder, in the apparent absence of vocal misuse. However, the concept of 'vocal misuse and abuse' (Van Thal, 1961) may also be properly regarded as a functional problem. It is obviously essential, in the management of voice disorders, to be clear what we mean by the term. To complicate the issue still further, functional is frequently used synonymously with hysterical, but as Van Thal observed, 'strictly speaking, hysterical aphonia is one form of functional voice disorder, and not all functional disorders are hysterical'.

The fact that the term hysterical is mentioned rather rarely in current literature on dysphonia, reflects a considerable shift in the appraisal of functional voice disorders and the changing attitudes on the subject of hysteria. It is interesting to note, for example, that Greene (1980) in the first edition of *The Voice and its Disorders*, wrote a chapter on 'Hysterical aphonia and dysphonia' (1964). In the third and fourth edition of the same book, the chapter is retitled 'Psychogenic disorders: anxiety and hysterical states'. Such changes in terminology represent a more careful approach to factors underlying so-called functional voice disorders. It is unfortunate that the term 'hysterical' should still be applied by therapists and ENT surgeons, with all its negative implications and connections. Luchsinger and Arnold (1965) suggest that it is better to avoid the term hysterical 'because of its derogatory characterological and sociological connotations'. It is all too easy to label a condition as 'neurotic' or 'hysterical' when it fails to respond to traditional treatment methods. Three or four decades ago, there was a parallel in the 'neurotic' lisp (lateral sigmatism). This form of articulatory deviation was labelled as a symptom of neuroticism in the absence of any evidence more convincing that the difficulties encountered in trying to correct the error sound (neurotic resistance!), and perhaps because the aesthetic qualities of lateral substitutions tend to provoke negative reactions in the listener. Very few therapists at the time possessed the necessary expertise to evaluate the oral morphology and motor abilities of the child, or the knowledge of skills acquisition which might have made their intervention programme more effective. We have seen the same changes taking place in stuttering, which is now seldom regarded as a primary neurosis. Conditions which fail to respond to treatment create anxiety in the therapist, and it is easy to understand how failures came to be blamed on concepts such as secondary gain and hysterical states. There are undoubtedly parallels here in voice therapy — we need to develop our understanding of vocal behaviour and improve our expertise in both the assessment of voice disorder and in the evaluation of the many variables which tend to predispose, precipitate and maintain it.

We have seen that the terms 'functional', 'psychogenic' and 'hysterical' have been used synonymously, and have been applied to those patients who exhibit a voice problem in the absence of any apparent organic symptoms on indirect or direct laryngoscopy. The use of the word 'apparent' is important: as Freeman (Chapter 11 of this volume) has stressed, increased knowledge of laryngeal function and the physical effects of stress, have made us aware of the need to investigate for hitherto unexpected causes of laryngeal dysfunctions.

We know, for example, that dysphonia (manifest by a lowering of pitch and a roughness of quality) is an early symptom of hypothyroidism which may be overlooked on laryngeal examination. Damsté (1967) has warned that the administration of androgens and anabolic steroids can result in vocal symptoms, such as 'unsteadiness of timbre', before changes are revealed by laryngoscopy or even stroboscopic examination. In a four-year period (1962–66) 10 per cent of women referred to the ENT clinic at the University of Utrecht had disturbances of vocal function due to virilising agents. It is not difficult to imagine that a label of psychogenic dysphonia could easily be applied to a group of menopausal women, with all the domestic and emotional problems associated with middle age! So the therapist must be aware of possible discreet physical changes which are not visible on what may have been a superficial examination (for example, indirect laryngoscopy of a patient whose larynx has been difficult to view).

In summary, functional is an umbrella term which can be used to describe a number of vocal behaviours:

(1) It can refer to those cases where abuse and misuse of the vocal mechanism is clearly indicated.
(2) We may propose that it is used for all 'learned' patterns of maladaptive vocal behaviour (for example, a compensatory mode of voice production which develops during a period of acute infective laryngitis).

(3) The umbrella must be large enough to cover an apparently psychogenic cause where there is a cumulative history of emotional stress and tension, but the patient does not present with a recent history of vocal fold pathology or evidence of misuse. Sudden onset can be associated with emotionally traumatic events.

We might further divide such apparently psychogenic cases into two groups:

(a) Patients who present with a (sometimes long) history of psychosomatic conditions and a positive psychiatric history, who seem to be particularly vulnerable to physical and emotional stress;
(b) Patients who appear to have a stable personality, and an absence of psychiatric history, but where the voice problem is a reaction to prolonged and increasing stress and tension in their domestic or work environment.

It is not within the scope of this chapter to discuss the possible mechanism of sudden or even more gradual voice loss in psychogenic voice disorder, or to consider the personality and physical variables involved in response to stress. It is obvious, however, that we need to be very clear in our own mind what we mean when we describe a voice case as functional, since this will inevitably have considerable implications for treatment. Quite apart from the problems involved in obtaining appropriate and effective psychiatric treatment, many patients would be distressed or defensive about such a referral. We must therefore be sure that we are not dealing with a case where careful management in terms of environmental modification, counselling and vocal remediation by the therapist is not the more appropriate course of action.

It has been demonstrated that the functional/organic dichotomy is not an entirely satisfactory form of classification. As Murphy (1964) said, they represent 'an untenable dichotomy'. He went on to say, however, that it is a convenient classification despite the imprecision of the terms, since most therapists recognise that in many functional cases subtle organic factors exist, and that in most, if not all, organic cases functional factors can be found[7].

Figure 1:1 below may help us to view this interaction more clearly and enable us to examine a patient's voice problem at any point on the triangle:

Figure 1.1

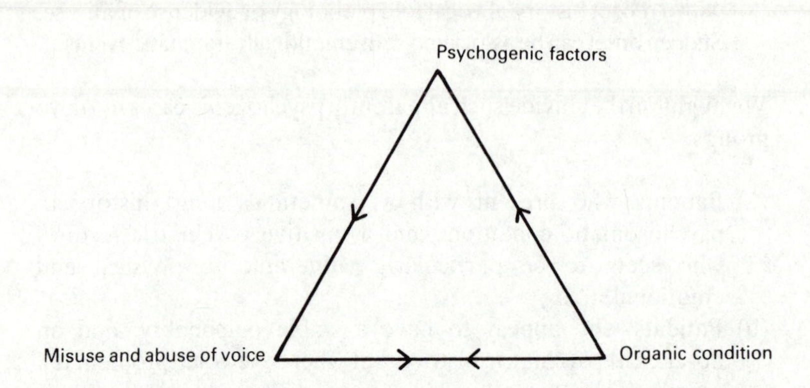

With this concept of a triangle in which organic processes, misuse and abuse and psychogenic factors interact, we may establish a kind of 'flowchart' which may aid our understanding of the several predisposing, precipitating and maintaining factors in all cases of dysphonia.

Hyperfunctional and Hypofunctional Voice Use

Some attempts have been made to classify voice on a continuum of overadduction or underadduction. Greene (1980) prefers the term hyperkinetic which she equates with vocal strain. Brackett (1971) introduces the concept of hypovalvular and hypervalvular phonation, which can clearly be used synonymously with hyperfunctional and hypofunctional and hyperkinetic and hypokinetic. He describes optimal laryngeal valving as a degree of valving which 'offers sufficient resistance to air flow to accomplish unhampered vibrations of the vocal folds at the desired intensity for speech'.

Luchsinger and Arnold (1965) use the term hypokinetic to describe inefficient laryngeal movements, 'reflecting the passive breakdown of laryngeal function'. Hyperkinetic refers to excessive laryngeal movements, which 'express the subconscious, aggressive protest of the patient against the difficulties encountered in his life'. They view both these problems as dysphonias of psychogenic origin.

Aronson (1980) uses the term kinesiologic for this form of classification, and comments that although this idea is not without merit, if used exclusively it 'oversimplifies the complexities of the laryngeal pathologies, placing excess emphasis on the degree of appropriation of the vocal edges rather than on the multiple causes of such approximation defects'.

The Aetiological Classification of Voice Disorders

A classification which looks at the causes of voice disorder 'encourages the deepest understanding of dysphonia or aphonia' (Aronson, 1980). Such a form of classification, based on the physical condition of the larynx, tends to have been developed by laryngologists. It implies the need for a careful investigation of the physical factors which may be involved, involving such diverse disciplines as otolaryngology, neurology and endocrinology. Indeed, while referrals normally come via the ENT department, both surgeons and speech therapists need to be alert to the possibility of both endocrine and neurological pathology as causative factors. Freeman (see Chapter 11 of this volume) emphasised that apparent absence of observable signs cannot always be assumed to indicate a psychogenic voice disorder.

Simpson's (1971) classification of voice disorders is given by Evans (Chapter 18 of this volume) and will therefore not be detailed here. It provides a systematic and comprehensive framework for the study of voice disorders and has clearly facilitated co-operation between laryngologists and speech therapists. Simpson wrote that 'dysphonia in the absence of gross laryngeal pathology has in the past received scant attention from the orthodox laryngologist, whose very training has concentrated his interest on gross pathology and life-threatening disease'. Such a statement has been less true in other parts of Europe, with emergence of the specialist area of medicine known as phoniatrics. Most, but not all, phoniatrists were originally otolaryngologists with a special interest in voice.

Luchsinger and Arnold (1965) give the following system of classification:

(1) Dsyplastic dysphonia: voice disorders of constitutions origin
(2) Vocal nodules and polyps: primary dysphonia and secondary laryngitis
(3) Endocrine dysphonia: vocal disorders of endocrine origin
(4) Paralytic dysphonia: vocal disorders from laryngeal paralysis
(5) Dysarthric dysphonia: vocal disorders of central origin
(6) Myopathic dysphonia: vocal disorders of myopathic origin
(7) The influence of neurovegetative system on the voice (in which they included vasomotor monochorditis and contact ulcers)
(8) Traumatic dysphonia: vocal disorders following laryngeal injury
(9) Alaryngeal dysphonia: voice without larynx
(10) Habitual dysphonia: vocal disorder of habitual origin
(11) Psychogenic dysphonia: vocal disorders of emotional origin

Aronson's aetiology of voice disorders is broken down under three main headings: organic and psychogenic, and those of indeterminate aetiology (under which he wisely places spastic dysphonia!). Under the organic heading: he lists the following causes:

Congenital disorders
Inflammation
Tumours
Endocrine disorders
Trauma
Neurological disease

The psychogenic voice disorders are listed as follows:

Emotional stress — musculoskeletal tension
Voice disorders without the secondary laryngeal pathology
Voice disorders with secondary laryngeal pathology (vocal nodules and contact ulcer)
Psychoneurosis
Conversion reaction — mutism, aphonia and dysphonia
Psychosocial conflict — mutational falsetto (puberphonia), dysphonias associated with conflict of sex identification
Iatrogenic

His classification of psychogenic voice disorders tends to assume causes which may not be demonstrated so easily — puberphonia may have a number of causes, and psychosocial conflict is not necessarily one of them! Not everyone would accept that hyperfunctional voice use should be classified as psychogenic. Aronson's classification remains, however, a useful and simple way of classifying voice disorders, devised by an experienced speech pathologist.

The aetiological classification attempts to locate the precise area of breakdown in the vocal mechanism, and the cause of that breakdown. It is the most essential aspect of assessment of vocal dysfunction, since we may find that there is a condition which requires medical and surgical treatment. Management of the voice disorder may therefore be irrelevant in some cases, or follows only after appropriate treatment from a laryngologist or endocrinologist.

Conclusions

Perhaps we have worried too much about getting the words right. Finally it is the patient and those who have to listen to him who will judge whether the voice is normal or not, whatever the 'experts' may say about the matter. The experts, however, continue to discuss the problem of describing voices, and continue to search for a more satisfactory way of doing so. We have seen that it is possible to look at voice disorders in a number of different ways: happily these are not mutually exclusive and each one may yield not only different information about the voice disorder but also a different way of looking at it. Perceptually we may describe the acoustic features of voice production in terms of pitch, intonation, intensity and quality; we recognise the variables involved in the development of voice disorders by attempting to describe the cause as functional or organic; the concept of underadduction or overadduction indicates the degree of tension involved, which has important implications for treatment procedures; and finally, it is the laryngologist and other medical specialists who give us a precise account of what is wrong (if anything) with the condition of the larynx and provide an essential opportunity to assess the efficacy of our treatment.

References

Aronson, A. E. *Clinical Voice Disorders: An Interdisciplinary Approach* (Thieme-Stratton, New York, 1980)
Boone, D. R. *The Voice and Voice Therapy* (Prentice-Hall, Englewood Cliffs, NJ, 1977)
Bowler, N. W. 'A Fundamental Frequency Analysis of Harsh Vocal Quality', *Speech Monograph*, 31 (1964)
Brackett, I. P. 'Parameters of Voice Quality', in L.E. Travis (ed.) *Handbook of Speech Pathology and Audiology* (Appleton-Century-Crofts, New York, 1971)
Brodnitz, F. S. *Vocal Rehabilitation*, 4th edn (American Academy of Ophthalmology and Otolaryngology, Rochester, Minnesota, 1959)
Damste, P. H. 'Voice Change in Adult Women Caused by Virilising Agents', *Journal of Speech and Hearing Disorders*, 32, 2 (1967)
Greene, M. C. L. *The Voice and its Disorders* (Pitman Medical, Tunbridge Wells, 1980)
Luchsinger, R. and Arnold, G. E. *Voice — Speech — Language — Clinical Communicology: Its Physiology and Pathology* (Constable, London, 1965)
Moore, G. P. 'Voice Disorders Organically Based', in L.E. Travis (ed.) *Handbook of Speech Pathology and Audiology* (Appleton Century-Crofts New York 1971)
Murphy, A. T. *Functional Voice Disorders* (Prentice-Hall, Englewood Cliffs, 1964)
Peacher, W. G. 'Neurological Factors in the Aetiology of Delayed Speech', *Journal of Speech and Hearing Disorders*, 14 (1949)
Perkins, W. H. 'Vocal Function: A Behavioural Analysis', in L. E. Travis (ed.) *Handbook of Speech Pathology and Audiology* (Appleton-Century-Crofts, New York, 1971)
Reed, C. G. 'Voice Therapy — A Need for Research' *Journal of Speech and Hearing Disorders*, 45, 2 (1980)
Simpson, I. C. 'Dysphonia: The Organisation and Working of a Dysphonia Clinic', *British Journal of Disorders in Communication*, 6, 70 (1971)
Thurman, W. L. 'Restructuring Voice Concepts and Production', in M. Cooper and M. H. Cooper (eds) *Approaches to Vocal Rehabilitation*(C. C. Thomas, Springfield, Illinois, 1977)
Van Riper, C. and Irwin, J.V. *Voice and Articulation*. (Prentice-Hall, Englewood Cliffs, New Jersey, 1958)
Van Thal, J. H. Dysphonia, *Speech Pathology and Therapy*, 4, 1 (1961)
Wilson, D. K. *Voice Problems of Children* (Williams and Wilkins, London, 1979)
Wynter, H. 'An Investigation into the Analysis and Terminology of Voice Quality and its Correlation with the Assessment Reliability of Speech Therapists', *British Journal of Disorders in Communication*, 9 (1974)

2 ASSESSMENT OF THE DYSPHONIC PATIENT

Margaret Gordon

Introduction

Dysphonia is usually the first and most obvious symptom of laryngeal disease but may also occur in a variety of disorders where vocal dysfunction is a secondary feature resulting from abnormality of the respiratory, nervous, endocrine or psychological systems and, in many cases, with no organic disease present. Most dysphonias of short duration are of simple inflammatory origin caused by viral or, less commonly, bacterial infection and do not justify formal investigation and assessment, but where the main symptom of hoarseness persists for no apparent reason, expert opinion must be sought without delay to exclude serious pathology or permit its early treatment.

This usually means that the patient is referred to an otolaryngologist as it is essential that the larynx should be examined visually to exclude inherent disease of the vocal cords, or other evidence of organic malfunction. Where no disease that requires surgical intervention or medical treatment is found, the case is usually left in the hands of the speech therapist who assesses the functional disorder and is responsible for subsequent management and treatment. However, many hospitals in the United Kingdom now operate joint consultative dysphonia clinics using the combined expertise of a laryngologist and speech therapist, requesting assistance from a neurologist, endocrinologist, or psychologist when appropriate, perhaps as signs and symptoms of the underlying disease develop or become modified with time (Simpson, 1971).

The laryngologist has, in general, received a training in his surgicopathological specialty which concentrates attention on gross pathology and life-threatening disease. The importance of dysphonia to him is essentially its value as an indicator to laryngeal and associated pathology, but the study of laryngeal physiology and its dysfunction has not been regarded as within the purview of the orthodox specialty other than simple referral of the case for speech therapy.

The speech therapist, with a multidisciplinary training which includes the study of pathology, physiology, linguistics, acoustics and psychology, is uniquely qualified not only to assess the functional disorder, while being aware of the pathological aspect of the dysphonia, but also to describe and grade the various characteristics of the perceived voice for the purpose of planning future management, as well as judging the results of treatment.

Most speech therapy clinics rely upon a purely subjective method for the description and assessment of dysphonia and in the hands of experienced therapists, using the same criteria, the results are surprisingly reliable and reproduceable, given the inexact terms such as 'harsh', 'breathy' and 'asthenic', which are open to different interpretation in character and degree (Kelman *et al.*, 1981).

A few specialist clinics supplement traditional assessment with precise physiological and acoustical measurement techniques to investigate the various components of the dysphonic voice, allowing the clinical syndrome of dysphonia to be defined in terms of altered laryngeal or association function. Thus, the dysphonic voice can be analysed in terms of physical parameters which can be measured repeatedly and their validity subjected to the scrutiny of statistical examination. Serial measurements can be compared as an indication of progress or the lack of it in treatment.

Assessment of the dysphonic voice must therefore begin with clinical examination of the larynx and proceed to a full investigation of the presenting symptom with a history of the disorder, psychological evaluation of the patient where appropriate, subjective description and appreciation of the method of voice production and scientific measurement of functional performance.

Methods of Laryngeal Examination

All methods of laryngoscopy allow good visualisation of the larynx at rest, given a co-operative patient without gross congenital or acquired structural defects which might interfere with instrumentation, and all permit the ready detection of laryngeal pathology. Some of the methods can be used during laryngeal action so allowing visual evaluation of phonatory function during selected phonation or continuous speech, and are thus of greater value for the detection of physiological dysfunction in the absence of gross pathology.

Indirect Laryngoscopy

The standard clinical examination is by indirect laryngoscopy. This requires a round laryngeal mirror of about 21 to 25 mm diameter angled on a long slender handle and a bright light source, which can be a light worn by the laryngologist on his forehead or more usually, an external light on a movable stand which shines on to a head mirror worn by the laryngologist.

The patient is seated on a low stool opposite to and at the same level as the laryngologist. If the patient wears dentures these must first be removed. The patient is then instructed to open his mouth and protrude his tongue, which is covered by a swab and held by the surgeon. The mirror, warmed sufficiently to avoid condensation but not uncomfortably hot, is introduced into the patient's mouth and pressed gently but firmly against the soft palate elevating it to improve the view of the larynx. Light is directed via the head mirror on to the laryngeal mirror illuminating it, and the laryngeal mirror can be manoeuvred to reflect the different structures of the larynx. The vocal folds are viewed in the abducted position during respiration and also when adducted during phonation of the vowel 'ee'. If the patient shows undue signs of discomfort, or a tendency to repeatedly gag, a xylocaine spray can be used to anaesthetise the tongue and pharynx.

Gross abnormalities are readily identified by this means but, as the folds vibrate rapidly in phonation in the approximate range of 100–160 Hz for males and 220–290 Hz for females, the often associated inherent disorders of laryngeal function are not easily detected. Secondary functional disorders arising from abnormalities in tension or deficiency of respiratory support may go unrecognised if vocal fold movement cannot be studied in sufficient detail to allow visualisation of all phases of the glottic explosion. This is clearly impossible using continuous lighting but can be achieved if only a stroboscopic light source is employed.

Stroboscopic Indirect Laryngoscopy

The use of a voice-synchronised stroboscope as a light source for indirect larynoscopy allows detailed scrutiny of the larynx. This enables detection of even slight abnormalities in structure or vibratory pattern by employing the optical illusion of slow motion or even the apparent stopping of the folds during phonation, so that all phases of the glottic explosion can be studied in detail.

The stroboscope works on the principle that an object moving rapidly and periodically is illuminated by an intermittent light with the same periodicity so that both are synchronous. Thus the object is illuminated at the same point in its trajectory on each flash and the eye cannot detect the movement, so the object appears to be stationary.

By synchronising the light flash with the frequency of vibration of the vocal folds, the cords appear to be standing still. The moment of lighting can be changed in relation to the phase of glottic explosion and the cords examined serially throughout the period of a single vibratory cycle.

If the frequency of the intermittent illumination is then changed so that it is no longer perfectly synchronous with the folds, the illusion of slow motion vibration is obtained, so that the shape, position and excursion of the folds is seen throughout phonation. This can permit the early recognition of very minor degrees of organic disease or physiological dysfunction, which may be completely missed by steady light indirect laryngoscopy.

The Stationary Image Examination. This allows scrutiny of the folds in any position of the vibratory cycle and thus scrutiny of any cord lesion. An imperfect stationary image with blurring results from asynchrony of vibration as seen in early oedema of the cord when the oedematous mucosa meets in advance of the true ligamentous cord and vibrates out of synchrony with the fold.

The amplitude of excursion of the vocal folds can be measured by noting the number of degrees through which the point of flash is moved when illuminating the folds, first in the completely adducted position and then at the point of fullest abduction. The amplitude of excursion varies significantly in disorders of function, and reduced amplitude is a reliable indicator of excessive tension in phonation.

The Slow Motion Effect. The illusion of slow motion allows observation of the movement of the cords throughout vibration. In oedema of the folds the mucosa can be seen meeting in advance of the ligamentous cord, and with cord edge nodule the two portions of the cord can be seen vibrating at different frequencies by varying the speed of the intermittent light source to synchronise in turn with each part of the cord.

The new modified stroboscope from Bruel and Kjaer has a

built-in automatic frequency tracking filter, a liquid crystal display (LCD) of fundamental frequency and is supplied with rigid and flexible fibreoptic cables. The rigid light probe can be used with an endoscope and also incorporates a laryngeal mirror holder thus allowing good visualisation with the advantage of stroboscopic lighting without the need for an external light source. The flexible cable combines the advantages of fibreoptic laryngoscopy with stroboscopic lighting. The laryngeal view can be recorded and displayed on a video screen (Figure 2.1).

Figure 2.1: Stroboscopic Fibreoptic Laryngoscopy

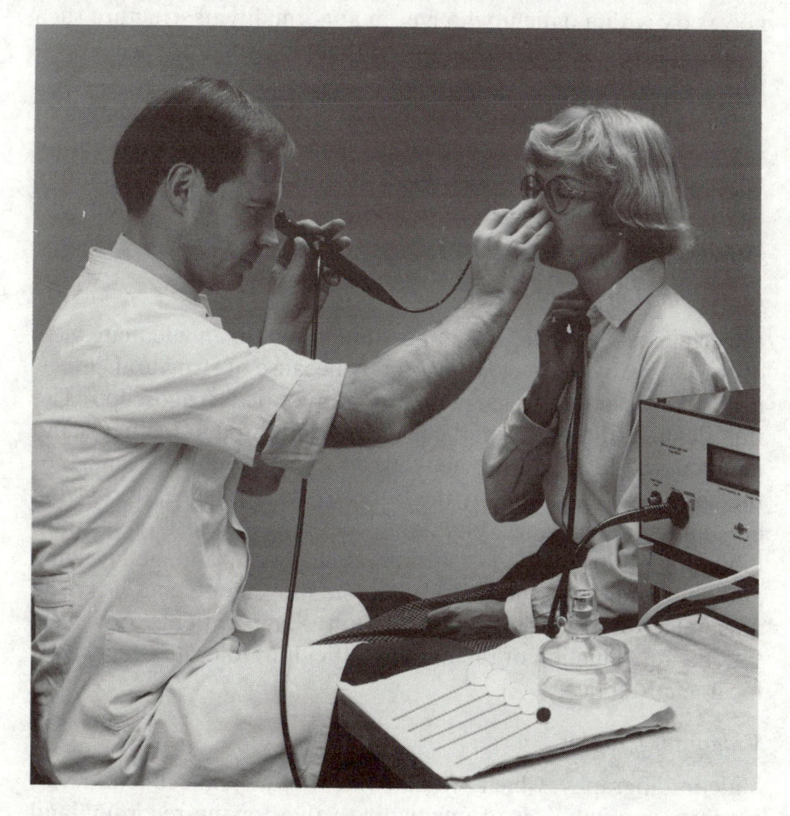

Source: Bruel and Kjaer, Denmark

The mirror examination suffers the usual constraint of any indirect laryngeal examination in that phonation is limited to a restricted range of vowel sounds and the larynx cannot be visualised during continuous speech — a disadvantage that is largely overcome when the flexible fibreoptic cable is introduced through the nares as described below.

Direct Laryngoscopy

Direct laryngoscopy is of value to the surgeon in diagnosis of pathology of the larynx, affording a clearer view than can be achieved using a mirror in the indirect examination. It may be necessary with a patient who has an abnormality of structure such as an undeveloped mandible or overhanging epiglottis which restricts the view of the larynx.

A general anaesthetic is usually required for the introduction of the laryngoscope into the pharynx and phonation is therefore impossible, so this examination is of little value in determining laryngeal function, but is an absolute necessity when a biopsy is required.

Fibreoptic Laryngoscopy

In certain cases, where it is impossible to obtain an adequate view of the larynx by indirect laryngoscopy because of structural defect, it may be desirable to use a flexible fibreoptic laryngoscope. The thin flexible fibreoptic bundle is introduced through the nares and manoeuvred into position above the larynx, so that the image of the larynx is transmitted by the fibres to the eye piece, thus giving an uninterrupted view. Phonation and speech are largely uninhibited, and this method of examination allows prolonged viewing and photography of the rapid vocal fold movements, but lacks the advantage of stroboscopic illumination. Some patients, however, find the introduction of the bundle difficult to tolerate even with a local anaesthetic.

Videoradiography

Videoradiography, which combines x-ray of dynamic function with synchronous sound, is of unequalled value for the recording and analysis of gross pharyngeal movements. Significant contributions have been made in the evaluation of alaryngeal speech (Simpson, Smith and Gordon, 1972) using this technique.

Videoradiography provides good feedback for the patient, but the method has the disadvantage of cumulative exposure to radiation, which limits the technique as a routine form of therapy. The lateral viewing position and poor soft tissue differentiation makes it inappropriate for detailed viewing of the larynx.

Xeroradiography

The term xeroradiography is applied to a technique that employs a comparatively high kilovolt (kV) x-ray production to enhance contrast in soft tissue which improves clarity of the image. There is a widespread misconception that the term is derived from the similar sounding prefix zero — thus implying a low-dose technique when in fact it is quite the reverse. The prefix xero is derived from the Greek *xeros* meaning dry. Xeroradiography is an x-ray imaging system in which an electrostatic image is produced on a xerographic plate by the effects of x-rays on an electrically charged plate, rather than on silver halide crystals or intensifying screens as in conventional radiography. Xeroradiography exhibits a specific type of image contrast called 'edge enhancement' in which a sharp demarcation occurs between two different broad areas of density.

A similar effect giving a clear definition can be attained by using a high kV x-ray discharge with a filter at the tube to homogenise the beam and thus enhance contrast at a lower dose of radiation and without the unnecessary employment of an extremely expensive technique.

Xeroradiography has been used to investigate the vocal tract dimensions during phonation. Data on pharyngeal anatomical parameters are assessed in conjunction with laryngographic recordings, and the combined technique has been termed xeroradiography-electrolaryngography (XEL) (MacCurtain, 1981).

It is claimed that aberrant vocal tract movements create aberrant sounds, but this has not been substantiated by sonagraphic analysis of laryngograph signals. Gordon (1977, 1980) and Kelman (1977) demonstrated by a comparison of sonagraphs of the LX and voice outputs that harmonic abnormalities in voice outputs were also detected in the LX outputs. The aberrant sound was thus shown to originate with irregularity of vibration of the vocal folds which might on some, but by no means all, occasions be caused by variance in the configuration of the vocal tract caused by tension.

When XEL assessment was applied to dysphonic voice in a

clinical setting (Berry *et al.*, 1982) the findings confirmed subjective assessments made by speech therapists, but did not add to the knowledge of physiological function in deviant voice, and no evidence was produced for the modification of treatment.

Xeroradiography-electrolaryngography is potentially a useful research technique, but in clinical use caution must be exercised, as with all radiological techniques, to ensure that the patient is not exposed unnecessarily to x-ray dosage. The annual dose limit for members of the public to the thyroid area is near to 3 rad, and must therefore exclude repetition of the examination as is necessary for comparison at various stages of treatment. This seriously limits the application of this technique for which safer and cheaper alternatives are readily available.

This procedure does not therefore meet the criteria for regular clinical use. Comparable information on the relatively gross pharyngeal movements studied can be obtained by using the high kV system described above or by using a 70 mm or 105 mm camera taking three to five exposures per second using conventional low dose radiography. Good differentiation can also be achieved using medichrome film with orange and yellow filters to vary the contrast and this is often adequate for clinical use. In a comparison of methods of laryngography, Landman (1970) concluded that disorders of laryngeal *function* can be most clearly visualised radiologically by means of cinelaryngography.

Speech Therapists' Assessments

Any assessment of the dysphonic patient must allow for flexibility of approach and an experienced therapist will continuously evaluate throughout the assessment session, varying the form of assessment and the time spent on individual sections according to the type of dysphonia presented. The assessment should be carried out in a relaxed and friendly atmosphere with, if possible, a pleasant environment and every effort should be made to put the patient at ease. The procedure described here is not intended to provide a rigid framework for evaluation, but is presented as a guide to the identification of the most distinctive and diagnostically differentiating features occurring regularly in association with dysphonic voice. The format for recording the information (Figure 2.2) was devised by the author and has been in

Figure 2.2: Case Sheet Report Form used in the Victoria Infirmary, Glasgow

VOICE ASSESSMENT

Name .... Date ....

Number .... Age ....

Clinical History (Onset and Constancy)

Onset

gradual ☐ following specific incident ☐ sudden for no apparent reason ☐

Constancy

	always present	increasing	intermittent	decreasing
History:	☐	☐	☐	☐
During Interview:	☐	☐	☐	☐

VOICE DESCRIPTION:

Pitch:	Normal	☐	High	☐	Low	☐	Unstable	☐
Pitch range:	Normal	☐	Diminished	☐				
Intensity:	Normal	☐	Loud	☐	Quiet	☐		
Breathiness:	Normal	☐	Excessive	☐				
Observed tension in voice:	Normal	☐	Excessive	☐	Diminished	☐		
Roughness:	Normal	☐	Excessive	☐				
Types of Hoarseness:	Tense	☐	Rough	☐	Breathy	☐		
Nasality:	Normal	☐	Hypo	☐	Hyper	☐		
Severity of Dysphonia:	Slight	☐	Moderate	☐	Severe	☐	Very Severe	☐

VOICE PRODUCTION:

Glottal attack:	Normal	☐	Soft	☐	Moderately Hard	☐	Very Hard	☐
Phonation time: on vowel /a/	Normal 8-16 secs	☐	Short 0-8 secs	☐	Long 16 Secs +	☐		
Air Support:	Normal	☐	Good	☐	Inadequate	☐		
Breathing Method	L/Costal Deep	☐	U/Costal Shallow	☐				
Environment in which voice is used:	Normal	☐	Noisy	☐	Quiet	☐		

Description of Larynx ____

Any Known Medical Condition/Drugs ____________________ Muscular weakness/ throat clearing ____________________

Articulatory Deviations ____________________ Personality and apparent emotional balance ____________________ regular use, with minor modifications, in the Victoria Infirmary, Glasgow, and associated hospitals since 1968.

For convenience, the assessment may be considered from three different aspects: the history of the dysphonia, the description of the dysphonic voice, and the physical production of the voice.

History of the Dysphonia

Onset. Upper respiratory tract infections amongst other physical causes and psychological pressures are recognised causative and perpetuating agents of dysphonias and the circumstances surrounding the onset of the dysphonia are, therefore, investigated.

Gradual onset. Dysphonia of slow, almost imperceptible onset, is generally a symptom of habitual misuse or abuse of voice, in other words mechanical dysphonia.

Onset following a specific incident. A common cold or other upper respiratory tract infection causing inflammation and/or oedema of the vocal folds (laryngitis) may result in a period of acute dysphonia which will resolve when the inflammation subsides but can be the initiating cause of mechanical dysphonia if voice rest is not observed. By adapting voice production, the patient compensates for the irregularities in the cord edges and lowered pitch due to inflammatory thickening of the folds, usually by increasing tension and raising pitch, and so may develop a habitual faulty pattern of voice production.

A single episode of shouting, which ruptures a minor vessel in the mucous membrane covering the folds can have the same long-term results.

Sudden onset. Dysphonias or aphonias developing suddenly for no apparent reason, or following an emotional shock, are generally of psychogenic origin.

Constancy. In some types of dysphonia the symptom itself is extremely variable with periods of remission when the symptom is completely absent, or periods when the severity is diminished. The variability may not only be evidenced in the history of the disorder, but also extends to the clinical session.

Increasing severity. A history of increasing severity is usual with mechanical dysphonia, but rapidly increasing severity during the clinical session may be a sign of fatigue in patients with neurological disorder.

Intermittent symptoms. A history of intermittency of the symptom is a feature of dysphonia of psychogenic or neurological origin. The psychogenic dysphonic may report several episodes of dysphonia with complete remissions in between and remissions also occur in some neurological disorders. In the dysphonia of psychogenic origin, the severity of the symptom often *decreases* during a sympathetic interview, whereas that of neurological origin increases, due to fatigue, as the interview proceeds. In evaluating the significance of constancy, the personality of the patient must be taken into account.

Relevant Medical History

Past medical history may at times give a valuable lead to the nature of dysphonia and this is clearly more probable where there is a history of a disease affecting the respiratory tract or neck, although more generalised disorders of the endocrine and nervous systems may also prove relevant.

Chronic bacterial infections, such as syphilis and tuberculosis, may specifically affect the larynx, and bronchogenic carcinoma may cause recurrent laryngeal nerve paralysis with resultant dysphonia. Myxoedema characteristically affects the voice, as might imbalance of the normal sex hormones as a result of menopause, disease, or treatment with oestrogens or androgens as may be necessary in certain tumours.

A physiological dysphonia is of course well known and entirely normal at male puberty with the breaking of the voice, but where the transition is prolonged or inhibited by psychological pressure, dysphonia may become a permanent feature requiring correction.

A history of recurring colds and sore throats may predispose to mechanical dysphonia, and factors such as smoking, working in a smoky environment or in the presence of irritant fumes are clearly of relevance. Past history of psychological disorders might indicate continuing emotional instability related to the dysphonia.

Psychological Evaluation

As the history of the disorder and the personality of the individual are closely linked and usually interdependent, psychological evaluation is of fundamental importance and is a continuous process throughout the assessment and any subsequent treatment. Some dysphonias are of purely psychogenic origin and, in all dysphonias, the patient's personality is an important factor in the management and eventual outcome of the case. In a study carried out in the Victoria Infirmary, Glasgow, 15.6 per cent of cases referred were aphonias found to be of purely psychological origin and therefore pure conversion symptoms, 12.8 per cent were found to be of mainly mechanical origin, but with some psychological factor causing stress and contributing to the perpetuation of the dysphonia, while 44.7 per cent were of mechanical origin only, and 7.3 per cent of neurological origin (Gordon, Morton and Simpson, 1978). In the majority of cases where there is a psychological problem, this is successfully resolved through counselling by the speech therapist, although collaboration with a psychologist may be desirable when there is evidence of a behavioural disorder or phobia.

The patient's attitude to the voice is important, both diagnostically and in the planning of the treatment, and motivation for recovery is an important factor in prognosis.

Nevertheless, the contribution of a psychological element in voice disorders must not be overrated and must never be accepted as a diagnosis without first excluding as far as possible organic causes. Particular care must be taken in differentiating between disorders of psychological origin and those where early neuromuscular disorders presents with dysphonia or dysarthrophonia as the first symptom. The speech therapist is perhaps in the unique position of recognising the earliest stages of these disorders and can then alert the medical staff to the possible neurological nature and occasionally the specific diagnosis.

Environment

The patient's environment may be a primary or secondary factor in the acquisition of dysphonia.

Atmospheres which are over dry, with high levels of dust, fumes or tobacco smoke contribute to laryngeal irritation, as does excessive consumption of alcohol which also irritates the pharyngeal mucosa.

Occupations involving teaching, preaching and beseeching (street trading) predispose an individual to dysphonia unless care is taken to produce voice with adequate air support. Singers are another group prone to vocal abuse, either as a result of excessive demands made over a prolonged period, or of deviant voice production in some of today's pop singers, who lack a trained voice capable of withstanding the demands made in production of the ubiquitous falsetto and harsh cacophony of sounds comprising much of the pop scene.

Voice Description

Habitual Pitch. The normal fundamental frequency for a male voice lies between 100 and 160 cycles per second (cps) and for a female between 230 and 290 cps. Frequency can be measured in cps by using a frequency analyser or an appropriate tuning fork, but for the purpose of clinical assessment this type of measurement is not essential as pitch anomalies are obvious even to the untrained ear.

Optimum pitch is usually the fourth note above the lowest comfortable note and can be gauged by asking the patient to hum up a scale from the lowest comfortable note. In many cases of mechanical dysphonia, by the time a patient is seen by the speech therapist a stage has been reached when the former optimum speaking level can no longer be easily attained and this type of assessment is unproductive. Natural pitch is readily established by asking the patient to phonate breathily on a vowel sound following a maximum inspiration as in sighing. This is the basis of the 'accent' method of vocal rehabilitation developed by Svend Smith (1980) and Kirsten Thyme (1981).

Lowered Pitch. In most cases of mechanical dysphonia the patient will give a history of a gradual lowering of pitch which has probably occurred as a result of some thickening of the cords. An increase in the mass of the cord causes it to vibrate at a lower frequency, as a result of which the patient may subconsciously increase glottal tension to raise the pitch again to that which his ear is accustomed. The increase in tension causes more damage to the cord with further increase in mass and lowering of the pitch establishing a vicious circle of increasing severity and persistence. Deliberately acquired, or assumed lowering of pitch, is not uncommonly found, having been adopted by the speaker as a more 'influential' sounding voice and 'creak' is often a feature of this voice. Over a period this type of misuse can result in the development of contact ulcers or interarytenoid inflammation but is rarely found in this country, although common in North America. Lowered pitch is frequently associated with low air flow rate (personal observation).

Elevated Pitch. Conversely, habitual elevation of pitch above the optimum for the patient can also result in damage to the cords with accompanying dysphonia. This occurs more often than has been recognised in the adolescent male and is very easily corrected in the early stages. If, however, it is allowed to persist past puberty it can become associated with excessive tension and over a period can give rise to secondary organic effects of oedema or nodules and ultimately, tensor weakness with resulting bowing of cords. The patient with bowed cords often presents in late middle age, having sustained a raised pitch mode of phonation since adolescence. Thickening of the cords may have 'masked' the abnormal phonation for a period, but with the development of tensor weakness the patient at last seeks help. Optimum pitch in these cases is often a resonant and beautiful bass which surprises no one more than the patient himself. The condition is associated with low air flow (Gordon, Morton and Simpson, 1978).

Unstable Habitual Pitch. Persistent fluctuation or frequent shifts in habitual pitch can be as a result of neurological or psychological abnormality, injury to the folds or a symptom of mutation in the adolescent.

Unstable pitch may also occur transiently in simple acute infective laryngitis, or when the subject is exposed to emotional stress.

Pitch Range. A reduction in pitch range can be an early indication of mechanical dysfunction and may be the first symptom the patient has noticed. This is especially so with singers. The amount of reduction in pitch range is often related to the severity of the dysphonia.

Pitch range may be estimated by asking the patient to sing or hum a scale accompanied by a piano or other instrument, or simply by the therapist. Some patients may feel awkward doing this, as singing scales is associated with musical ability and they might find it easier to follow a square wave tone which has itself a dysphonic sound. Visual feedback, such as is provided by the Royal National Institute for the Deaf (London) 'Visispeech' display is a useful aid to establishing pitch range.

Intensity. Exact measurement of intensity is unnecessary as significant variations from normal accepted levels of sound will be obvious to the listener and can be readily brought to the attention of the patient.

Habitual excessive loudness results in an increase of tension in the larynx with a longer closed period in the vibratory cycle of the vocal folds. A sustained period of vocal abuse of this type can contribute to cord thickening, nodules and singer's nodes in children, through mechanical irritation.

A decrease in intensity can be significant for differential diagnosis, and can be of psychological origin or related to neuromuscular hypotonia as in Parkinson's disease.

Breathiness. Excessive breathiness is due to incomplete adduction of the vocal folds and can be a psychogenic, neurological or other organic manifestation, such as a nodule or nodules on the cord edge interfering with the glottic explosion, a neoplasm restricting the movement of the vocal fold, or paralysis due to recurrent laryngeal nerve damage which may be a result of thyroidectomy or associated with bronchial carcinoma.

Excessive breathiness of psychogenic origin is associated with pseudoadductor palsy or posterior glottal 'chink', that is, incomplete closure of the cords in phonation.

Neuromuscular hypotonia can also result in excessive breathiness and is usually associated with restricted breathing pattern, particularly where the condition is of long standing and in the latter stages of a disorder such as bulbar palsy.

Excessive breathiness is rarely a feature of bowed cord phonation due to tensor weakness as, although incomplete adduction of the vocal folds is evident, airflow rate is so reduced that breathiness is not observable, even if the voice sounds 'asthenic'.

Tension. Hyperkinesia in voice can be simply a habitual increase of intensity or it can result from increased vocal effort of simple mechanical origin — a result of the vicious circle of vocal strain as previously described in connection with anomalies of pitch. Unconsciously, the patient tries to raise the pitch of the voice which has lowered due to cord thickening, thus increasing tension. In addition he may consciously increase intensity.

Excessive or fluctuating tension can also be of psychogenic origin (increased tension is clearly visible in body position, mandibular movements, shoulders, arms and neck muscles and in elevation of the larynx on phonation) and can be the most disturbing feature of the dysphonia as in spastic dysphonia where fluctuating tension gives the spasmodic bursts of 'creak' or 'fry' which typify this voice.

Hypokinesia, that is insufficient observable tension in the voice, is associated with:

1. Bowing of cords, occurring as the end result of prolonged vocal misuse and usually habitual elevation of pitch.
2. Psychological states.
3. Neurological degeneration, producing neuromuscular hypotonia.

Roughness. This is related to irregularities in the duration of sequential cycles of vocal fold vibration, giving rise to frequency shifts and double harmonics. The loss of regular periodicity can be caused by asymmetrical mass distribution such as a lesion on one fold or by asymmetrical tension of the folds due to abnormality in the laryngeal musculature or nerve supply. Asymmetric vibration generates subharmonics giving rise to the phenomenon of diplophonia, the double voice which can also be caused by overactive false cords pressing on and obliterating the ventricles. There is no way of accurately judging roughness without using acoustic measurement instrumentation.

Severity. The severity of the perceived dysphonia should be noted and a record kept, either on tape or on a language-master strip or, best of all, a sonagraphic print as a subjective estimation cannot be easily compared with subsequent assessment.

Nasality. The presence of hypernasality should alert the therapist to the possibility of myopathic dysphonia such as myasthenia gravis, motorneurone disease or bulbar palsy, as an early manifestation of these disorders can be hypernasal dysphonia with or without articulatory involvement. The severity of the hypernasality, the time since onset and any change that has occurred may all be of significance.

The prime causes of *hyponasality* are nasal airway polyps, deviated septum, catarrh and enlarged adenoids in children, all of which would have been noted in the laryngologist's report.

Voice Production

Glottal Attack. Normal glottal attack is dependent on the maintenance of a delicate balance between the tension in the vocal folds and subglottic air pressure, so that when the folds are adducted at the onset of phonation, the pressure below the glottis is sufficient to overcome the tension in the folds and initiate vibration, normally reaching maximum amplitude after several cycles. Abnormal glottal attack can be either excessively hard or soft and, if not immediately obvious, can be assessed by asking the patient to repeat a list of words with vowels initially, or a sentence such as 'Arthur went out every afternoon with Amy, Olive and Ian'.

Hard attack. This occurs when excessive tension in the vocal folds exerts a resistance which is too great for the subglottic pressure, causing delay in initiation of vibration until sufficient pressure is built up to overcome the tension. This results in a prolonged closed phase in the vibratory cycle which can be heard as an increase in intensity or, when severe, as a stop. Hard attack is a common feature of mechanical dysphonia but can also be heard in hyperfunctional dysphonia of psychogenic origin, spastic dysphonia, and should not be confused with the strong vocal attack of a trained singer when the cords are extremely elastic and have an exceptionally fast closing time, perfectly balanced by a controlled air supply capable of generating the higher harmonics which give the extremely resonant pleasing quality to the voice.

Soft attack. This results when there is insufficient tension in the vocal folds and occurs in psychogenic and myopathic dysphonias, in severe mechanical dysphonias when there is tensor weakness and in senescence. It is often associated with asthenic voice quality.

Phonation Time. An individual's phonation time has been shown to bear an inverse relationship to the severity of some types of dysphonia and is, therefore, significant (Arnold, 1955). It can be measured with a stopwatch and is the length of time phonation can be maintained without breaks following a maximum inspiration and may vary within a range of 10–35 seconds. It is dependent upon a combination of phonation volume, airflow rate and elasticity of the folds. The norms for clinical assessment are considerably shorter than those obtained under stringent research conditions when subjects can be trained to maximise phonation time by increasing inspiration volume and reducing airflow (personal observation).

Short phonation time is associated with most types of dysphonia. Organic manifestations which may, or may not be secondary to the misuse of voice, inhibit vibration causing voice break. Lack of air support or failure to maintain adduction of the folds due to psychogenic or neurological cause has a similar effect.

The exception to the rule is in certain types of mechanical hyperfunctional dysphonia when airflow is low and the patient is capable of habitually producing excessively long phonation times. Even when tensor weakness has occurred, flow may remain low and, in these cases, there is usually a history of prolonged use of elevated pitch.

Breathing Method. The patient's breathing method should be noted. The physiologically correct breathing pattern is lower costal/diaphragmatic where inspiration is initiated by a strong contraction of the diaphragm resulting in forward extension of the abdominal wall and is accompanied by an upward swing of the lower ribs. Shoulders are relaxed and respiration even and rhythmic making full use of lung capacity. Expiration is effected by controlled contraction of the intercostal muscles and abdominal wall.

An upper costal breathing pattern is found in about 50 per cent of patients with dysphonia of mechanical origin (Gordon, Morton and Simpson, 1978). This method is usually accompanied by excessive tension. The shoulders are raised on inspiration and the rib cage elevated allowing expansion of the upper one-third of the lungs only. This method cannot support professional or extensive use of voice and, if practised by serious singers over a period, can result in permanent deformity of the chest.

Air Support. Air support and vocal fold tension are interdependent and inadequate air support can have far-reaching consequences, being the most frequently occurring causative factor in mechanical dysphonia. Poor air support results in hypertonicity of the vocal folds if the vocal intensity is maintained when airflow drops below the optimum level. Loss of the Bernoulli effect where air accelerating through the narrowed glottis exerts a lateral force on the folds drawing them together, results in slower cord movement in the closing phase and a reduction in generation of the higher harmonics which shows as deterioration in voice quality. Available air support is closely related to breathing method and is assessed by asking the patient to take a maximum inspiration then to exhale on a sibilant, usually /s/ and measuring the time with a stopwatch (25–30 seconds). Functional air support is estimated by asking the patient to exhale on /s/ over a period of several respiratory cycles. If adequate, the patient will be able to sustain a moderately intense /s/ for at least 12 seconds on each exhalation, with little variation in the sound from cycle to cycle. Air flow rate is directly related to resonance and deficiencies result in inadequacies in resonance.

Observations should be made of the patient's conversational speech during which persistent creak, use of low pitch, or breathlessness is an indication of poor air support. The use that is made of available air is more important than the volume which the patient can inspire.

Evaluation of air support is one of the most important sections of a voice assessment, but it is most unlikely to produce a reliable result when a subjective assessment is made. Where possible, observations should be supported by air flow measurement.

Throat Clearing. Excessive throat clearing and reported globus hystericus with a feeling of a 'lump in the throat' are frequent symptoms accompanying dysphonia of mechanical or psychogenic origin. Smoking and alcohol, particularly if combined, can irritate the mucous membrane causing the folds and pharyngeal lining discomfort which can lead to throat clearing.

Articulatory Deviations and Muscle Weakness. Dysarthria, dyspraxia, difficulty in walking and writing are all significant when arriving at a differential diagnosis. Difficulty in walking and articulation, slurring for example, may indicate a dysphonia of neurological rather than psychogenic origin when many of the other symptoms are similar and the dysphonias are easily confused.

In an assessment such as this the voice is described in terms which can be easily understood by each therapist and laryngologist who has to attend to the patient. A clinical description is necessarily subjective and must be made in terms such as described. Although reliable when carried out by an experienced therapist, the imprecision of these assessments is widely acknowledged and many attempts have been made to devise a universally acceptable system of voice description and it is useful here to consider contributions which have influenced present-day thinking.

Pike (1943) isolated five significant factors of voice and used a system of opposites (bipolar factor system) to describe the condition: tension — tense versus relaxed; stricture — small throat opening versus large throat opening; pitch — normal versus falsetto; phonation — whispered versus voiced; sound — breathy versus clear.

Osgood, Suci and Jannenbaum (1957) advocated a semantic method, essentially again a scale between opposites to measure the voice as described by abstract adjectival words often ascribed to voice, for example, soft . . . hard; dark . . . bright.

Much of the present-day work on vocal profiles is based on these early studies. Isshiki and Von Leden (1964) used a similar approach to isolate and highlight the four factors which are prime contributors to the perceived dysphonia. These factors are rough (R), breathy (B), asthenic (A) and normal (N) (or sometimes D for degree). The factor profiles were correlated with laryngeal disorders to produce a rule of thumb differential diagnosis, for example, a B(R) type was related to vocal cord neoplasm, while R(N) was associated with laryngeal nodule. Although the method has severe limitations in differential diagnosis it is a useful beginning because the number of descriptive terms is limited to generally recognised essential features of the dysphonic voice.

A five factor analysis, introduced by Fritzell, Hammarberg and Wedin (1977) is essentially an updated modification or variation on Pike's theme, with each factor representing a group of phonation types, thus: (I) steady/unstable; (II) breathy/overtight; (III) hypokinetic/hyperkinetic; (IV) light/coarse; (V) chest register/head register. Significant correlation was found by the authors between the factors and acoustic data. Differentiation between factors might prove difficult in practice and with factor analysis there is a danger of oversimplification unless this is used in combination with a fuller assessment taking account of other fundamental contributory factors.

Catford (1964) recognised this when he recommended a kinaesthetic auditory exploration technique to classify normal phonation types and took into account a wider range of factors including type of stricture, location of stricture, vertical displacement of larynx, upper laryngeal constrictions, vocal fold length, thickness and tension, with much of this being verified by laryngoscopic examination.

The vocal profile produced by Laver (1980) owes much to this early work. While bearing resemblance to the traditional speech therapists' assessment, the profile stresses supralaryngeal features, many of which are of little consequence when applied to patients with mechanical hyperkinetic dysphonia, or psychogenic dysphonia categories which make up two-thirds of the case-load in a dysphonia clinic. A major part of the profile is a scale on which degrees of normality versus abnormality are scored for supralaryngeal and laryngeal features, with what are termed 'dynamic' factors, that is pitch and loudness, and what are called 'temporal organisation factors', that is breath support, rhythmicality and rate, included in a less well-researched section at the end. The profile falls somewhere between a descriptive profile and an assessment, giving a useful evaluation of aspects of dysarthrophonia but is insufficient for a complete assessment. In common with all clinical assessments it is subjective and heavily dependent upon the experience of the assessor. Training courses are typically provided for therapists intending to use the Vocal Profiles Analysis (VPA)scheme.

The practising clinician's assessment must be succinct, selective, show high correlation when used by other members of the team (otolaryngologists and other speech therapists) and be sufficiently structured to provide for comparability of reassessment after a period of treatment, all of which criteria are met by the Victoria (Glasgow) assessment (Kelman *et al.*, 1981). A diagnostic profile as suggested by Isshiki and Von Leden (1964) can be easily extracted from the Victoria assessment (Table 2.1).

Table 2.1: Suggested Diagnostic Profile

Assessment Profile	*Diagnostic Indication*
Breathy, hypotense: B + (T −)	neuromuscular or psychogenic
Breathy, hypotense, quiet, hypernasal: B + (T−) + (I−) + N	neuromuscular
Breathy, hypotense, decreasing or intermittent severity: B + (T −) + (S −)	psychogenic
Breathy, rough: B + R	neoplasm
Breathy, rough, tense, low pitch: B + R + T + (P −)	vocal nodule, Reinke's oedema, etc.
Breathy, rough, tense, high pitch: B + R + T + (P +)	hyperkinetic dysphonias

If increasing severity these are likely to be of mechanical origin and if fluctuating, of psychogenic origin.

Instrumentation and Objective Measurement

The use of instrumentation to provide objective measurements of voice production parameters is fully justified in that measurements can be repeated at intervals throughout treatment and an accurate record of progress can be kept. Areas requiring attention can be identified and therapy directed to these rather than using an empirical approach to treatment.

Certain criteria govern the regular use of investigative techniques in the clinic. The procedure must not subject the patient to discomfort or risk, must not be invasive, and the information extracted must be worth the time and money spent. The procedure must be easily carried out under clinical conditions and be readily repeated for evaluation of treatment. The research worker has slightly greater freedom than the clinician and, on occasions, may use techniques which could not be permitted in the clinic, if no other method is available which can provide the necessary information.

The following investigative methods meet the *clinical* criteria.

Figure 2.3: Sonagraph Display of Phonation of Sustained Vowel: (a) Magnification of narrow band showing 'shift' which is perceived as voice break; (b) section of same phonation with voice break shown as noise in the first formant with loss of distinction in harmonics; (c) wide band display of the same phonation

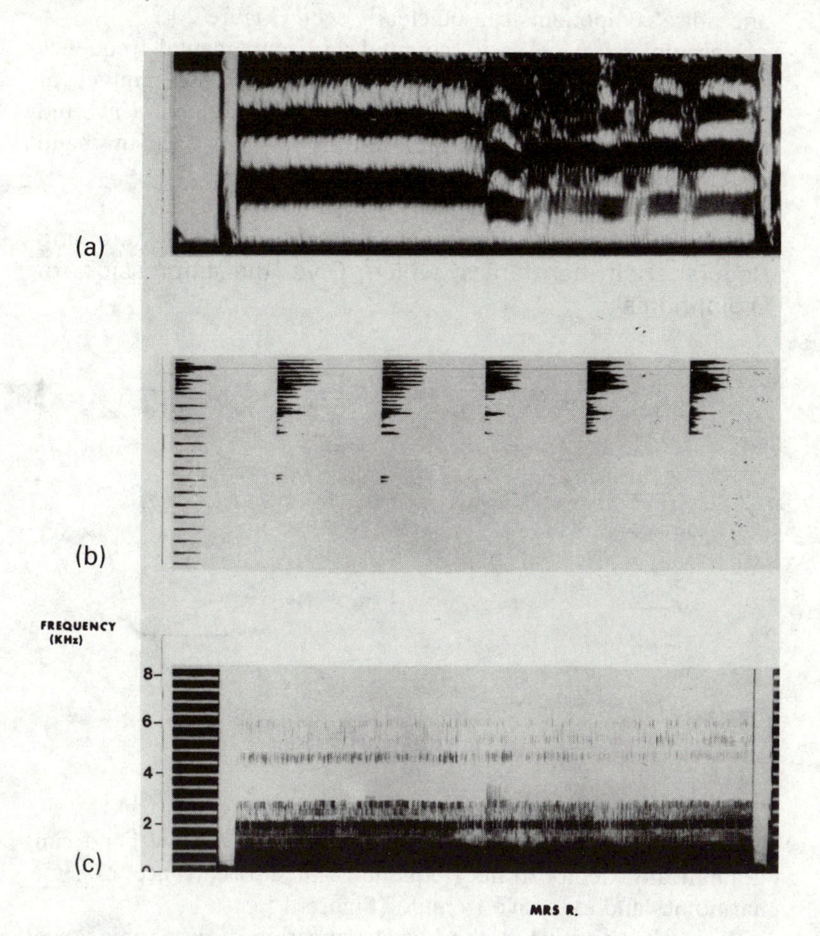

Sonagraphic Analysis

Analysis can be made of any voice output and can be carried out in the absence of the patient using tape recordings of phonation.

Modes of display are varied and can be wide-band, narrow-band, contour or section in any chosen frequency range and magnification (Figure 2.3).

In wide and narrow band display the intensity of the harmonics is shown as density and the frequency plotted against time. In section display the intensity of the harmonics is plotted against frequency. Using a narrow band section, formants, subharmonics and noise components can be clearly seen (Figure 2.4).

Harmonics can be easily counted and fundamental frequency established by dividing a given frequency by the number of harmonics. The section can be displayed with frequency inverted thus allowing it to be superimposed on a wide or narrow band display and facilitating comparison.

Figure 2.4: Section Display of Sustained Vowel, Showing Regular Half harmonics which Give the Impression of Diplophonia

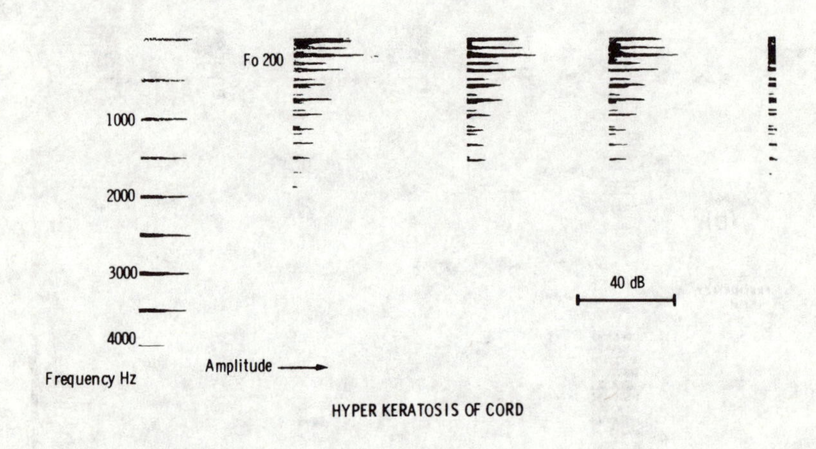

Magnification of the first formant in wide or narrow band can dramatically demonstrate frequency shifts, occurrence of subharmonics and excessive tremulo (Figure 2.5).

A purely objective method of classification of dysphonic voice using sonagraphic analysis was described by Yanagihara (1967) and warrants further exploration and use. Four degrees of dysphonia were classified according to degree of severity of dysphonia, the premise being that harmonic components disappear to be replaced by noise with the fourth formant being

Figure 2.5: Sustained Vowel Showing Excessive Tremulo: (a) wide band display of excessive tremulo; (b) magnification of the first formant

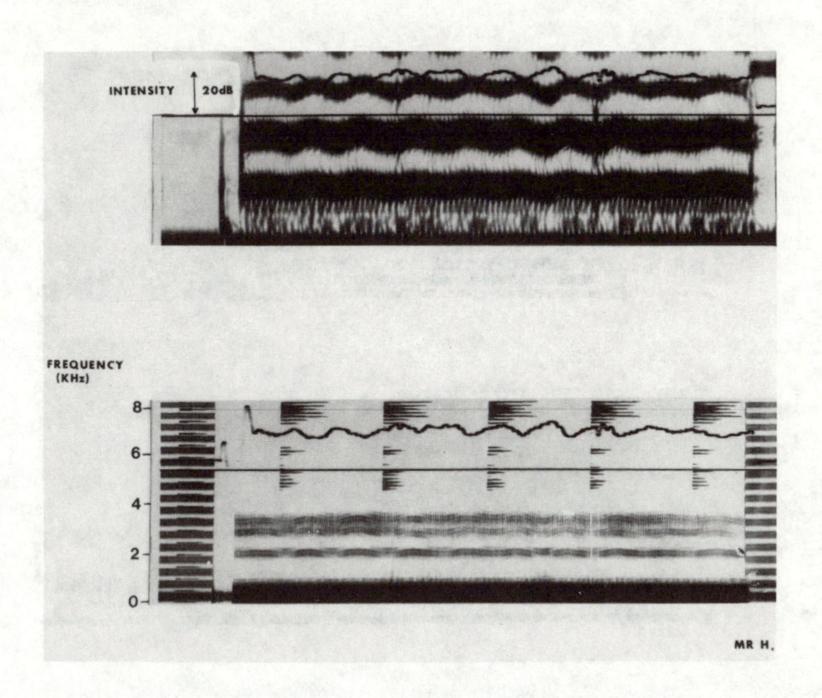

affected first and the lower formants as severity increases with the first formant affected only in the most severe dysphonias (Figure 2.6).

Laryngograph and Voiscope

The laryngograph developed by Fourcin and Abberton (1971) is a completely safe and non-invasive instrument, ideal for routine clinical use. The instrument provides information on the vibratory pattern of the vocal folds (LX) for the clinician and biofeedback information for the patient. The frequency/time mode (FX) incorporated in the voiscope, shows fundamental frequency changes in real time, giving information on pitch. Two electrodes are placed externally on the neck over the wings of the thyroid and an AC

Figure 2.6: Sustained Vowel; Higher Formants are Affected Early in Phonation but the First Formant Only When the Voice Break Occurs

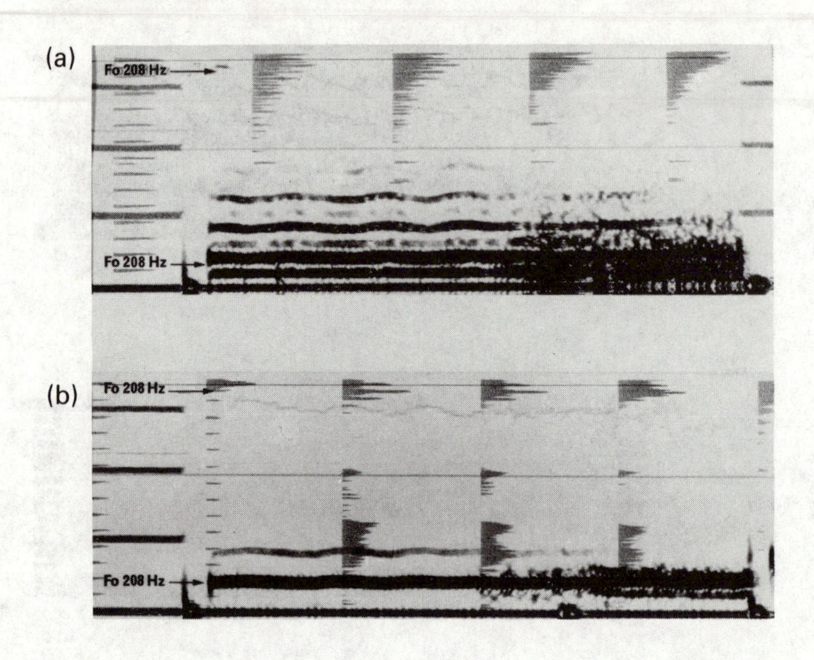

current is passed between them. The impedence varies with the movement of the vocal folds, decreasing when they are in contact and increasing when apart. The electrical signal can be stored on tape and viewed on an oscilloscope and consists of three parts; a sharp rise produced by a decrease in impedence while the folds are rapidly closing is followed by a gradual fall as the folds part and impedence increases and a flattish base corresponds to the interval when the folds are out of contact (Figure 2.7).

Variations in the shape of the signal have been shown to bear a relationship to certain types of voice and pathological conditions (Fourcin and Abberton, 1971) (Figure 2.8). Normally the closing phase is short when compared to the opening and open phases, and is of great importance to the phonatory process as it corresponds to the time of maximum excitation of the vocal tract.

Figure 2.7: Typical LX Output as Seen on Oscilloscope

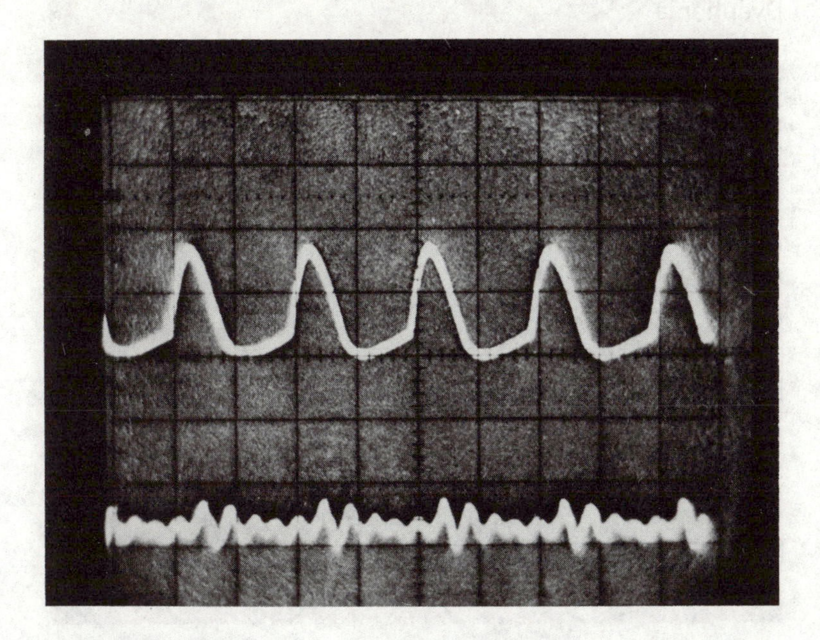

Spectral Display of LX Recordings using a Kay Sonagraph in the Section Display Mode

The frequency spectrum of the LX can be displayed in section using the sonagraph, and the effect of the LX waveform on the LX has been investigated; the gradient of the spectrum is shown to be governed by the closing time. Thus closing time can be calculated from a knowledge of the gradient of the spectrum or from the fine structure of the spectrum (Gordon, 1977; Kelman, 1977; Figure 2.9).

A short or fast closing time, with *relatively longer period when the cords are in contact*, shows a steep gradient on the spectrum and generates more higher harmonics than a slow closing time.

The short closing time is, therefore, capable of exciting more response in the resonators and producing a more resonant voice. This should not be confused with the stiff long closed period in the hyperkinetic voice.

Figure 2.8: LX Output Obtained from Patient with Spastic Dysphonia

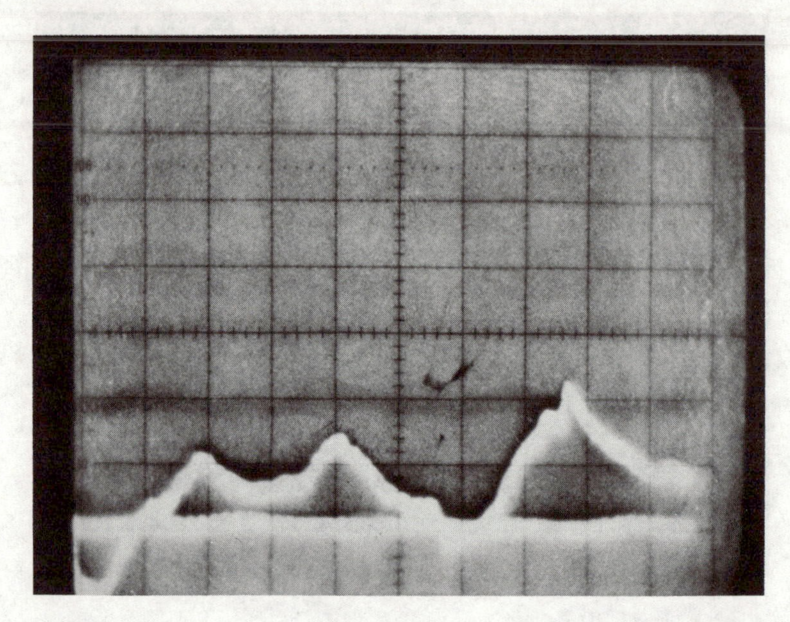

Figure 2.9: Section Display of LX of Sustained Vowel Showing Decrease in Gradient as Voice Deteriorates

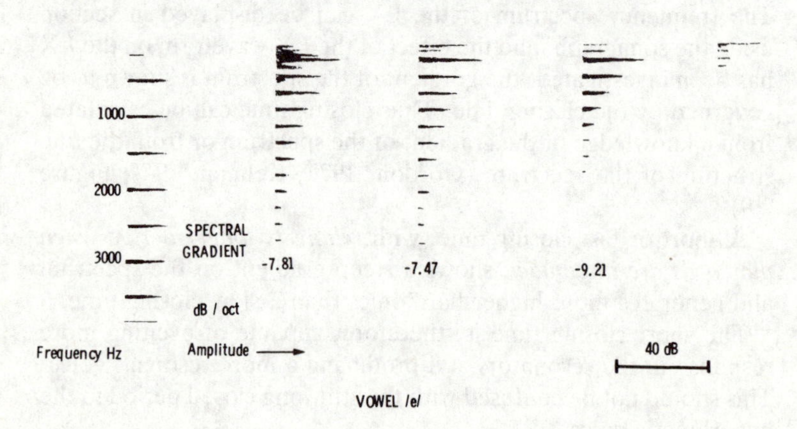

Rapid closing is facilitated by the Bernoulli effect when air flow is adequate. Sonagraphic analysis of voice output and LX output during a voice 'break' can demonstrate that the abnormality arises in the larynx as seen in the LX output, and although enhanced by the resonators is found to be virtually unchanged in the voice output when the two are compared.

The perceived 'break' can arise from a shift in frequency of the lower harmonics with sometimes a loss of higher harmonics or the intrusion of half harmonics or even thirds between the true harmonics in the first formant (Figures 2.10 and 2.11).

Figure 2.10: Voice Output Spectra Showing Half Harmonics at Voice Break

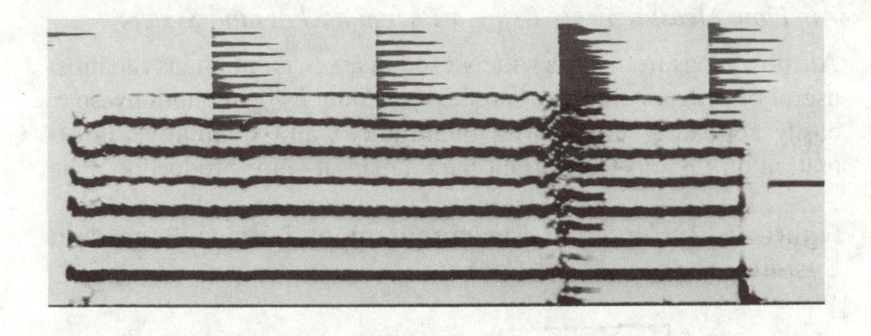

Figure 2.11: LX Output of the Same Phonation Showing the Break Again with Identical Half Harmonics

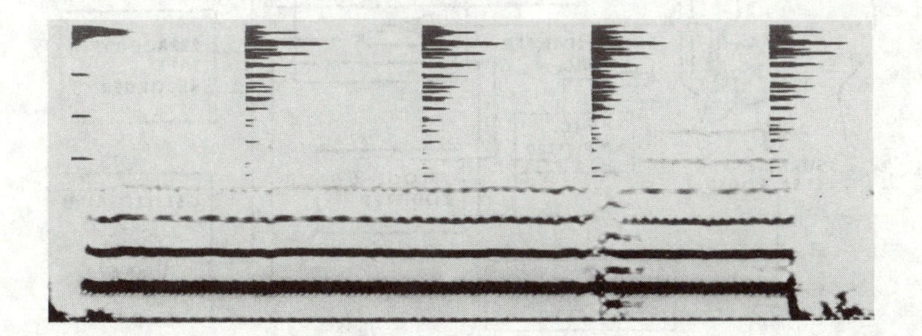

Visispeech

The Visispeech display was developed by the Royal National Institute for the Deaf and is now computer-based with visual display on a VDU monitor screen. The system operates by simple commands via a microcomputer keyboard (Apple II or BBC(B)) and provides the means of accurately measuring and describing aspects of dysphonia related to frequency, such as pitch range, habitual pitch, optimal pitch. Measurements are also made of intensity and phonation time. This is an extremely useful adjunct to assessment which also provides attractive feedback for therapy (Macgillivray, 1984). Maximum and minimum frequencies and intensities can be plotted from hard copy to produce a phonetogram as described by Schutte and Seidner (1983).

Air Flow Measurements Using a Pneumotachograph System

Air flow measurement is widely used in assessment and is the most useful of instrumental measurement techniques being non-invasive, easily repeated, and giving quantitative and qualitative information on the most important parameters of voice production. The

Figure 2.12: Air Flow Measurement and Voice Recording System

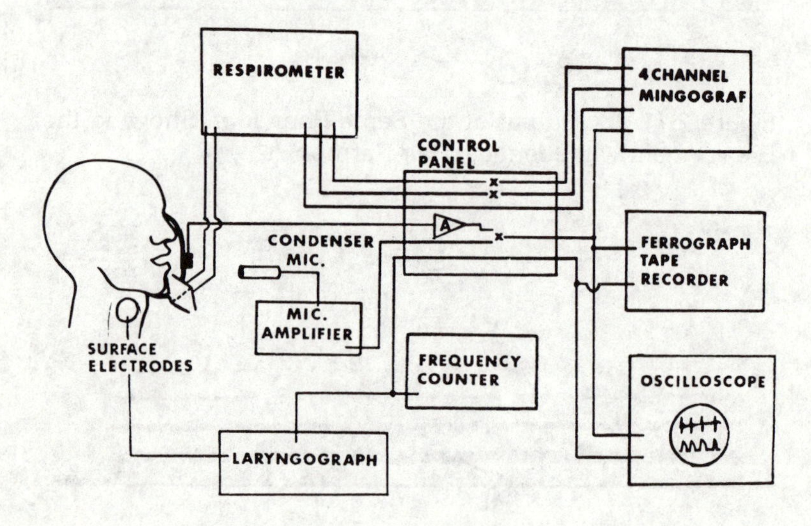

pneumotachograph system incorporates a respirometer, a flow head with a wire gauze mesh separating the two halves and, usually, a pen recording system with at least four channels; it has been described by the author elsewhere (Gordon 1977, 1980; Gordon *et al.*, 1978; Kelman *et al.*, 1975; Figure 2.13).

As the subject breathes into the flow head a pressure difference is generated across the gauze which is proportional to the air flow rate. An electrical output signal is obtained using a differential pressure transducer. The flow rate is integrated with time to give volumes and measurements can thus be made of tidal volumes and the time taken for each respiratory cycle and inspiration fraction of the cycle so assessing the regularity and efficiency of respiration at rest (Figure 2.13).

During phonation the volume of air used on a particular phonation can be measured (*PhV*). The mean rate of flow of that

Figure 2.13: Diagrammatic Representation of Air Flow Recording During Respiration at Rest and During Phonation

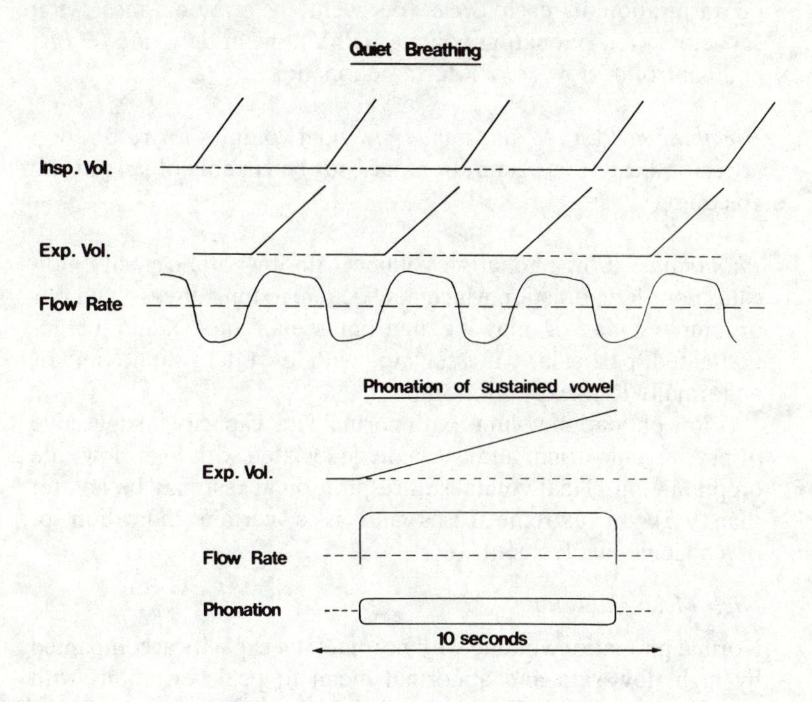

volume of air (*MFR*) of the flow can be compared to the peak flow *M*/*P*, thus giving a measurement of the regularity of the expelled air and, therefore, regularity of vibration of the folds. A vocal velocity index (*VVI*) the ratio of *MFR* to vital capacity (*VC*) is computed (Koike and Hirano, 1968) and used as a measurement of laryngeal resistance (tension) in the evaluation of laryngeal dysfunction.

The efficiency of respiration and of phonation can thus be measured and compared with subsequent assessment of the same patient or with different patients. Abnormal patterns have been identified and quantified using a binary scoring system (Kelman *et al*., 1975; Figure 2.14).

The assessment has proved useful in monitoring the effect of therapy for all categories of voice disorder. Specific aspects of disordered function have been identified for treatment thus avoiding a time-consuming empirical approach.

The significant measurements are regularity of tidal volumes and of rhythm of breathing at rest (period) the relative time spent on inspiration in each cycle (per cent inspiration time), vital capacity (*VC*), phonation volumes (PhV), mean flow rate (*MFR*) and control of flow (*M*/*P*) during phonation.

Breathing at Rest. Abnormally low tidal volumes for respiration at rest indicate that respiration may not be capable of supporting voice use.

Phonation. Low phonation volume with low vital capacity indicates poor lung function which may be due to lung disease, tumour or emphysema, or may be neuromuscular and should be investigated, particularly if associated with low tidal volumes and/or abnormally long expiration time.

A low phonation volume with normal vital capacity is suggestive of psychogenic origin and is usually associated with high flow rate on phonation. Tidal volumes in respiration at rest may be greater than *PhV* in extreme cases and is a certain indication of psychogenic involvement.

High Mean Flow Rate

Normal phonation volume with normal vital capacity accompanied by high flow rate and abnormal mean to peak variations with uncontrolled flow indicates possible pathological changes in the

Figure 2.14: Air Flow Record Used with Binary Score: 0 = Within Limits of Normality; 1 = Outside Normal Limits

Name ________ Unit No. ________ Date ________

RESTING RESPIRATION ________

% VARIATIONS IN. (Normal Limits)	INSP. (16%)	EXP. (16%)	PERIOD (14%)	% INSP. TIME (14%)
SCORE				

TOTAL ________

MEAN TIDAL VOLUME ________	VITAL CAP. ________ B.V.C. ________	R VC/BVC ________ (Normal Limits Above 0.70)	SCORE

PHONATION

	NORMAL LIMITS	NPa SCORE	HPa SCORE	LPa SCORE
Pitch	Fo 120			
	Fo 240			
Phonation Time	12 - 16 secs.			
Phonation Volume	(See template) + 0.9			
Mean Flow Rate	5 - 11 l/min.			
Mean/Peak	Above 0.65. Low - Irreg. High - No irreg.			
Vocal Velocity Index	Low - Tense High - Phonatory loss			

	SCORE
VC/BVC	
PH.V	
MFR	
MP	
TOTAL	

SONAGRAPH ANALYSIS ________

STROBOSCOPE ________

DIAGNOSIS ________

cord which could be tumour, oedema, nodule or paralysis. In cases of cord palsy where there is no compensatory movement of the opposing cord, mean flow rate may be so uncontrolled that it is unmeasurable, but measurement can be obtained from the very distinctive and transitory peak. The patient with hyperkinetic dysphonia of mechanical origin is likely also to show irregularity in tidal volumes in quiet respiration.

Low Mean Flow Rate

This can result from increased glottal resistance or reduction in respiratory effort. Where *VC* is normal and phonation volume normal, this is most often found in hyperkinetic phonation, even when tensor weakness has occurred and cords are bowed. Low air flow results in poor resonance.

Table 2.2: Diagnostic Profile for Further Investigations

Respiration at Rest	*Diagnostic Indications*
Tidal volumes irregular	Most frequently found associated with mechanical dysphonia or hyperkinetic psychogenic
Low volumes	Poor lung function with organic or neuromuscular origin; occasionally found in dysphonias of psychological origin
Timing irregular	Short inspiration time with long expiration time but otherwise regular indicates elasticity of lungs (eg. possibly emphysema);
	The total score out of four indicates severity of disorder of respiration
Air flow in Phonation	
Low *VC* and *PhV*	Poor lung function — emphysema or neuromuscular in origin
VC normal and low *PhV*, with possibly, high flow rate	Psychogenic, especially when associated with high flow
MF high, *M/P* irregular, *VC* normal, *PhV* normal	Oedema, nodule or other organic manifestation
MF low	Hyperkinetic phonation
	The total score out of four indicates the severity of the dysphonia.

Although obviously of value in providing a differential diagnosis, the results of air flow measurement procedures specifying aspects of respiratory performance which require modification also have a direct effect on treatment, particularly when evaluated in conjunction with the speech therapists' subjective assessment. A rule-of-thumb diagnostic profile can also be used to indicate areas for further investigation (Table 2.2).

With a complex disorder such as dysphonia, to which there can be many contributory factors, it is tempting to extend the history and accumulate a multiplicity of facts of varying degrees of relevance.

Accurate and easily applicable instrumental procedures for measurement and analysis of dysphonic voice are becoming cheaper and more available, and the speech therapist must welcome any technology which will increase her understanding of the disorder and thus enhance the patient's treatment. Nevertheless, discretion must be exercised in the selection of useful techniques and care must be taken lest the patient is overwhelmed by a battery of tests which arouse anxiety and confusion where one has intended to heal.

History, subjective assessment and physiological measurements should be confined to features significant to differential diagnosis and to the selection of treatment regimes. A combination of assessment procedures ensures that accurate diagnosis is made and effective treatment is selected and applied where malfunction has been clearly demonstrated.

In particular a combination of the speech therapists' subjective assessment and airflow measurement have been found by the author to be effective in diagnosis disorders, and formulating treatment in difficult cases.

References

Arnold, G. E. 'Vocal Rehabilitation of Paralytic Dysphonia. Acoustic Analysis of Vocal Function', *Archives of Otolaryngology,* 62, 593 (1955)

Berry, R. J., Epstein, R., Freeman, M. MacCurtain, F. and Noscoe, N. 'An Objective Analysis of Voice Disorders', *British Journal of Disorders of Communication* 17, 77 (1982)

Catford, D. C. 'Phonation Types. The Classification of Some Laryngeal Components of Speech Production', *In Honour of Daniel Jones*. (Longmans, London, 1964)

Fourcin, A. J. and Abberton, E. 'First Application of a New Laryngograph', *Medical and Biological Illustration*, 21, 172 (1971)

Fritzell, B. Hammarberg, B. and Wedin, L. 'Clinical Applications of Acoustic Voice Analysis', *Swedish Transmission Laboratory Reports*, (1977)
Gordon, M. T. 'Physical Measurements in a Clinically Orientated Voice Pathology Department', *Proceedings of 17th Congress, International Association of Logopaedics and Phoniatrics and Phoniatrics*, Copenhagen (1977)
—— 'Air Flow Rates and Vocal Cord Closing Time in Phonation', *Proceedings 18th Congress, International Association of Logopaedics and Phoniatrics*, Washington (1980)
—— Morton, F. M. and Simpson, I. C., 'Air Flow Measurements in Diagnosis, Assessment and Treatment of Mechanical Dysphonia'. *Folia Phoniatrica (Basel)*, 30, 161 (1978)
Isshiki, N. and Von Leden, H. 'Hoarseness: Aerodynamic Studies', *Archives of Otology* 80, 206 (1964)
Kelman, A. W., Gordon, M. T., Simpson, I. C. and Morton, F. M., 'Assessment of Vocal Function by Air Flow Measurements', *Folia Phoniatrica*, (Basel), 27, 250 (1975)
Kelman, A. W., 'A Study of Voice Production in Normal and Dysphonic Subjects, *PhD Thesis. University of Glasgow* (1977)
—— Gordon, M. T., Morton, F. M. and Simpson, I. C., 'Comparison of Methods of Assessing Vocal Function', *Folia Phoniatrica (Basel)*, 33, 51 (1981)
Koike, Y. and Hirano, M., 'Significance of Vocal Velocity Index'. *Folia Phoniatrica*, 20, 285 (1968)
Landman, G.H.M. *Laryngography. Cinelaryngography* (Excerpta Medica, Amsterdam, 1970)
Laver, J., *Phonetic Description of Voice Quality* Cambridge University Press, Cambridge, 1980)
MacCurtain, F. *Pharyngeal Factors Influencing Voice Quality* (London University Press, London, 1981)
Macgillivray, M. 'Letter to the Editor', *Bulletin of the College of Speech Therapists*, May (1984)
Osgood, C. E., Suci, G. J. and Jannenbaum, P. H. *The Measurement of Meaning* (University of Illinois Press, Urbana, 1957)
Pike, K. L., *Phonetics* (University of Michigan Press, Ann Arbor, 1943)
Schutte, H. K. and Seidner, W., Recommendation by the Union of European Phoniatricians (UEP):Standardising Voice Area Measurement/Phonetography', *Folia Phoniatrica (Basel)*, 35, 286 (1983)
Smith, S. 'The Accent Method', Proceedings of the 18th Congress, International Association of Logopaedics and Phoniatrics, Washington (1980)
Simpson, I. C., The Organisation and Working of a Dysphonia Clinic. *British Journal of Disorders of Communication* 6, 70 (1971)
—— Smith, J. C. S. and Gordon, M. T. 'Laryngectomy. The Influence of Muscle Reconstruction on the Mechanism of Oesophageal Voice Production', *Journal of Laryngology and Otology*, 86, 961 (1972)
Thyme, K. 'Trials of the Accent Method', Proceedings of the 18th Congress, International Association of Logopaedics and Phoniatrics, Washington (1980)
Yanagihara, N. 'Significance of Harmonic Changes and Noise Components in Hoarseness', *Journal of Speech and Hearing Research* 10, 531 (1967)

3 LARYNGEAL DISORDERS IN ADULTS

Andrew Johns

Introduction

The aim of this chapter is to present the ENT surgeon's approach to the management of disorders of the larynx (Ballantyne and Groves, 1981). Chapter 4 has been devoted to the particular problems found in children. There is of necessity some overlap of the chapters as there is no clear division between pathology and its manifestations in the adult and child.

Disease processes affecting the larynx reveal themselves to a greater or lesser extent by disorder of the various functions of the larynx. As part of the upper airway and its role of protection to the lower air passages, the larynx has a vital function. Its use in phonation is essential for the chief method of human communication. When life is threatened by airway obstruction or by incompetence of the laryngeal sphincter, the surgeon can overcome the problem by way of an opening made into the trachea through the tissues of the front of the neck — *tracheotomy*. Indeed this 'essential' organ can be removed — *total laryngectomy* and respiration continues through a permanent opening of the trachea onto the neck — *tracheostomy*. The airway and food passages are thus completely separated such that a sphincter mechanism (that is, the larynx) is obviated.

Clearly such a major interference with the larynx will have profound effects on phonation. Communication by speech is one of the features that distinguishes man from the other primates, and its loss produces a severe alteration in customary way of life. The immense power of man's adaptability plays a large part in overcoming this handicap, aided by surgeon and speech therapist. Some diseases manifest themselves chiefly by alteration of the voice, and their management must be carefully tailored to remove causative factors and improve phonation without embarrassment to the other role of the larynx as airway protector. The balance between adequate removal of disease, the achievement of an acceptable voice and the maintenance of a safe airway will be a theme pursued in this chapter. By way of illustration, this is well demonstrated by bilateral abductor vocal cord palsy. The two cords, immobile in the adducted position, produce a good voice but an inadequate airway. Surgery to widen the glottic opening to improve the airway will have a reciprocal detrimental effect on the quality of the voice.

Presentation

A patient with a hoarse voice of recent onset, who visits his family doctor, will often be given treatment for an acute inflammation of the larynx. This is a presumptive diagnosis but a concurrent cold or sore throat makes the diagnosis probable. If the voice does not return to normal within two weeks, or if the dysphonia is of longer duration at presentation, a firm diagnosis of the cause must be made. The importance of the symptom of persistent hoarseness cannot be overstated because of the possibility of a malignant cause. Diagnosis requires adequate inspection of the larynx (which usually means referral to an ENT department) and, where necessary, the examination histologically of a sample of tissue from any abnormal area.

A partially obstructed airway produces a noise called stridor. As a life-threatening situation it demands emergency referral to an ENT department for relief of the obstruction and diagnosis and treatment of the cause.

Most laryngeal disease presents with an altered voice. Stridor forms a small group; other symptoms that may be encountered are pain and discomfort, which may be experienced as earache (referred pain), cough, swallowing difficulties or the feeling of a lump in the throat.

History

These symptoms, their duration, fluctuation or progression will be elicited by a carefully taken and recorded history. Other relevant information will be obtained with regard to vocal use and abuse, smoking and alcohol consumption and the work and home environments.

Examination

Inspection of the interior of the larynx is achieved in most patients by the method of *indirect laryngoscopy* (see also p. 19). The patient's tongue is grasped firmly and gently pulled forward, while a warmed laryngeal mirror is held in the back of the throat, pressed against the soft palate. The angle of the mirror allows visualisation of the larynx and hypopharynx, illumination being provided by a lamp positioned above and behind the patient's shoulder and reflected from a mirror worn on the examiner's forehead. A patient who does not tolerate this procedure at first may do so after the application of local anaesthetic to the mucous membrane of the throat. The particular advantages of indirect laryngoscopy are the simplicity of the technique and the ability to observe movements of the vocal cords during respiration and phonation.

An alternative to mirror examination is the fibreoptic laryngoscope (see p. 22), passed through the nose into the pharynx, both of which have been anaesthetised. This method, which again may not always be tolerated, is useful when, for anatomical reasons, the mirror gives an inadequate view. It also has the advantage of allowing recording of the findings by still photography, or concurrent and future display by video recording, particularly useful for teaching.

The clinical examination is completed by palpation of the neck, paying particular attention to the mobility of the larynx and the presence of enlarged lymph nodes. The rest of the upper respiratory tract is inspected noting the state of the teeth, mouth, throat, nasal airway and any evidence of sinusitis. The general physical state is assessed for poor nutrition, weight loss and lung and heart disease. It may also be relevant to assess hearing.

As a result of this examination patients can be assigned to one of the following groups.

Group I	Inadequate view of larynx
Group II	Structural abnormality
Group III	Impaired vocal cord movement
Group IV	Combination of II and III
Group V	Normal appearance of larynx

Group I: Inadequate View of Larynx

For those few patients who do not tolerate mirror examination or fibreoptic examination (if available), or in whom the larynx just cannot be seen, inspection will be performed under a general anaesthetic – *direct laryngoscopy* (see p.22). A rigid laryngoscope is passed through the mouth and the larynx visualised through the lumen of the laryngoscope. The pharynx is also examined, and inspection of the trachea and bronchi (*bronchoscopy*) and the oesophagus (*oesophagoscopy*) may be indicated.

It is not easy to be certain of vocal cord movement at direct laryngoscopy under general anaesthetic but usually patients can be classified into one of the remaining groups. Where endoscopic surgical procedures are required as discussed in group II, it will usually be possible to do them under the same anaesthetic as this diagnostic laryngoscopy.

Group II: Structural Abnormality

This group contains those patients in whom the inspection, whether by indirect laryngoscopy or direct laryngoscopy, has revealed an abnormality of the lining of the larynx. This may be a surface lump, irregularity, ulceration or colour change, or a swelling of the subepithelial tissues. In many cases the appearance is so typical that a specific diagnosis is suggested. In the majority of cases it will be necessary to confirm this histologically and often the treatment of the lesion includes its removal. One exception is early 'classical' vocal cord nodules which may regress with vocal training, so avoiding surgery. To obtain the specimen for examination a direct laryngoscopy is performed and a sample (*biopsy*) or all (*excision biopsy*) of the lesion is removed. Where all the lesion is removed, as would be the case for some of the benign conditions such as polyps and cysts, the laryngoscopy is best performed with the aid of the operating microscope – *microlaryngoscopy*. This allows clear visualisation of the laryngeal interior and the precise excision of the lesion using microsurgical instruments. The laryngoscope is held by a suspension apparatus, which releases both the surgeon's hands for the manipulation of the instruments.

The processing of the specimen takes a few days and usually the report confirms the clinical impression. Treatment is then planned on the basis of the pathology and the overall clinical picture.

Pathology

The most urgently awaited aspect of the histology report classifies the lesion into a malignant or a non-malignant type. The classification is not quite so clear cut and there has to be a third group to contain those lesions which, while not being frankly malignant, are recognised as having the potential to become malignant. Such patients must be maintained on a regular review list for frequent reassessment including further biopsy as necessary.

Malignant Lesions

The larynx is composed of structural tissues such as cartilage, fibrous connective tissue, blood vessels etc. and lining epithelium. Malignant change can occur in any of these tissues but by far the commonest (95 per cent) are of the epithelium. These are the carcinomas and irrespective of the site of the lesion in the larynx they are nearly always of the squamous cell type. This indicates that in those areas of the larynx lined by respiratory type epithelium there has been a change of cell type to the squamous cell.

The histology report also gives information as to the degree of differentiation of the malignant cells, that is how closely they resemble the normal cells. To a certain extent this is an indication of the aggressiveness of the cancer.

The behaviour of malignant cells is to spread, at first by local increase in number and invasion of the surrounding tissues. Eventually, if untreated, the cells gain access to the lymphatic channels and blood vessels which leads to widespread distribution of the malignant cells throughout the body. In the case of carcinomas this distant spread occurs mostly via the lymphatics and the first clinical sign of this spread is the appearance of enlarged lymph nodes in the neck. This takes place most readily from those regions of the larynx richly supplied with lymphatics. These are the supraglottic and subglottic regions. The glottis itself has a surface epithelium that is tightly bound down to the underlying fibrous structure of the vocal cord, there being very little submucosal tissue spaces and therefore a relative deficiency of lymphatics.

The picture emerges that malignant disease of the larynx is not a single disease. Lesions of the vocal cord will give rise to a symptom, such as hoarseness, very early in their natural history and moreover this symptom is usually acted upon by patient and doctor. Second, distant spread by lymphatics is a late occurrence in relation to the onset of symptoms. Finally, they are usually well or moderately well differentiated and therefore not highly aggressive. Contrasting this with other sites in the larynx, hoarseness does not occur so early, spread takes place more readily and is more likely to have done so at diagnosis. These are the important factors in considering the prognosis, and it is not surprising that glottic tumours have a much higher cure rate than those tumours arising elsewhere in the larynx.

Malignant disease of the larynx is found mostly in males (in a ratio of males:females 8:1). It usually occurs in the later years of life and there is a definite relationship to smoking.

Benign Lesions

Inflammation. The majority of benign laryngeal lesions are due to inflammatory processes. Inflammation is described as acute or chronic. In the latter there is persistence of the irritative cause maintaining the inflammation, while the tissues also attempt a healing response with the formation of granulation and fibrous scar tissue. Typically acute inflammation of the larynx (acute laryngitis) is a viral infection, part of a generalised upper respiratory tract infection. The cardinal features of acute inflammation, redness, swelling, heat, pain and loss of function are well demonstrated. The throat is sore, there is fever, aphonia or dysphonia, and indirect laryngoscopy will show red and swollen vocal cords.

Many factors are potential irritants to the larynx and include smoking, alcohol, vocal abuse, dirty and dry atmospheres, poor dental hygiene, mouth breathing and chronic sinusitis. Following an acute laryngitis the presence of one or a combination of these factors may allow the persistence of inflammation into a chronic state, producing the clinical picture of chronic laryngitis. The changes in the laryngeal lining may be generalised and this is particularly seen in male smokers. The appearances are of a swollen, thickened, reddened mucous membrane coated with sticky secretions. Attention must be paid to any irregular, white areas as these are indistinguishable to the naked eye from early carcinomas. In the case of chronic laryngitis, histological examination after biopsy shows these white patches to be areas of squamous epithelium in which an excess of keratin is produced. This process is called hyperkeratosis, and where it is found in areas of the larynx not normally lined by squamous cells the change in cell type is called metaplasia. The significance of these changes is that they may represent early steps in the development of a cancer and hence these cases require careful follow-up examinations.

The localised lesions are polyps, nodules, cysts and contact ulcers. Polyps are oedematous areas of the surface epithelium, particularly affecting the free edge of the vocal cord, often bilaterally. This lesion is more common in females and usually occurs after the menopause.

Vocal cord nodules arise as a result of vocal abuse. This occurs in professional voice users if the voice is untrained or overused, and in others with excessive use or misuse of the voice. There may be other irritant factors present producing a more generalised change in the larynx, but most often nodules are seen as an isolated lesion within an otherwise normal-looking larynx. The nodules are usually bilateral and symmetrically placed on each vocal cord, one-third of the way back from the anterior commissure. They begin as an area of oedema but in time this becomes organised into a fibrous nodule.

Cysts develop when a mucus-secreting gland becomes blocked and the continued secretion produces the recognisable grey swelling.

A less common lesion is the contact ulcer. This is again a feature of vocal abuse, the trauma occurring at the point of contact in adduction of the vocal processes of the arytenoid cartilages within the posterior third of the vocal cords. There is superficial ulceration and attempts at healing may produce a granuloma.

Trauma. External injuries to the neck may involve the larynx and this is most often seen as part of a road traffic accident. The mechanism of injury may be a direct blow, a laceration or a whiplash. This may result in bruising or tears to the mucosa, fractures and disruption of the cartilaginous skeleton of the larynx and injuries to the laryngeal nerves. Very often there are multiple injuries, any of which may take precedence for treatment, but these severe laryngeal injuries usually produce airway obstruction necessitating urgent relief by tracheotomy.

The long-term result of trauma is the formation of scar tissue which can interfere with phonation by fixation of the vocal cords, or by formation of a web, and can narrow the airway (stenosis). These effects can best be avoided by the earliest possible repair of the mucosal tears and the accurate repositioning and fixation of fractured cartilage. In order to prevent stenosis some injuries require a stent or mould to be left in the lumen of the larynx while healing is taking place. The tracheotomy can be closed once the stent has been removed and the intralaryngeal swelling has subsided. Injuries to the laryngeal nerves are considered in a later section (p. 65).

The larynx may also be damaged by internal injury. An endotracheal tube passed through the larynx is frequently used in general anaesthesia. The short duration of most general anaesthetics rarely traumatises the larynx, but on occasion ulceration may occur with subsequent formation of a granuloma. Long-term intubation is part of the management of respiratory problems requiring mechanically assisted ventilation. Trauma is much more likely to occur and to avoid this a tracheotomy is performed.

Surgical procedures on the larynx, particularly those performed endoscopically, require extreme care to avoid residual scarring. The use of the operating microscope makes such procedures more precise. Recently the advent of laser surgery performed at microlaryngoscopy allows pinpoint excision of diseased tissue with minimum damage to normal tissues. One area in the larynx to which special care must be applied is the anterior commissure. Trauma here may result in a web of scar tissue, a very troublesome situation to reverse.

Endocrines and Ageing. One feature of hypofunction of the thyroid gland (myxoedema) is a hoarse voice due to thickening of the submucosal tissues of the vocal cords. The appearances are similar to chronic laryngitis and the cause is suspected when other features of myxoedema are present. The condition is corrected by replacement therapy with thyroxine tablets.

The larynx is also under the influence of the sex hormones, obvious changes in the voice occurring at puberty. The development of vocal cord oedema and polyp formation after the menopause has already been mentioned. Androgenic hormones are sometimes used in the treatment of gynaecological conditions and as a side-effect there may be an alteration in the female voice.

The ageing process affects the tissues of the larynx, such that they become lax and less elastic. The voice may change in pitch and lose its strength.

Papillomas. The benign lesions so far described are not true neoplasms. Benign neoplasms are the non-invasive, non-spreading counterparts of the cancers. Symptoms are produced by the local effects of the swelling. They are rare in the larynx compared to the other benign lesions and the malignant lesions. The commonest true benign neoplasm is the papilloma which has the appearance of a wart. In adults they are often solitary making removal relatively easy, but careful follow-up is required for they may recur.

Benign neoplasms arising from other tissues such as glands in the epithelium (adenoma), fibrous tissue (fibroma) and cartilage (chondroma) are much rarer and if large will require excision via a laryngofissure (see below, p. 64).

Congenital Conditions. These are described in Chapter 4.

Treatment of Malignant Lesions

First and foremost, patients with laryngeal cancer require sensitive, lengthy and repeated counselling. There will be fears that need to be allayed, in particular that cancer has an inevitable and fatal outcome. Explanations of the effects of radiotherapy and surgery are not readily taken in and therefore need reinforcing by doctor, nurse and speech therapist. An excellent account of the management of laryngeal cancer is given in the book *Laryngectomy* (Edels, 1983). What follows is a brief outline of the principles of treatment.

There are two modalities of treatment that may be used to effect a cure. They are radiotherapy and surgery. In this country the majority of patients are first treated by radiotherapy. This has the benefit of retaining the patient's normal method of breathing and speaking. The curative success with small glottic tumours is very high (more than 90 per cent). Larger tumours is the supraglottic and subglottic regions do less well but some are cured with retention of laryngeal function. Very careful review of the patients is required during the radiotherapy and after to identify residual or recurrent disease at the earliest time. Radiotherapy itself has effects on the normal tissues of the larynx, in some cases producing marked oedema of the mucosa. The restoration of a satisfactory voice after radiotherapy may be helped by speech therapy, but the therapist must be on guard for any sign of deterioration of the voice. This could indicate recurrence of the cancer and urgent referral to the ENT surgeon is needed.

A therapeutic dose of radiotherapy usually cannot be repeated as the effects are additive, even with a gap of years, and the neck tissues will be damaged excessively. Surgery is the choice of treatment for those cases which do not respond to radiotherapy, or which recur or which are so advanced at outset of treatment.

Total Laryngectomy. The surgical procedure most widely used is the total laryngectomy, an operation which predates the development of radiotherapy. The principle that governs cancer surgery is that to overcome the invasive nature of the disease a sufficiently wide margin of healthy tissue surrounding the tumour must be removed. Applying this principle to the larynx requires an operation to be devised that will not jeopardise the adequate removal of disease, yet leave the patient able to perform the functions of respiration, swallowing and phonation. With total laryngectomy the first two are achieved at the expense of the latter.

This operation is usually well tolerated physically and has its major effects on the person rather than the body. It is this aspect of management that requires most sympathetic and optimistic counselling.

The operation may be performed through a U-shaped incision in the skin of the neck. The larynx is mobilised by division of the strap muscles, division and ligation of the neurovascular pedicles, and division of the thyroid isthmus. One or both thyroid lobes are removed with the larynx if to leave them would inadequately clear the cancer. Transection of the trachea and its suture to an opening in the skin of the neck creates the permanent tracheostomy. The final excision of the larynx leaves an opening into the pharynx which is repaired. The patient is fed via a nasogastric tube for 7–10 days while healing of the pharynx takes place and then normal swallowing can be re-established. This also heralds the time at which vocal rehabilitation can be started. Occasionally healing is delayed and a fistula between the pharynx and neck skin forms. This can take months to heal and may take several surgical procedures to effect closure. The commencement of speech therapy must await healing.

Vocal Rehabilitation. The standard method of vocal rehabilitation is the teaching of one of the techniques to produce a pseudovoice. These rely on the outflow of air taken into the pharynx to vibrate the pharyngo-oesophageal sphincter, so producing a noise that can be developed by the resonators and articulators of the remaining vocal tract. Because of the difficulties in learning the techniques, and the variable quality of the voice obtained, attempts have been made to surgically overcome the problem. Many of these have achieved little success due to the complexity of the apparatus, the introduction of infection, the inadequate removal of the cancer and difficulties associated with swallowing.

A recent line of approach has been to create a tracheo-oesophageal fistula maintained by a prosthetic valve (for example, the Blom–Singer Valve and Panjé Button). This combines surgical speech rehabilitation with the techniques for acquisition of pseudovoice by directing air from the lungs into the pharynx for phonation. The one-way action of the valve is designed to prevent reflux of saliva or food from the oesophagus into the trachea. The simplicity of the idea and the relative ease with which the valves can be fitted bodes well for their success in aiding speech rehabilitation.

Other Surgical Procedures. Other surgical procedures such as the partial laryngectomies, either supraglottic or vertical, and the reconstructive techniques of Staffieri and Serafini have found only limited application in this country. In many cases previous radiotherapy makes the healing after such operations suspect and other cases are too advanced to make anything less than a total laryngectomy possible.

Not all patients are cured. Professional skills are required to meet the physical needs of the patient, in particular the relief of pain. Special human skills are required of all members of the treatment team to maintain the patient's dignity during the terminal phase of the illness.

Treatment of Benign Lesions

The treatment of these lesions can be considered under three headings.

(1) Excision of the lesion.
(2) Elimination of causative factors.
(3) Follow-up.

Excision of the Lesion. Many of the discrete lesions are easily recognised at indirect laryngoscopy. The majority require excision and this can be performed at microlaryngoscopy. The excised tissue is sent for histological examination.

Occasionally a large benign lesion is encountered that requires removal via a *laryngofissure*. In this procedure the larynx is exposed through the front of the neck and then split vertically along the angle of the thyroid cartilage. The inside of the larynx can then be inspected and the lesion excised. A tracheotomy is needed during the operation and for the postoperative recovery period.

A particularly difficult problem is the long-term scarring following trauma. The tendency is for the surgical excision of one scar to be replaced by another. The reconstruction of a stenosed larynx is one of the most challenging in laryngology.

Elimination of Causative Factors. This largely is the role of the speech therapist and is described in Chapter 10. In the case of vocal cord nodules speech therapy may precede surgical excision as some early cases may regress. However, if they do not regress surgical treatment is indicated followed by further speech therapy. In many cases of benign lesions faulty voice production occurs and speech therapy is required even if vocal abuse was not the prime cause of the lesion.

The advice that would need to be given to correct the factors producing a chronic diffuse laryngitis is often not followed. It is unrealistic to expect a man to give up his pleasures and his work! A source of chronic infection in the upper respiratory tract such as the sinuses or poor dental hygiene can receive attention, as can a cause of nasal obstruction. The vocal abuse can be relieved by providing a deaf relative with a hearing aid.

Follow-up. It is mandatory that some cases are kept under long-term regular review. These are the patients with chronic laryngitis where the histology has shown changes that are premalignant.

In other cases, once the voice has returned to normal, the patients need not be seen regularly but can be asked to return if their symptoms recur. Unfortunately there is a high incidence of relapse in these conditions.

Group III: Impaired Vocal Cord Movement

Impairments of mobility of the vocal cords will affect the swallowing, respiration and phonation functions of the larynx to a varying degree, depending on the movements that are paralysed and the static position adopted by the cords. The nerve supply to the larynx contains both motor fibres to the muscles and sensory fibres to the mucosa. The protective function of the larynx is equally dependent on an intact sensory input as it is on the motor response to complete the reflex.

Interference with the nerve supply is the major cause of abnormal movement of the vocal cords, but the rare muscle disorders and fixation of the cricoarytenoid joints need to be borne in mind. The former may be encountered in a generalised muscle disorder such as myasthenia gravis, and the latter as a result of trauma to the joints or as part of a generalised arthritis such as rheumatoid. Joint fixation may also develop after long-term immobility of a paralysed cord.

Management of patients with vocal cord palsy consists of three aspects. Investigation to identify the cause, treatment of that cause, if possible, and correction of the laryngeal dysfunction. These will be considered in relation to the various clinical presentations.

Unilateral Recurrent Laryngeal Nerve Palsy

The commonest lesion is a paralysed cord which adopts a position in or close to the midline. This is the effect usually of a recurrent laryngeal nerve palsy. There is no universally agreed explanation to account for the position taken up by the paralysed cord, but a reasonable explanation is that the position is produced by the unopposed adduction exerted by the cricothyroid muscle (nerve supply is external laryngeal nerve).

For many cases no cause can be found despite careful investigation. Some will recover spontaneously although this may take many months. In other cases the cause is obvious, such as those due to trauma. An unfortunate cause of trauma is that of surgery to the thyroid gland, but injuries to the neck or thorax may also damage the recurrent laryngeal nerves. The course of the left recurrent laryngeal nerve takes it into the chest and being longer than the right is more liable to damage. In the chest the nerve may be involved in malignant growths of the bronchus or oesophagus, or malignant lymph glands at the hilum of the lung. In the neck oesophageal, thyroid, tracheal and laryngeal malignancies may paralyse the nerve. The investigation includes palpation of the neck, chest x-ray, a barium swallow x-ray and endoscopic examination of the larynx, trachea, bronchi, pharynx and oesophagus.

Oesophageal and bronchial malignancies are usually so advanced when they produce a vocal cord palsy that the chance of cure is small. Thyroid, and particularly laryngeal malignancies, offer a much higher success rate. Trauma to the nerve will recover if it was bruised and the nerve sheath remained intact, although recovery may take many months. Complete division of the nerve is unlikely to recover.

The laryngeal dysfunction of this lesion is confined to a voice change of a rough quality with some weakness, air-escape and a tendency for the voice to deteriorate with tiredness. In cases where the paralysed cord is in the midline there may be virtually no alteration in the voice, and in others there is compensation by the non-paralysed cord which overadducts to meet the paralysed cord in phonation. This compensation can be encouraged by speech therapy, but such treatment must not be expected to influence the recovery of movement in the paralysed cord.

Bilateral Recurrent Laryngeal Nerve Palsy

When the condition described above occurs bilaterally the clinical picture changes dramatically. With both cords in a position near to the midline, and unable to abduct, the airway is imperilled. This is an uncommon occurrence and the most frequently encountered cause is thyroid surgery. It is usually necessary to relieve the obstruction by tracheotomy, but on occasion the airway is not so severely embarrassed.

The situation is observed for at least 12 months as spontaneous recovery of movement of one or both cords may occur. If after this time there has been no recovery, a decision is made between the retention of the tracheotomy and a surgical procedure to widen the glottis. A tracheotomy tube fitted with a 'speaking-valve' allows a good voice as in this condition the vocal cords are approximated and have smooth edges. The 'speaking-valve' must not be confused with a vibrating mechanism. It is simply an hinged flap inside the entrance of the tracheotomy tube which opens on inspiration and closes on expiration. The expiratory air is directed around the tube and out through the larynx, vibrating the cords for phonation. (Inspiration is not possible through the larynx as the attempt to draw in air sucks in the soft tissues of the larynx, exaggerating the obstruction.)

In order to close the tracheotomy the glottis must be widened by a cordopexy procedure. Various methods are available from the complete excision of a vocal cord, the removal of one arytenoid cartilage, to the stitching of one vocal cord into an abducted position. It will be appreciated that this will have a detrimental effect on the voice, but for social purposes it may be acceptable. There is a large degree of self-decision by the patient as to the management, taking into consideration the importance of voice in work and the desire to lose the tracheotomy.

Vagus Nerve Damage

Some injuries or disease processes affect the vagus nerve before it has given off its laryngeal branches. Tumours of the vagus nerve and related structures and their surgical treatment, and intracranial neurological conditions, are some of the causes. The voice is often very weak and hoarse with air escape, and examination of the larynx shows the immobile cord to be in a more abducted position than is the case with a pure recurrent laryngeal nerve palsy. This can be explained by the added paralysis of the crico-thyroid muscle, and the cord adopts a position midway between full adduction and full abduction. The mobile cord is less able to compensate, hence the more marked voice change.

Following investigation of the cause, treatment is first directed to that. Speech therapy may be given during the period of waiting for spontaneous recovery (although this rarely happens in these cases). If the voice does remain poor (and for those cases of recurrent laryngeal nerve palsy in which the voice is unsatisfactory) improvement can be gained by adding bulk to the paralysed cord to place it near the midline such that the mobile cord can now meet it. This is most simply performed by the endoscopic injection of Teflon paste into the substance of the immobile cord. Judgement is required neither to overcorrect nor undercorrect, but the procedure can be repeated as required to maintain a good voice.

There is some risk in this condition of a partial incompetence of the larynx due to the loss of a large area of sensory input from the epithelium and the inability to completely close the glottic sphincter. There may be some difficulty experienced in swallowing, but this can usually be overcome by the patient taking extra care, and the situation will also be improved by the Teflon injection.

Bilateral Vagus Nerve Damage

A dangerously incompetent larynx results when both cords are paralysed in a semiabducted position. This rare occurrence is usually the result of a serious brain-stem lesion, for example, a vascular accident or tumour. These lesions often have a fatal outcome, but the few patients who survive present a most difficult management problem. There is no stridor but the airway is compromised by the inability to prevent food and liquids entering the trachea and lower airways. This can be managed (temporarily) by a tracheotomy using a tube with an inflatable cuff to protect the lower airways during swallowing. This is unsatisfactory in the long term and one drastic solution is a total laryngectomy, which separates the airway from the upper digestive tract. An alternative is to suture the epiglottis over the laryngeal inlet, thereby affording the necessary protection to the airway, but the tracheotomy may continue to be required for respiration.

External Laryngeal Nerve Damage

Following thyroidectomy some patients notice a voice change but indirect laryngoscopy reveals fully mobile vocal cords. This has been attributed to damage to the nerve supply to the cricothyroid muscle. The described appearance of a wavy edge to the vocal cord is rarely seen.

Group IV: Combination of Groups II and III

Some cases are seen in which there is impaired movement of the vocal cords and in which a structural lesion is visible. Malignant laryngeal disease will be responsible for some of these, indicating advanced local disease with fixation of one side of the larynx. Second, as a result of trauma, there may be a combination of scarring within the larynx and paralysis of the motor nerve supply, or fixation of the cricoarytenoid joint. The principles of management are given in the relevant sections above.

Group V: Normal Appearance of Larynx

In this group the surface lining of the larynx is normal in appearance. The cords appear to be fully mobile during the phases of respiration and they adduct fully on coughing. Adduction may not occur completely or be maintained for phonation, but this is often difficult to see and essentially the mirror examination shows a normal larynx.

Provided the examiner is confident in the indirect laryngoscopy findings, then it is likely that the voice disturbance, either aphonia or dysphonia, is functional. These conditions are seen most frequently in females, often in the younger age groups. Rarely is there a severe psychiatric condition but rather a superficial emotional upset, perhaps of a recurrent nature. It is, however, not often possible to elucidate the particular factors during a busy outpatient clinic, even though they may be suspected. It is of great benefit to the patient's recovery to be reassured that there is no serious pathology. A fear of cancer often superimposes itself and overshadows the original psychogenic disturbance.

Referral is to the speech therapist. A few cases do not respond, or the speech therapist may notice a deterioration in the voice. These cases must be re-examined by the ENT surgeon. In the rare instance where a deepseated psychiatric disturbance is suspected referral to a psychiatrist is required.

Occasionally a pubertal or post-pubertal boy is referred to the ENT surgeon for investigation of a dysphonia or the persistence of a high-pitched voice. These boys have usually developed normally in all other physical respects, as those cases with a definite hormone deficiency have had previous referral to a paediatrician or endocrinologist. Examination of the larynx is typically normal but in some cases of dysphonia the false cords are seen to take a prominent part in phonation. Again referral is to the speech therapist and in most cases the voice disturbance can be quickly corrected.

Conclusion

The causes of voice disorders cover the full range of pathological processes. Their management from diagnosis to treatment is an important aspect of the ENT surgeon's work. A close working relationship between speech therapist and surgeon is helpful. Joint consultation is particularly beneficial and the results of treatment are very rewarding.

References

Ballantyne, J. and Groves, J. *Scott Brown's Diseases of the Ear, Nose and Throat*, 4th edn (Butterworths, London, 1981)

Edels, Y. (ed) *Laryngectomy: Diagnosis to Rehabilitation* (Croom Helm, London, 1983)

4 LARYNGEAL DISORDERS IN CHILDREN

Andrew Johns

Introduction

The management of laryngeal disorders in children is as much the management of the child as it is the diagnosis and treatment of the laryngeal pathology. Close co-operation between specialists of varying disciplines ensures that both the child and the whole family environment are not ignored by too narrow a consideration of what may be a rare and fascinating disorder. Speech therapist, ENT surgeon, paediatrician and, for those children requiring hospital treatment, nursing staff and anaesthetist are the primary team members.

An important hallmark of childhood is growth and its accompanying changes. Development, at its most rapid before birth, continues apace and stages labelled as neonate, infant, toddler, child and adolescent soon pass. This constantly changing and growing environment has important bearings on the manifestation of disease processes and calls for fine judgement in their management.

What follows does not consist of a list of the many varied conditions affecting the child's larynx. A detailed description of a particular condition can be found in other reference works. Rather it is hoped that the reader will obtain an overview of the presentation and management of the disordered larynx in children. Various conditions will therefore received mention under the different section headings. Some will be given greater attention than others, the more common disorders being dealt with in most detail. Cross-reference should also be made to Chapter 3 on laryngeal disorders in adults, where, in order to avoid too much repetition, some topics are given greater emphasis.

Presentation

In a textbook devoted to voice it is perhaps insensitive to assign priority to the functions of the larynx. It is often written that the oldest and primary function of the larynx is as a sphincter to protect the lower air passages, and that phonation is a secondary function which makes use of this sphincter mechanism. When both these functions perform without hindrance they assume equal importance, indeed the one carries on unnoticed while the working of the 'voicebox' is apparent to all. Rather than rank being given to the functions of the larynx, priority can clearly be assigned to disorders of these functions. An obstructed or unprotected airway has consequences not shared by an absent or altered voice.

The Obstructed Airway

Air passing through a narrowed or partially obstructed airway produces a noise. When the obstruction is in the pharynx the noise is rasping and bubbly-sounding and is called *stertor*. An example is the Pierre Robin syndrome. In this congenital condition the small lower jaw does not allow sufficient room for the tongue, which falls backwards to obstruct the pharynx, unless the baby is nursed in a prone, head-down position. Often there is an associated cleft palate.

Stridor is the name given to the noise when it is produced by an obstruction in the larynx or trachea. Some indication of the level of the obstruction can be obtained by assessing the phase of respiration in which the noise maximally occurs. Supraglottic and glottic obstructions produce stridor of somewhat musical quality maximal in the inspiratory phase. This is well demonstrated by the condition of laryngomalacia, and when a baby with this congenital condition is examined under general anaesthesia the soft tissues of the supraglottis can be seen to fall inwards during inspiration and the stridor becomes audible as the anaesthetic lightens.

A noise produced in both phases of respiration usually indicates an obstruction in the subglottis or upper trachea. Congenital conditions occurring in this situation are subglottic stenosis and subglottic haemangioma. These lesions produce similarly obstructed breathing but the latter would be suspected if there is a cutaneous haemangioma present, usually found on the face or trunk.

An essentially expiratory noise occurs when the obstruction is in the intrathoracic portion of the trachea or the main bronchi and their subdivisions. The larger air passages may be blocked by inhaled foreign bodies, which most commonly lodge in the right main bronchus. The peanut is a notorious offender in young children and is particularly unpleasant due to the intense local mucosal inflammatory reaction to the vegetable oils in the nut.

Other mechanisms of tracheal narrowing include compression by surrounding structures or collapse due to a deficiency of its cartilaginous support.

Varying degrees of airway obstruction occur. Severe narrowing will demand a much increased respiratory effort manifested by a raised respiratory rate and indrawing of the suprasternal and intercostal soft tissues. This extra effort can only be sustained temporarily and unless the obstruction is relieved the respiratory and cardiovascular systems will start to fail as evidenced by the onset of sweating and cyanosis. Complete upper airway obstruction is incompatible with life unless immediately recognised and relieved. This situation can arise if a large foreign body impacts in the lumen of the larynx. Rarely a baby may be born with total airway obstruction due to failure of the formation of a lumen in the larynx called laryngeal atresia. Near total obstruction may be caused by bilateral abductor cord palsy, a condition usually associated with other neurological abnormalities. It must always be remembered that in a neonate with severe upper airway obstruction the obstruction may lie in the nose, usually due to posterior choanal atresia.

Lesser degrees of obstruction will often produce a loud stridor, understandably worrying to the parents, but without causing any constitutional upset to the child.

The Unprotected Airway

The larynx is not simply an air passage but it is the mechanism which prevents ingested liquids and solids from entering the lower airways. When the larynx is incompetent to perform this function, swallowing is impossible due to the risk of inhalation. This situation is rare in children but as described in the next section minor degrees of feeding difficulty often accompany laryngeal disorders. A posterior cleft larynx is a rare congenital malformation in which the larynx is incompetent due to a deficiency of its posterior wall.

Feeding Difficulties

As a protector of the lower airway the larynx plays an important role in swallowing. The neonate is confronted with an entirely liquid diet which the larynx must prevent from entering the trachea. Complex reflex movements are required, dependent on co-ordinated nerve and muscle function. Immaturity in this can lead to slow feeding and difficulties such as a tendency to cough and choke during feeds. Any laryngeal disorder in infancy may have an associated feeding problem, but a typical example is the commonest cause of congenital stridor, laryngomalacia, in which the stridor is often more marked during feeding. This can sometimes be overcome by thickening the feeds and the early introduction of a solid diet. The thicker food has less tendency to enter the laryngeal lumen and is more easily directed into the lateral food channels.

Dysphonia

Impaired phonation may be due to an irregularity in the larynx, especially of the surface of the vocal cords, which disturbs the airflow or which prevents the approximation of the vocal cord edges. It may also be due to vocal cords whose mobility is impaired by a neuromuscular failure or by fixation at the cricoarytenoid joints. Such abnormalities may manifest themselves as a weak or absent cry in a baby. The severe laryngeal disorders, in which the cry may be feeble, are likely to also give rise to the more serious problem of an obstructed airway.

Harshness, hoarseness and breathiness are qualities in the voice indicative of laryngeal pathology. A congenital laryngeal web may present with obstruction, if large enough, and also with dysphonia. The webs are most commonly situated in the anterior glottis and may consist of just a thin membrane or may extend down into the subglottic region (Wilson, 1979).

Pathological Processes

Diseases may be the result of genetic factors or the body's response to abnormal environmental influences. In any individual the particular manifestation of disease is the result of the combination of the inherited genetic constitution and the external influences. These factors may operate before birth giving rise to congenital abnormalities — these are often multiple, so a baby born with a disordered larynx may have an abnormality of another system.

Abnormal Development

It is out of place here to give a detailed account of the embryology of the larynx. However, in order to understand how some of the congenital abnormalities arise, it is relevant that early in its formation the entrance to the larynx ends blindly. Failure of canalisation to occur would produce atresia of the larynx, if complete, and a laryngeal web or a narrowed subglottic lumen, if partial (Pracy, 1983).

Growth and development of the larynx continue after birth until the adult structure is attained. The infant larynx lies higher in the neck than the adult larynx, being tucked under the base of the tongue. The epiglottis is often easily visible when inspecting the child's throat with a tongue depressor. The normal neonatal larynx is of a size adequate to meet the oxygen needs of the baby but the ratio of the glottic area to body surface area is smaller in the neonate than the adult. There is therefore less margin for narrowing to occur before the onset of symptoms of obstruction. On occasion the entire larynx is too small but most often it is only the subglottic region that has failed to form an adequately sized lumen.

The most noticeable difference in appearance of the infant larynx from the adult, apart from overall size, is the shape of the laryngeal inlet. The aryepiglottic folds are short and the epiglottis more curled. The commonest cause of congenital laryngeal stridor is laryngomalacia, indeed in early textbooks the terms congenital laryngeal stridor and laryngomalacia are used synonymously. The name suggests that the laryngeal cartilages are soft and give inadequate support to the larynx. Compared to adult cartilage the cartilage of all infants' larynges is soft. The failure of development in laryngomalacia appears to be a delayed lengthening of the aryepiglottic fold tissue. Because this is short the edges of the soft epiglottic cartilage are pulled in, creating the exaggerated curve described as 'omega'-shaped (Ω) and the arytenoid cartilages are tilted forward. On inspiration the arytenoid cartilages prolapse further forward and the epiglottis flops inwards. On expiration the flow of air pushes the same structures apart and hence this phase of respiration is quiet.

Some congenital disorders arise from the chance coming together of the particular sets of genetic material from the parents. Faults may also occur in the genetic material itself. One such example does affect the larynx to produce the cri-du-chat syndrome; characterised by a feeble mewing cry, there are other abnormalities which lead to severe physical and mental retardation.

Inflammation

Acquired disease is usually a response to damage from an external agent such as physical, chemical, living organism or dietary deficiency. The most frequently encountered response to tissue damage is the inflammatory reaction, which attempts to nullify the damaging agent and initiate repair of the damage. The acute infections of the larynx demonstrate the inflammatory reaction. There is an increased blood flow through the inflamed tissues and the blood vessels become leaky allowing fluid to enter the tissue spaces. Thus white blood cells, antibodies and circulating antibiotics, if administered, reach the damaged area. One effect of this is to produce swelling and within the lumen of the larynx there is little spare room. In the case of acute supraglottitis (acute epiglottitis) the inflammatory process is confined mainly above the vocal cords, where because of the lax mucosal tissues the swelling is marked and the obstruction to breathing is quick in onset. A temporary artificial airway is required to prevent suffocation. The inflammatory reaction in laryngotracheobronchitis is essentially below the level of the vocal cords, and as there is often less swelling of the tissues many cases can be managed without an artificial airway. If there is already an underlying congenital abnormality such as laryngomalacia or subglottic stenosis, even a mild infection producing little swelling may be sufficient to cause severe breathing difficulty. The parents of children with such disorders are warned of the potential danger of minor upper respiratory tract infections and the possible need for temporary hospital care.

Most acute inflammations are followed by restitution of the tissues to normal. When the damaging process is not quickly relieved or removed then the persisting inflammation leads to repair processes which do not return the tissues to normal. Scar tissue, consisting of dense fibrous material, is laid down. An illustration of this is trauma to the larynx from prolonged peroral or pernasal endotracheal intubation. Modern methods of ventilatory support requiring the use of endotracheal tubes have produced a dramatic reduction in perinatal and neonatal mortality but this is sometimes at the expense of laryngeal damage. The trauma to the larynx by a tube remaining *in situ* for many weeks results in inflammation, ulceration and subsequent scarring both to the glottis and the subglottis. This may eventually produce a web or an acquired subglottic stenosis.

Change in Cell Character

Under certain external influences the character and behaviour of cells may change. They may alter in appearance and change type and growth rate. This is dealt with in more detail in Chapter 3. Metaplasia and neoplasia are rare in childhood but one condition that should receive mention is juvenile papillomatosis. In this condition the external factor is believed to be a virus. The papillomata, which have a warty appearance, consist of a core of vascular fibrous tissue covered by layer upon layer of well-differentiated squamous epithelial cells. The distressing feature of these papillomata is their tendency to recur after removal and to spread throughout the respiratory tract.

Management of Laryngeal Disorders in Children

Management consists of diagnosis and appropriate treatment. It is customary medical practice to delay commencement of treatment until the diagnosis has been made, but there are certain *symptoms*, severe stridor being one, that demand immediate treatment before the diagnosis of the cause of that symptom is made (Ferguson and Kendig, 1972).

Urgent Management

By this is meant cases where treatment takes precedent over diagnosis. When an assessment is made that the airway is severely obstructed so as to be life-threatening urgent relief is required. This necessitates the use of an artificial tube to bypass the obstruction and in the case of laryngeal disease this may be achieved by a tracheotomy or by a tube passed via the nose or mouth through the larynx into the trachea. Most obstructions can be temporarily relieved by this latter method of endotracheal intubation. This will be satisfactory for those conditions, such as the acute inflammatory laryngeal diseases, which are quickly resolved by appropriate medication. Children managed with endotracheal tubes do require the immediate availability of skilled nurses, anaesthetist and a surgeon competent to perform paediatric tracheotomy.

Tracheotomy

Long-term relief of an obstructed airway is better achieved by a tracheotomy. This is usually performed under general anaesthesia and consists of an incision in the neck skin, separation of the tissues overlying the trachea and a vertical slit made in the anterior tracheal wall. The patency of this fistula is maintained by a tracheotomy tube.

Although tracheotomy has a morbidity and a mortality, the necessary nursing skills can be taught to parents so that these children can live at home. Vocalisation will occur if air is able to escape around the tracheotomy tube through the larynx on expiration. Children learn the trick of partially occluding the opening of the tube with their chin or finger on expiration to increase this flow of air through the larynx. Alternatively a valved tube can be used, the valve of which opens on inspiration and closes on expiration. Provided the other parameters (such as normal hearing) are intact, language and speech will be acquired unaffected by the presence of a tracheotomy.

Methods of Diagnosis

The only sure diagnostic method is inspection of the larynx. Some indication will have been gained from the mode of presentation. X-ray techniques may add useful information and a neonate or infant with stridor should have a barium swallow x-ray to exclude the presence of an abnormally placed blood vessel compressing the trachea and oesophagus. Apart from this, diagnosis depends on visualising the larynx, which in the neonate is possible without anaesthesia. This will be performed at the same time as an endotracheal tube is passed to relieve the breathing difficulty.

After the first few weeks of life, to inspect the larynx directly requires a general anaesthetic. This demands particular skills of the anaesthetist and surgeon, who are both seeking access to the larynx. The operating microscope gives a magnified view of the larynx seen through a rigid laryngoscope passed via the mouth. This is the technique of microlaryngoscopy. Attention is paid both to the size and appearance of the laryngeal structures and to movement. As the anaesthetic wears off the dynamics of the larynx are revealed allowing assessment to be made of the vocal cord movement in order to diagnose a vocal cord palsy or view the characteristic appearance of laryngomalacia. If necessary, surgical procedures may be carried out as described below. The trachea and bronchi are usually inspected under the same anaesthetic.

It is surprising how young a child will allow examination of the larynx with a mirror held in the back of the throat. This method of indirect laryngoscopy is particularly useful where vocal cord nodules are suspected. This allows the diagnosis to be made without a general anaesthetic and the child can be referred for speech therapy. Although technically easy to remove the nodules (by one of the methods outlined below), it is likely to be of little value unless the vocal misuse can be corrected. Once this has been achieved, should the nodules remain, surgery can be hoped to be worthwhile. The occasion will arise when diagnosis is made under general anaesthetic and the opportunity may as well be taken to remove the nodules, but unless vocal retraining is quickly learnt the nodules are likely to return.

General Health and Development

Attention must continually be paid to the development of a child with a laryngeal disorder. An airway that is adequate at birth may fail to grow to keep pace with the increased needs of the growing child and the demands of exercise. The result will be retarded physical and mental development.

The rest of the upper respiratory tract must not be overlooked and disease of the tonsils, adenoids and sinuses may require treatment.

Surgical Treatment

Endoscopic Surgery

Using the technique of microlaryngoscopy described above it is possible to perform surgical procedures. Various tools are used to do this. Microsurgical instruments such as scissors and forceps allow surgery in the traditional manner to be performed. This also supplies samples of the lesion for histological examination. Other modes for removal of lesions include freezing with cryotherapy, burning with diathermy and vaporisation with the laser. As mentioned above it is often unnecessary to remove vocal cord nodules in children but this can easily be performed by microdissection or by using the laser.

The laser offers the best method for the treatment of juvenile papillomata. They can thus be removed with the least risk of spillage of cells reducing the chance of recurrence and spread. It also allows for very accurate removal of the papillomata with the minimum of residual scarring. In some cases this has to be repeated often and at short intervals in order to maintain laryngeal function. Tracheotomy is occasionally necessary but adds to the risk of dissemination of the papillomata into the lower airways. There is a natural tendency for the majority of cases to regress but the condition remains one of the most challenging to the paediatric laryngologist and many alternative treatments to surgery have been evaluated. Chemotherapeutic agents having antibacterial, antiviral and cytotoxic properties and the use of prepared vaccines have in individual cases proved successful but are not yet a universal solution to the problem.

Congenital subglottic haemangiomata have a life-cycle that leads to their regression by about the age of three years. Their situation, however, usually makes a tracheotomy necessary and in order to allow earlier decannulation attempts may be made to remove the haemangioma with the laser endoscopically or they can be dissected out at 'open laryngeal surgery'.

'Open' Laryngeal Surgery

It has long been held that to interfere with the cartilage of the growing larynx would lead to damage and deformity more troublesome than the laryngeal pathology that was being treated. A wait-and-see policy was adopted and the infant managed with a tracheotomy until such time as growth relieved the obstruction. In times past this policy had to be applied to relatively few children as babies with severe laryngeal abnormalities did not usually survive long after birth. With the advent of neonatal intensive care units many more infants do survive with tracheotomies and the need is much greater, in terms of numbers of children, to correct the lesion and so allow restoration of the normal airway. This particularly applies to the lesion of subglottic stenosis.

Methods have been devised to enlarge the subglottic lumen and may be carried out if examination under anaesthetic at three-monthly intervals has shown that there is insufficient growth occurring naturally. The surgery would then be performed at about the age of 18 months. The larynx is exposed through a neck skin incision. The thyroid cartilage is vertically split in the midline to open into the laryngeal lumen and the narrowed segment of the subglottis can be identified. This may be widened by slitting vertically through the narrowed portion and holding the two edges apart with a cartilage graft taken from a rib, or by performing a stepped incision through the narrowed segment and placing appropriate sutures to hold the edges apart (laryngotracheoplasty). In the latter case a supporting stent is placed in the lumen of the larynx and upper trachea and later removed after healing has occurred, usually six weeks postoperatively. By these means early decannulation of the tracheotomy is possible (Cotton and Evans, 1981).

Laryngeal webs may also be removed by an open technique. The substance of the web is dissected out, keeping intact the epithelial edge, which is used to reconstruct the anterior portion of one of the vocal cords. The raw edge of the anterior portion of the other vocal cord epithelialises naturally. Accurate positioning of the two cords is essential to create the anterior commissure. Failure to do this leads to persisting dysphonia. The use of the laser to remove webs endoscopically is being evaluated. The timing of surgery for laryngeal webs depends on whether the web causes obstruction sufficient to require tracheotomy. If so then early removal of the web is desirable to allow decannulation. If the laryngeal disorder is solely dysphonia, then treatment can be delayed but it is preferable to attempt to improve the voice before the child starts school.

Conclusion

The work of those managing disorders of the larynx in children aims to restore normal laryngeal function. Judgement is required to balance active intervention against the natural processes of growth and repair. Failure to act promptly in the severely obstructed larynx leads to disaster. Failure to recognise that a partially obstructed larynx is not providing for the needs of the infant will have long-term effects on physical and mental development. Overenthusiastic surgical intervention may produce permanent laryngeal deformities with consequent effects on the voice.

References

Cotton, R. T. and Evans, J. N. G. 'Laryngotracheal Reconstruction in Children: Five Year Follow-up', *Annals of Otology, Rhinology and Laryngology*, 90, 516–20 (1981)

Ferguson, C. F. and Kendig, E. L. *Paediatric Otolaryngology*, Vol 2 of *Disorders of the Respiratory Tract in Children*, 2nd edn (W. B. Saunders Co., Philadelphia, 1972)
Pracy, R. 'The Infant Larynx', *Journal of Laryngology and Otology*, 97, 933–47 (1983)
Wilson, D. K. *Voice Problems of Children*, 2nd edn (Williams and Wilkins, Baltimore, 1979)

5 THERAPY AND MANAGEMENT OF THE DYSPHONIC CHILD

Elaine Hodkinson

Introduction

The human voice reflects many aspects of a person's physical, social, cultural and psychological development and background. From the birth cry to voice mutation at puberty, and voice stability during adolescence, there are many influences upon the child's voice development.

When a child is unable to produce a voice that is normal for the age, stage of growth and maturation, the child should be identified as having a sign or symptom that requires investigation and assessment. In this way we can avoid, as far as possible, the child's use of vocal behaviour that can detract from the child's social and cultural interactions or psychological and educational development and achievement. Dysphonia can be described as disorder of voice which includes phonation and resonance.

At birth some syndromes are immediately obvious and it can be deduced that the child is 'at risk' and that amongst various problems the child may have disorders of phonation and/or resonance. In other chapters of this book the cerebral palsied and the deaf are presented. However, the child who is mentally handicapped with Down's syndrome, who has cleft lip and palate or laryngeal atresia is easily diagnosed.

Voice disorders can be caused by growths, structural laryngeal pathology or the child's voice can be abnormal because of neuromuscular weakness which interferes with the normal function of the larynx or resonators.

The speech therapist's work as a team member is to bring specialist knowledge about the production, development and effectiveness of voice production to the parents, medical and social workers and teachers. These interactions require knowledge and skills in counselling, informing and teaching, and require that professional communication skills are essential to the therapist. In working with the child all these roles have to be used so that both child and therapist can relate at the level of contact and communication appropriate to the child's most effective learning.

When a potential problem is identified and the team require the involvement of the speech therapist, as much as possible should be done to minimise the effects of diagnosed conditions upon the child's voice production as well as all other aspects of development. Parental support and counselling throughout the infant's early years can help produce the most satisfactory climate, not only for assisting the child to develop most effectively, but for preventing some of the problems acquired and demonstrated when parents are ill-informed, anxious or unsure of how to help their child. Careful and informed observation about where, when, why and how much information is required so that parents can absorb and understand what is happening. It takes a good deal of time for some parents to accept that their child has a particular problem. They must then understand the nature of the difficulty for the child and how they can assist in supporting and encouraging the child's progress. It may be that the therapist can be more effective in a preventive role when parents recognise the importance of human communication, and what is required of them to support the work of the multidisciplinary team of which they are a member.

Parents obviously are helped to understand that voice is part of the communication process and that speech, language and behaviour are also considered when looking at how best to find out about and help the whole child.

Identifying Problems in the First Year

In the first year of the child's life, the parents develop close contact with the baby, in holding, feeding, caring for the child and responding to his needs. Martin (1981) has spent some time in comparing the voices of babies as a significant feature in the child's development. The main signal used by the child is voice (Wolff, 1969); the larynx is used for crying, coughing and vocal play and the child's cries can be interpreted by the parents. It is an important agent in bonding. Wasz-Hockert *et al.* (1968) used spectrographic studies and listener judgement data based on 419 cries of 351 healthy infants. Four distinctive cries were identified from birth to seven months.

(1) Birth signal: short duration with a flat or falling melody, always strained or strident and containing glottal plosives.
(2) Pain signal: long duration, high pitched and strident with usually a falling melody.
(3) Hunger signal: pitch rising/falling with frequent glottal plosives.
(4) Pleasure signal: flat pitch with greater pitch variability than other types of cries, never strident and with rare glottal plosives.

Mothers appeared to have little difficulty recognising the cries of their own babies as demonstrated by Hollien, Brown and Hollien (1971) and Muller, Hollien and Murray (1974).

Infant cries and other vocalisations are found to be inseparable from associated facial expressions and bodily movements. Young and Decarie (1977) coded the facial/vocal behaviour and bodily movements of 75 infants into positive and negative vocalisations. These vocalisations were then categorised into babbling, cooing, laughing and squealing, wail, soft wail and harsh wail. It is from these voice sounds that children develop the language of their culture, and Lenneberg (1967) made distinctions between the early appearing sounds of crying and vegetative activity and later voice behaviour of cooing and babbling.

It is obvious that parents are much influenced by the voice of the baby and that the family relationships and interactions are built up and affected by even subtle changes of phonation and resonances as infancy becomes childhood and then puberty. The parents have expectations of how this growing up should be achieved and deviations from an orderly process can cause tension and anxiety and other negative reactions.

Voice Problems in Older Children

Some children are particularly in need of special care which has to be monitored throughout their childhood, and the professionals looking after the child should share relevant information with each other of practical or theoretical importance. This information can range from research into environmental characteristics, considering cultural factors, attitudes and social influences on the basic competencies. In this way the total world of the child and its influence upon him, as well as his interaction with the environment can be considered.

Where the child has an obvious organic syndrome such as papillomata it is hoped that the speech therapist will be involved at an early stage for voice and speech assessment. Where the child has had early surgical intervention there will be investigative and supportive work to encourage the child to be an effective communicator. In the case of the child with tracheostomy there is a role in ongoing management in that the child learns to occlude the opening of the tube on expiration and projects air through the larynx. These children can be encouraged to be more effective in their non-verbal skills, so that eye contact, smiling, facial expression and gesture can enhance their effective communication. It is important for the speech therapist to understand the medical and surgical treatment programme so that any information that needs to be passed on is accurate and relevant. If the child is on new treatment such as interferon therapy for papillomatosis, the therapist is one of the members of the team who, in monitoring progress, can report on the child's attention, mood, behaviour and general communication as well as specific laryngeal performance (Goepfert, 1982).

The work of the speech therapist with congenitally handicapped children is important in aiding development and effective use of voice as the child matures physically and cognitively. Each new situation requires voice to be adapted depending upon the acoustics and the psychological variables influencing the child.

The child with structural change to the vocal tract will normally be referred to the speech therapist by the appropriate consultant surgeon or physician. Assessments and diagnoses will be made regarding the anatomical and physiological condition of the larynx and resonators. However, children are not so easily classified by having a diagnosis of 'vocal nodules', 'misuse and abuse of voice' and much care in investigating the child and his life and behaviour is required to help the child to unlearn the voice behaviour that has produced a traumatic result. Voice samples of voice disorders are found in Stemple (1984). A young girl with congenital web and monotonous pitch, and a hoarse and breathy dysphonia in a girl with bilateral nodules are found on the record in his book.

Classification of Voice Problems

Wilson (1979) classifies voice problems into (1) voice quality problems, (2) resonance problems, and (3) loudness and pitch problems. Aronson (1980) suggests that the following voice parameters are the elements of voice:

(1) Pitch: the perceptual correlate of frequency
(2) Loudness: the perceptual correlate of intensity
(3) Quality: the perceptual correlate of complexity
(4) Flexibility: the perceptual correlate of pitch, loudness and quality variations
(5) Voice is described as audible sound produced by phonation
(6) Phonation is the physical act of sound production by means of vocal fold interaction with the exhaled airstream

The causes of voice problems in children have been classified by Wilson (1979) as (1) organic, (2) organic changes resulting from vocal abuse and misuse, (3) functional, and (4) factors contributing to the voice problem. He suggests that voice problems exist on a continuum with organic at one end and functional at the other. It is a two-way path because a pathology can result in a poorly functioning voice mechanism, or a poorly functioning mechanism can result in organic changes or conditions.

The four variables rated by Boone (1977) on a nine-point scale are (1) pitch, (2) phonation quality, (3) loudness, and (4) resonance quality. This is a voice screening outline in which pitch level considered normal for the child's age and sex would be rated 1 or 2, and pitch level much higher and lower than peers would be rated 8 or 9. Phonation quality is rated according to the presence or absence of hoarseness, breathiness or harshness with 1 or 2 rated normal and 8 or 9 with deviations in quality. Quality disorders require careful observation according to Boone as they often are the first symptoms of a nodule or papilloma. It may be that persistent quality disorders confirmed by parent or teacher will initiate laryngoscopic examination to confirm diagnosis.

Screening evaluation of loudness in an artificial situation is difficult as the testing environment inhibits the child. Sometimes the test can be carried out at the nursery group or school and rated when the child interacts normally with other children. It is easier to compare the voices of the peer group in this way.

The Buffalo Voice Profile of Wilson (1979) is considered a useful seven-point rating scheme indicating severity of phonation problems in 12 descriptive items. More recently a vocal profile analysis protocol has been developed by Laver, Wirz and McKenzie (1982). This is particularly useful when a full evaluation of all articulatory as well as laryngeal parameters is to be assessed. Imaging techniques to demonstrate what vocal gestures are being performed by the vocal tract can give clear information of what the child is doing on phonation to the larynx and supraglottic resonators. The work of MacCurtain (1982) gives information not only to the doctor and speech therapist, but allows both parents and child to gain insight into what happens when the child uses voice.

Clinical Examination of Voice

A scientific approach to clinical examination of voice is outlined by Hirano (1981). Diagnostic procedures determine:

(1) The cause of the voice disorder
(2) The degree and extent of the causative disease
(3) The degree of disturbance in phonatory function
(4) The prognosis of the voice disorder as well as that of the cause of the disorder
(5) The establishment of a therapeutic programme

Hirano classifies ways in which direct or indirect assessment, observation and/or measurements can be made. Physiological and physical parameters are listed which regulate vibratory patterns of the vocal folds.

The following areas suggest the many investigations that may need to be made.

(1) History-taking
(2) Physical examinations
(3) Neurological examinations
(4) Function tests
(5) Endoscopy
(6) X-ray examinations
(7) Electromyography

(8) Aerodynamic measurements
(9) Histological examinations
(10) Microbiological examinations
(11) Endocrinological examinations
(12) Blood and serum examinations
(13) Observations during surgery
(14) Behavioural tests
(15) Psychological examinations

The speech therapist uses this medical information to clarify organic problems. The site and extent of the lesion is noted as is the aetiology and pathology of any diagnosed condition. There will be discussion by the team of the preferred approaches to management and treatment policy and careful follow-up to assess progress.

Voice Programme for Children

A voice programme for children has been produced by Boone (1980). Two manuals are available which describe (a) screening, evaluation and referral, and (b) remediation. An additional help to the clinician are the forms available which allow detailed analysis of the history of the disorder and the health of the child. Other sections allow evaluation reports on hearing, respiration, oral examination and voice rating scales. The organisation of the voice team and the various tasks each specialist should undertake are outlined by Wilson (1979). The speech therapist assesses vocal behaviour formally and informally when the child is alone with the therapist and aware of the evaluation. The therapist also observes group play and how the child uses voice either with abuse or effectively. The voice screening profile of Wilson and Rice (1977), is advocated in which laryngeal tone, voice pitch, loudness and resonance with overall voice efficiency are rated from normal to mild, moderate and severe problems.

Boone's remediation manual may be found helpful by clinicians who appreciate a clear and formal treatment structure.

The areas for new learning by the child incorporate ear training, yawn-sigh, new mouth movements and altering tongue position. The facilitating approaches develop new kinaesthetic awareness in the child as well as improved auditory perception. The visual materials in the manual also hold the child's attention and interest and give guidelines for sequences in therapy.

An overall picture of the child in his family should be developed, and the help of the family encouraged and supported by the speech therapist. Once the child is at nursery or junior school, the class teacher or specialist singing or drama teacher may need to understand the overall management plan. In some school settings teachers who are interested in reinforcing good voice production can help the dysphonic child by planning class activities that allow the group to practise voice programmes that are beneficial to individual children in many ways. The careful rehearsal of reading out loud, singing and role play can help the children understand what they are doing in performing these activities. Appropriate parts can be given to the children to practise different voices in a variety of characters in plays. There are many aspects of voice work that the teacher can support much more naturally at school than the parent at home or the therapist in the clinic. Once teachers see the need for healthy vocal behaviour they are only too ready to seek information on the many strategies open to them. They also begin to suggest seeing other children whose voice and speech they believe not to be normal. There are still problems to be overcome in promoting the classroom teachers' understanding of speech disorders (Wertz and Mead, 1975).

Speech Therapy

Parents and teachers have to believe that learning can be fun in therapy. Sometimes they think it is the serious work of the therapist, and they forget all they know in the normal context of the child's life that play or wanted activity is what best assists the child's desire to achieve or accomplish an aim. There are ways of communicating ideas to children that are appropriate to a particular age or stage of growth. Therapy should be tailored to the child's existing mode of gaining awareness, understanding his own present behaviours and setting and achieving objectives. These cognitive factors should be represented in natural everyday activities chosen or accepted by the child. He should be encouraged to participate actively in the learning process (Bruner, 1972).

Speech therapy can be described as the sharing of work which identifies and allows clear understanding of the communication problems to be dealt with, and strategies and techniques that will facilitate learning and change. All modalities of perception can be used and some children react to and prefer sensory experience from vision, taste or smell at one stage to tactile or kinaesthetic at another time. Auditory perception and discrimination is often the latest to refine and requires maturity of the child before they can be self-monitoring. It is essential that the therapist has knowledge of a wide range of toys and equipment that can be called upon to illustrate an area of work that requires attention or can promote an activity. The practice of a game or the repetition of an interesting task gives the child an opportunity to develop awareness and skill. The therapist has to be able to provide appropriate materials, outline the possibilities that exist and can be created by the child in engaging in the process of therapy, and monitor with the child developments and future objectives.

Treatment Approaches

The following ideas are examples of treatment approaches for the child with voice disorders that follow the well-described areas of what is required for effective voice production – relaxation, posture and movement, respiration, phonation, resonance and articulation. The therapist's skills are first called upon to make the child feel comfortable and relaxed and encourage a relationship in which the patient trusts and enjoys what the therapist has to offer.

It is from the rapport that develops, that aims and objectives can be negotiated with the child and a contract outlined that identifies expectations on both sides. A sequence of activities or exercises can be described and noted. A variety of materials are shown and types of work agreed with the child. In this way a plan is discussed with the child and others and a time sequence organised with the objectives in mind. Therapy thus has a focus and clear aims and does not just proceed in an unstructured way.

Assessment of the child and the type and extent of voice disorder will continue throughout treatment. Most children enjoy activity and movement and it is necessary to observe how the child habitually responds when offered tasks. Each child reacts in his or her own unique way demonstrating habit patterns, imagination and skills. Some children respond to movement from observations of reality – swimming movements or dance or skating. Television has given pictures of free falling from aeroplanes or walking on the moon. Other children respond to the ideas of 'beaming down' in postures of all kinds, or aspects of movement such as slow motion or particular rhythms. Dramatic interpretation is often displayed when children work through postural changes from puppets on strings, statues moving, sea flowers opening, or interpretations of a variety of animals or objects standing, sitting, jumping, eating or sleeping. Children loosen up and laugh in these 'dramas' and will take on new impressions and ideas for posture and movement that underpin improved relaxation and posture for efficient respiration and phonation. Music, mime, drawing pictures and patterns give opportunities to listen and do things and take the emphasis off necessarily using voice. It is part of the work to give space for silence even though quiet activity, such as drawing, is in progress. Quiet time with the therapist is required for assimilation of ideas and new skills to take place.

The therapist may therefore be painting or doing a puzzle with the child, but the key task is to assist the child to relax.

For many overactive children with misuse and abuse of voice this is a new experience. From this baseline work can proceed to painting masks or mirrors with faces that depict mood or characterisation. A well-tried favourite is a story painted or a collage depicted on a freeze. This allows a continuity of events in the child's life or a description of adventures of a chosen character in which a variety of sounds and voices are encouraged. Sweeney (1981) advocates 'encouragement' as an essential element in the helping process. He quotes the Adlerian model that in order for children to develop into self-confident healthy adults, they need to know that you have faith in their abilities and that you accept them for who they are, not only for what they do.

There are many natural phenomena to draw the child's attention to: the movement of the wind in the trees and the natural rhythm and sounds perceived; watching the way that water moves and perhaps fish swimming in water; imitating animal, bird and fish movements and suggesting sounds and voices associated with them; describing the movements of mobiles and kites, and shaping ourselves into these objects and images allows for consideration of breathing exercises that encourage deep capacity of breath and easy respiratory control in set tasks. How do birds breathe? What do whales do? If clouds were full of air and floating across the sky what would they do? In a garden of enchantment what lovely smells would there be?

These imaginative approaches allow the child to enjoy themselves and 'freewheel' in new and interesting ways. The therapist needs to think about presentation of these ideas and his or her own involvement in the exercises to support the child.

The therapist, in using imaginative strategies, can be effective in enabling the child to feel and think about understanding and accepting new behaviour. Freedom to learn gives permission for involvement, and feeling and use of self from which support and trust will grow (Rogers, 1969).

Following success in establishing appropriate posture and movement imaginative work on breathing patterns can be developed. These activities require practice and can be essential elements in building up appropriate phonation. Continuous assessment of the child's developing competence and confidence is required so that voice exercises are selected in exactly the right situation to promote, reinforce and be effective. Exercises and games can incorporate changes in loudness and pitch: these tasks can be as far apart as singing gently to dolls, chanting or using puppet voices to timing by stopwatch, continuous phonation in high, medium or low pitch range. Some children particularly enjoy the use of instrumentation to control their own work. The auditory training unit allows the patient close listening to his own voice. He may model sounds from the therapist, particularly intonation patterns, but often the child wishes to take the initiative and invites the therapist to copy his voice patterns. During these exercises it is helpful to enjoy vocal play that can be shared. In my own clinical work 'voice painting' can be utilised, and shapes and pictures drawn and coloured through voice sounds. It is in this developing voice work that changes of resonance can also be noted and used. Auditory perception and discrimination has to be further refined so that therapist and child are agreed about what are the desired sounds to achieve, how the voice manages to produce loudness and softness, high and low pitch and changes in resonance. Kinaesthetic awareness can then anchor the ability to retain the skills necessary for a range of appropriate intonation patterns. Books and stories can give the child opportunities to utilise new voice skills. It may be that reading out loud assists the child in not only use of voice but in confidence and self-regard for his achievements.

Integration of Communication

As communication is a complex activity, it is necessary for the therapist to keep integrated all positive aspects of non-verbal communication with the developing voice. The use of eye contact, observation of gaze and pupil dilatation can give clues to the child's involvement and excitement. Encouragement of smiling and easy laughter, with modification of facial expression according to context, can also give satisfaction and credibility to overall speech. The physical appearance of the child may change as he becomes more relaxed and confident. It may be necessary to decide with parent and/or teachers how to bring about these changes. Discussions with parents can cover a range of subjects. Not only can they discuss haircuts and clothes, but also bedtimes, pocket money and how a child has learnt to blow his nose. With children who are dysphonic, it is often necessary to clarify the best ways to clear the throat or inhibit shouting.

This chapter has attempted to draw upon a general understanding of the treatment and management of the dysphonic child. The human voice is part of the unique characteristics of a person, and in this way it is the child who requires the care and commitment of all those involved in his education. Speech therapy offers understanding of the process of development of communication, and how lack of development or breakdown of good voice production alters relationships with those involved with the child. Participation in therapy through this educational and counselling approach increases the success of speech therapy intervention, allows for the child's own pattern of learning to be considered, and encourages the development of insight and self-esteem.

References

Aronson, A. E. *Clinical Voice Disorders* (Brian C. Decker/Thieme-Stratton, New York 1980)

—— Peterson, H. W., and Litin, E.M.

'Psychiatric Symptomatology in Functional Dysphonia and Aphonia', *Journal of Speech and Hearing Disorders*, 31, 115–27 (1966)

Boone, D. *The Voice and Voice Therapy*, 2nd edn (Prentice-Hall, Englewood Cliffs, NJ 1977)

—— *The Boone Voice Program for Children* (CC Publications, Oregon, 1980)

Bruner, J. *The Process of Education* (Harvard University Press, Cambridge, Mass. 1970)
—— *The Relevance of Education* (Penguin, Harmondsworth, 1972)
Goepfert, H. *et al.*, 'Leukocyte Interferon in Patients with Juvenile Laryngeal Papillomatosis', *Otology, Rhinology, Laryngology,* 91, (1982)
Hirano, M. *Clinical Examination of Voice* (Springer-Verlag, New York, 1981)
Hollien, H., Brown, W. S. and Hollien, K. 'Vocal Fold Length Associated with Modal, Falsetto and Varying Intensity Phoniatrics', *Folia Phoniatrica (Basel)*, 23, 66–78 (1971)
Laver, J. Wirz, S. and MacKenzie, J. 'Vocal Profile Analysis Protocol', *Vocal Profiles of Speech Disorders Research Project*, University of Edinburgh (1982)
Lenneberg, E. *The Biological Foundations of Language*, (John Wiley, New York 1967)
MacCurtain, F. 'Pharyngeal Factors Influencing Voice Quality', PhD thesis University of London (1982)
Martin, J. A. M. *Voice Speech and Language in the Child Development and Disorder* (Springer-Verlag, New York, 1981)
Muller, E., Hollien, H. and Murray, T. 'Perceptual Responses to Infant Crying: Identification of Cry Types', *Journal of Child Language*, 4, 321–8 (1974)
Rogers, C. *Freedom to Learn: A View of What Education Might Become* (Charles E. Merrill, Columbus, Ohio, 1969)
Stemple, J. C. *Clinical Voice Pathology — Theory and Management* (Charles E. Merrill, Columbus, Ohio, 1984)
Sweeney, T. J. *Adlerian Counselling: Proven Concepts and Strategies* (Accelerated Development Inc., Indiana 1981)
Wasz-Hockert, O. *et. al., The Infant Cry* (William Heinemann Medical Books Ltd, London, 1968)
Wertz, R. T. and Mead, M. D. 'Classroom Teacher and Speech Clinician Severity Ratings of Different Speech Disorders', *Language and Speech Hearing Services for Schools*, 6, 119–24 (1975)
Wilson, D. K. *Voice Problems of Children* (Williams and Wilkins Company, Baltimore, 1979)
Wilson, F. B. and Rice, M. *A Programmed Approach to Voice Therapy* (Learning Concepts Inc., Austin, Texas, 1977)
Wolff, P. H. 'The Natural History of Crying and Other Vocalisations in Early Infancy', in B. M. Foss (ed.) *Determinants of Infant Behaviour*, (Methuen, London, 1969)
Young, G. and Decarie, T. G. 'An Ethology Based Catalogue of Facial/Vocal Behaviour in Infancy', *Animal Behaviour*, 25, 95–107 (1977)

6 VOICE IN CEREBRAL PALSIED CHILDREN

Kay Coombes

Introduction

Cerebral palsied children have a multiplicity of problems: depending upon the extent of the brain damage, there may be intellectual deficit and sensory loss in addition to the motor disability. These, together with psychosocial factors, will influence communicative ability. Maximum development of a child's communication should be a principal goal for everyone concerned. Speech may be impossible for some children to achieve, and increasingly sophisticated augmentative systems are becoming available for some in this group. However, almost all children exhibit vocalisation of some sort at various times, and it is part of the speech therapist's brief to promote the most normal use of voice.

Conventionally, dysphonias in the cerebral palsies are analysed and described in accordance with restrictions imposed upon respiration, phonation and resonance, by hypertonic, flaccid or fluctuating muscle tone, and by involuntary movements due to released reflex activity, irradiation (overflow), chorea or tremor. Classical divisions are principally those of spasticity and dyskinesia (including athetosis and ataxia). Descriptions of associated vocal characteristics of each group include terms such as 'monotonous', 'laboured', and 'prolongation of vowels'. Athetoid and ataxic children are described as having 'pitch breaks', 'breathy', and 'inconsistent' voice; in other words, their vocal performance is seen to mirror their varied and variable neuromuscular co-ordination. Such descriptions are clinical shorthand, they are not inaccurate, but they are not precise or comprehensive and they do not immediately reflect the combination of symptoms which might be evident in any one child, or the way in which coexisting symptoms interact. There is no indication, for instance, of the significant effects that attempts to vocalise may have on posture and balance. This means that such descriptions are not descriptive diagnoses and they cannot indicate an appropriate point of intervention or therapy approach.

In these children, dysphonia is typically part of a wider pattern of dysarthria involving resonance and articulation. Several authorities on voice disorders and their remediation have been pessimistic about achieving success in treating this group. While it may be true that some forms of dysarthrophonia are 'resistant to modification' (Aronson, 1980) it may be particularly important to consider: (1) purposes of intervention at any one time and, associated with these, (2) criteria for success.

There may also be a number of ways to effect improvement more successfully than those typically employed; there has been too little evaluation of clinical methods to judge. However, timing, consistency and continuity of intervention may be as crucial as the selection of an appropriate clinical technique.

This chapter considers some treatment principles employed by speech therapists working with cerebral palsied children and their objectives. Objectives are necessarily defined according to each clinician's view of neurophysiological and psychological processes operating in normal and disrupted speech production together with his beliefs about potential opportunities and strategies for preventing aberrant behaviour or modifying existing behaviour. Clinicians who share the currently accepted view of phonation as part of a valved air-stream system of speech production (Darley, Aronson and Brown, 1975) will include oral articulation processes in their assessment of function and try to examine the relationship between all levels of valving. It is easy to misinterpret phonetic features in patients with central lesions, mainly because there are often many interrelated patterns of impairment due to the nature of the damage. For example, some misarticulations or omission of phonemes may be manifestations of inadequate phonation rather than the result of incompetent oral musculature. In turn 'dysphonia' may stem from difficulties below the glottis, rather than from laryngeal malfunction (Hardy, 1983). A six-year-old child with athetoid quadriplegia fails to make voice/voiceless contrasts: she voices all plosives, stops and voices labiodental fricatives in initial positions. Other fricatives are omitted. Does this reflect hearing loss, phonological disorder, an inability to inhibit voice by abducting vocal cord promptly, or does it demonstrate an automatic adaptation to economise on an inadequate supply of air pressure by reducing the demand? The picture presented possesses all characteristics of the classical chicken and egg syndrome. Part of the clinician's expertise lies in separating eggs from chickens in order to intervene in the right way at the right time. This has to involve close liaison with the physiotherapists concerned, but responsibility for making a differential diagnosis of voice, speech and language difficulties, incorporating appropriate physical management into the treatment of dysarthrophonia and monitoring progress, rests with the speech therapist. Satisfactory discharge of this responsibility demands a degree of communication and co-operation, both amongst professionals concerned and between them and the parents, which seems elusive for a number of reasons. Often there is too little contact between therapists to allow any real sharing of aims and attitudes, although this would seem essential for successful pursuit of function.

Intervention Routes by Therapists

There seem to be two main intervention routes used by therapists which can be termed: (a) facilitative, and (b) compensatory.

Implications of these approaches for the treatment of children who have dysarthrophonia (or who are believed to be likely to develop dysarthrophonia), are outlined below.

Facilitative Approach

This assumes that vegetative movements of respiration and feeding underlie movements of speech. Therapy, therefore, would be directed towards modifying abnormal at-rest breathing and promoting patterns of sucking and swallowing in infants and biting, chewing and mature swallowing in older children. But are vegetative functions and speech production directly related? Do movements of respiration and feeding impact on valving the vocal tract for speech and can proficiency at this basic level predict vocal performance?

Another assumption is that non-speech movements, such as yawning and gagging and also non-speech vocalisations, are associated with phonation and voice quality. Practising these non-speech activities is therefore expected to improve voluntary phonation. Again, however, it is not clear that such practice is helpful, although there may be intrinsic value in eliciting voice in terms of prelinguistic communication and enjoyment.

Finally, it is assumed that ability to produce isolated speech-type behaviours, such as consonant–vowel combinations, implies potential ability to produce intelligible speech. However, the extent to which practising isolated nonsense syllables, or even single words, may be expected to lead to improvement in the production of continuous speech is uncertain, although again there may be some intrinsic value in practising this kind of vocal exercise for other reasons.

The usefulness of oral exercises probably varies from individual to individual. Those with more involvement of oral musculature and less respiratory/phonatory paresis, or inco-ordination, may well benefit from an 'oral gymnastics' approach, and be able to incorporate learnt positions and movements of jaw, lips and tongue into their speech. There are certainly individuals who are not able to generalise such isolated learning, and they seem to be those who have more (or equal) involvement of thorax, pharynx and larynx, that is individuals with moderate or severe dysphonia. It appears fruitless to concentrate on oral movements for consonant production without regard for the interaction between respiratory, phonatory and articulatory mechanisms which has been comprehensively described elsewhere (Darley, Aronson and Brown, 1975; Mysak, 1980).

Compensatory Approach

In both these approaches, speech production can be viewed essentially as a system in which air pressure is generated and controlled by a series of valves, although therapists adopting either approach may differ in their opinions about the origins and development of the system. The compensatory approach, however, assumes little overlap of vegetative function, or any other non-speech activity and propositional speech. Neuromotor programming of speech is considered unique and separate from the non-speech functions described in the facilitatory model. Thus, intervention is aimed at modifying dysarthric speech itself, that is, the entire vocal output, by teaching the speaker strategies which accommodate his neuromotor limitations.

Strategies would include, for instance, adjusting to a short expiratory time associated with low respiratory (tidal) volume and air wastage by using short phrases (rather than aiming to alter the breathing pattern), by slowing the rate of speech using devices for stress, such as pausing before the emphasised word, and, at an oral level, using phonetic approximations in place of those phonemes which are impossible for the speaker to produce. Paradoxically, this approach which has been labelled 'compensatory', can become a form of facilitation in that devices or tricks such as those illustrated sometimes appear to influence breathing for speech, and facilitate the co-ordination of air flow and vocal cord movement. The way in which this comes about has not been satisfactorily explained and may vary between different individuals in various situations.

Merely providing the speaker with a strategy to use may reduce anxiety sufficiently to inhibit hypertonicity associated with stress, which has been overlaid on primary hypertonicity. The novelty of the consciously adopted manner of speech may be a helpful distraction, which serves to maintain this reduction of tone. Alternatively, or additionally, improvement may be the result of acoustic and kinaesthetic feedback due to the induced behaviour having provoked changes in neurophysiological organisation: repeatedly breaking a stereotyped sensorimotor pattern may allow integration at a higher level; in this case true motor learning is taking place (Mysak, 1980). For example, speech breathing is often impaired in individuals whether there is (predominantly) spasticity or involuntary movements. Air flow and pressure required for phonation is likely to be reduced in a speaker who has spasticity. Inefficiency results sometimes from impairment of inspiratory movements and often from difficulty in extending the exhalation, that is, an inability to adjust the breathing cycle for speech. In addition, air is wasted at laryngeal level by inefficient valving. Characteristically, there is a delay in adducting vocal cords so that air escapes through them prior to the onset of vibration and/or hyperadduction occurs so that greater force is required to blow the cords apart. This results in further air wastage as well as perceived features of harsh attack, loud initial volume, and so on. There may also be extraneous bodily movement or spasm associated with the effort of forced expiration for voice.

When the speaker practises short utterances at a *slowed* rate it seems to facilitate better co-ordination of respiration and phonation and so there may be less air wastage of the kind described at laryngeal level. Intrinsic laryngeal musculature appears better able to function given an increase in air flow. There is less effort and the reduction in hypertonicity increases mobility and reduces distortions of head and neck posture, which influences extrinsic laryngeal muscles directly and intrinsic laryngeal muscles indirectly.

Increased mobility of the neck permits independent head movement in individuals who have head control. This promotes a more normal postural relationship between head and upper trunk. Importantly, this may allow extrinsic laryngeal muscles to alter the position of the larynx vertically, thereby changing the length of the resonating column and enhancing pitch changes which might be obtained from the more mobile vocal cords.

Variations in pitch and stress help to make slowed speech acceptable. A slower rate of speech than normal is probably inevitable for spastic dysarthrophonic speakers; it is the even rate and monotonous voice which make it hard for listeners to accept the speaker's performance and truly listen to his output. A consciously slowed rate of speech may be presented as a specific goal to these speakers. However, it seems to be more effective to emphasise reducing effort by teaching the speaker to use exhaled air efficiently through: increased monitoring of the initiation of phonation, contrasting voiced and voiceless sounds, exploiting pitch changes and pausing. This results in slowing speech in a more acceptable way than concentrating on rate per se, which tends to produce a kind of syllable-timed reduction with less improvement of aesthetic quality or intelligibility.

This compensatory approach sounds attractively straightforward, since it tends to imply that informed and motivated speakers should achieve speech which is intelligible, albeit slow and aesthetically limited. It also suggests that effective remediation is more likely when children can actively co-operate in therapy. These conclusions are not usually supported by observation of children with moderate to severe involvement of trunk and head control who are trying to speak. Typically, you see and hear an obvious difficulty in initiating and sustaining voice and in controlling pitch and volume. These are probably the inevitable results of faulty learning.

Primary and Secondary Impairment and Sensorimotor Integration

Speech represents the highest level of sensorimotor integration. The highest level in the neurological organisation of speech production is the cerebral cortex, where sequences of sounds are programmed. Messages are transmitted by pyramidal fibres to respiratory, laryngeal and articulatory muscles via the motor cortex and motor nuclei in the brain-stem and spinal cord. Fine regulation of the system is facilitated by the extrapyramidal system (cortex, cerebellum and basal ganglia).

Any form of cerebral palsy is liable to involve diffuse neurological damage, predominant symptoms are taken as indicators of sites and combination of lesions. For instance, the impairment of extrapyramidal function is clearly evident in children with ataxia and athetosis where lesions primarily affect cerebellar and basal ganglia fibres respectively. Symptoms of athetosis and ataxia coexist in many children. In addition to the neurophysiological effects of brain damage on voice production, 'psychological states can affect any aspect of the entire sequences of phonation' (Hirano, 1981). This is certainly the case in many cerebral palsied children and effective management encompasses physical and psychological aspects. Speech activities become embedded in an abnormal tactile and kinaesthetic background produced by distorted muscle tone, posture and movement. The essential nature of speech, involving emotion and cognition, together with the neuromuscular demands of highly integrated synergies is liable to produce the most extreme distortions. It is during speaking attempts that the child is likely to experience the grossest divergence from normal patterns. In summary, there is likely to be primary sensorimotor impairment of respiratory, phonatory and articulatory function which will always limit potential performance. Secondary handicap is superimposed on primary disabilities when symptoms of the primary impairment (which may be evident in non-speech behaviour, but are typically aggravated by attempts to speak), are not modified by appropriate therapy.

The more voice and speech have been experienced without such modification, the more difficult it will be to unlearn the practised patterns and replace them with unfamiliar and therefore non-automatic (although 'more normal') ones. In addition, some children compound the problem by adopting a telegrammatic speech style, apparently in order to economise on air and muscular co-ordination. This maladaptive response tends to further reduce linguistic clues provided by redundancy and rhythm, and it probably makes speech less intelligible.

Aim for Intelligible Communication

Aiming for intelligible speech means directing therapy towards goals of prosodic adequacy rather than articulatory precision. This is not a new idea, it has been emphasised repeatedly in print at least since 1949 (Peacher, 1949). Phrasing, stress and intonation, together with associated communicative gestures of body and facial expression are recognised to be more significant than precise and consistent articulation of jaw, lips, tongue and palate. Many children who are not cerebral palsied, but appear neurologically normal, demonstrate a delay in acquiring a full repertoire of consonantal sounds. Nevertheless, they are often intelligible communicators because they do not have restricted intonation patterns or motor impairment. They transmit the message via appropriately intonated English vowel sounds and the odd consonant and emphasise it by gesture (pointing, arm waving and facial expression). Both these basic abilities are likely to be difficult for children with cerebral palsy. Nevertheless, they are fundamental elements: intonation patterns are normally manifested during the first year; non-verbal communication precedes speech, then proceeds to support and amplify it, and on occasion may take the place of speech.

Illustrations of the way in which infants combine prespeech utterances and non-verbal communication are recounted in the literature, together with comments on the similarity of some prespeech utterances and true words produced in parallel contexts. Stark (1978) cites the instance of an infant saying [ma] [mə] [mæ] as he reaches for something he wants. All those utterances bear some resemblance to 'more' and 'mine', words produced later with (probably) similar intent. However, a cerebral palsied child in a similar situation might show various difficulties of differentiated movement and co-ordination, such as extension of the reaching arm may elicit associated hyperextension of the jaw (and possibly generalised hyperextension of the whole body). The involuntarily (wide-open) oral position proscribes making the bilabial sound altogether and is likely to produce delayed production and distortion of the vowel sound(s). Treatment for this kind of difficulty would involve preventing jaw movement being associated with arm extension, and then the facilitating of graded (that is, controlled) jaw opening.

In this particular, case, the ultimate aim would be to precede the vowel with lip closure and voicing of the bilabial nasal /m/. This may best be achieved via a route in which phonation for the vowel sound is initiated, then channelled nasally by lip closure (using passive movement if necessary). The vowel–consonant utterance is repeated easily and rhythmically before attempting to initiate the utterance with /m/. Initiation of voice is often problematic for dysphonic patients, and although humming is still recommended in the literature, it tends to be difficult for many individuals. It may produce generalised flexion in those with flexor spasticity.

The child with any form of cerebral palsy is likely to have restricted and delayed development of early vocal patterns. His ability to initiate voice or experiment with pitch and rhythm in vocal play on his own, or in response to his parents, will depend upon people handling him in a way that minimises the effects of cerebral palsy. Retained startle responses, spasm, hypertonicity or hypotonicity all disrupt the infant's vocal activity and reduce or cancel the pleasurable associations which often accompany it. Although some authorities have recommended teaching consonant production in isolation, it is difficult to believe that skill developed in this way might be integrated into speech by a process of neurophysiological maturation. The theory is comforting, but clinical experience is cautionary.

Dysarthrophonia and its Management

Dysarthrophonia in children with developmental neuromotor dysfunction is different from the dysarthrophonias of acquired neurological lesions, with the exception of some acoustic features, and its management is necessarily different.

The most important differences are as follows.

First is the unavailability of any other sensorimotor experience for the cerebral palsied child. He has no personal comparison available and so he cannot aim at a remembered acoustic or kinaesthetic target.

Second, the child's dysarthrophonia is only one symptom of diffuse neurological impairment that delays and distorts behaviour and interaction in psychological as well as in physical ways. Children with any significant degree of dysarthrophonia have involvement of trunk and upper extremities and are likely to be diplegic or quadriplegic. They are therefore destined to be physically more dependent for longer than other infants. Their physical and emotional needs can be expected to bring forth predictable protective responses, which are moderated by other recognised parental responses associated with grieving, anxiety and exhaustion. These are expected in families who are coming to terms with disability, but there is a great divide between documented theory (and little of this is available) and delivery of practical help. Current theories of communication development acknowledge the importance of prelinguistic vocal and non-vocal interaction; developmental psychology journals contain descriptions of 'motherese' (Gleitman, Newport and Gleitman, 1984) and the emotional comfort afforded by physical contact between a child and its parents. The underlying processes of interaction and language development would seem to be universal (if not universally agreed) and a primary aim of therapy should be the fostering of infant–parent interaction. Therapists' descriptions of parents as 'over-protective', 'defensive', and otherwise inept in 'adjusting', probably testify to an inadequate supply of emotional support, information and specific treatment.

Timing Intervention

Early intervention is required. It entails counselling, explanation, demonstration and practice in communicating. Physical handling of the child facilitates the most normal and pleasurable experience of movement (establishing the kinaesthetic background described on p. 102)

Handling must also permit and promote eye contact with mother, and hand-to-face contact, as well as inhibiting abnormal physical responses to the exciting stimulus of the parent's voice. Such reactions interfere with early listening and associated behaviours, such as taking turns, etc.

Parents' intuitive behaviour is increasingly acknowledged by 'experts' like psycholinguists and speech therapists to be the most effective catalyst in the development of the child's language (Bruner, 1975). The way in which parents of children with learning problems accommodate their children's language difficulties has been described as conversational 'buffering' by Stanhope and Bell (1981) and illustrations of this behaviour appear in descriptions of mother–child interactions (see, for example, Bryan *et al.*, 1984). Intuitive behaviour of parents whose child is cerebral palsied can appear to be inhibited or depressed because the child's spontaneous signals, which would normally help to elicit parental behaviour are absent, infrequent, delayed or distorted. In addition, parents lack confidence, and are self-conscious, and anxious about the best way to manage when a persisting disability is suspected or confirmed.

Confirmation in early infancy is only likely when children are severely disabled, or when they show obvious hemiplegic asymmetry. Therapists should be involved before confirmation. As soon as any degree of disability is suspected there should be careful monitoring of progress; sensory input should include combining 'talking' (that is, mother's speech, and the child's early speech or prespeech vocalisations), with other activities, particularly those that are typically accompanied by mother–baby conversation, such as nappy changing, washing, dressing and eating. Positioning and moving the child therapeutically during these activities can exploit patterns of trunk extension, flexion and rotation. All these increase thoracic movement for respiration. Also, because the child is not static there tends to be more spontaneous (reflex) vocalisation than when children are held in fixed positions. This is not surprising: small children are normally noisiest during active movement, whether lying supine and kicking their legs, playing with their fingers, or engaged in rough and tumble play. This experience of automatic voicing is reduced or missing in many cerebral palsied children. Yet it is usually easy to elicit a variety of vowel sounds by making use of active movement or, if this is not possible, perhaps using passive movements. In both cases the therapist or mother accompanies the facilitated movement with her own vocal cue, or model and inhibits undesired associated movements. It is essential that the primary care giver (usually mother, and whenever possible, father too) learns to handle the baby in a way that facilitates vocalisation during daily activities.

Knowing that extension promotes inspiration and that subsequently flexing the child's legs (at knees and hips), particularly while leaning over the baby with a smile, is likely to produce vocalisation, is not only helpful in giving the child experience of vocalisation and social interaction, it enables the parents to feel successful and confident in their parenting ability. Vocalisation which is as normal as possible, and disrupts muscle tone as little as possible, contributes to more normal family relationships.

Just as the child learns from sensorimotor practice, parents need opportunities to put learning into practice under supervision.

The Relationship Between Infant Vocalisation, Voice and Speech

This is a controversial area. Developmental studies of vocal behaviour in normal and in neurologically impaired children have been interpreted differently by various authorities. Advocates of a neurodevelopmental approach to cerebral palsy, exemplified by the Bobath School (Bobath and Bobath, 1964; Mysak, 1959) view primitive reflex behaviours as natural precursors, and possibly prerequisites, of early speech development; neurological maturation results in suppression of reflex behaviours as higher brain centres are brought into operation. Differentiated and highly skilled movements result from the integration of earlier, more simple, activities. The process is facilitated by practice in combining and recombining sequences of movement similar to the way in which Bruner (1975) describes the acquisition of complex skills. Stark, Rose and Benson (1978) would seem to support this view, observing that babbling and children's first words normally appear to be governed by the same 'natural phonetic preferences'.

Jakobson (1968) disagrees: babbling is considered an essentially random activity; prespeech behaviour is seen as distinct and separate from first words. Lenneberg (1967) adopted a theory of compromise; he hypothesised that crying and vegetative sounds, such as coughing and burping, were unrelated to cooing and babbling, while conceding that the latter might be precursors of early speech development. However, two years later, Wolff (1969) concluded that cooing incorporated vocal features of crying, and later Bosma (1975), suggested that babies' feeding movements, that is, vegetative activity, influenced non-reflexive vocal output.

Features of Early Infant Behaviour

For the first two months (and possibly for much longer in the case of neurologically impaired children), the vocal tract is controlled by primitive reflexes. The infants' vocal output comprises crying and discomfort sounds, vegetative sounds (such as burps), and various grunting noises which accompany activity. It is difficult to be comprehensive and precise in describing these sounds, although speech therapists treating babies suspected of having brain damage usually make an attempt to observe and record them. Stark, Rose and McLagen (1975) devised a classification system based on auditory and spectrographic information identifying primary features, with various secondary features that were dependent on them. Primary features were: voicing; breath direction (egressive, ingressive or changing direction): 'vowel-like', that is, open tract, or 'consonant-like' (when some form of closure occurred).

Analysis of various behaviours showed interesting similarities and differences. For instance, crying and discomfort sounds shared primary features; both were typically voiced and vowel-like and produced mainly on an egressive air stream. Vegetative sounds were different; they tended to be voiceless and ingressive, and involved intermittent closure of the vocal tract which produced clicks, stops and friction noises. The infrequent consonant-like closures in crying and discomfort sounds on the other hand, were usually nasal continuants, such as /m/, liquids or stops, rather than clicks and friction sounds.

By the end of the second month, normal infants demonstrate increasing control over voicing. This development appears to be of paramount importance in the progression via vowel-like comfort sounds (at about six weeks), to subsequent 'cooing' or early babbling, at about eight weeks. At this stage, however, primitive reflex behaviour is unsuppressed. Early sound play possesses mixed elements of crying, discomfort and vegetative sounds: there is voicing, egressive breath direction, and consonant-type closure of the tract. A comparison of this performance with that of brain-damaged children reveals that some neurologically impaired infants may only be able to produce voice when distressed, for example, in response to pain (Benjamin and Stark (1974) in Stark 1978), and many continue to have difficulty in producing variations in vocal play.

Implications for Treatment

The controversy continues. Nevertheless, there is general agreement on the importance of achieving voluntary voicing in order to develop speech normally. Evidence that children with various forms of cerebral palsy fail to achieve adequate control of phonation is incontrovertible.

The typical oral patterns of eating have not been proved to be essential precursors of speech, but anyone who has observed normal children experimenting with sound play during eating, or listened to toddlers vocalising and finger feeding at teatime, must agree that meal times are vocal events rich in acoustic and tactile experience after infancy too!

The speech therapist is routinely expected to take special responsibility for assessing and treating feeding difficulties. While it is not clear that feeding contributes directly to the valving processes involved in effective phonation (see above), it seems to be the case that extraneous movement, including overflow or irradiation and released reflex activity which interfere with feeding in some children, also interrupts or delays the effective acquisition of synchronised respiratory phonatory patterns, the operation of the velopharyngeal port, and the position of the tongue. Tongue position is seen by some clinicians as essentially bound up with articulatory performance. However, since the position of the tongue influences air flow in both the pharynx and nasopharynx (so does the velum, of course), the division between articulation and phonation is seen as artificial. Tongue position, in the production of vowels particularly, is seen as part of both 'phonation' and 'articulation'.

Assessment of Voice and Related Function

Mysak's neurophysiological speech index (1981) and the prespeech assessment scales (Evans-Morris, 1982) are probably the most soundly based and comprehensive tools published to date. Their administration involves subjective clinical judgement, but both are practical and provide a clear rationale for the procedures employed, and the treatment indicated. There remains a desperate need for rigorous clinical weaponry that will enable therapists to evaluate function precisely, plan effective treatment more easily and also provide a method of measuring progress in subsequent reassessment. At the moment there is little equipment for any '-ography' (high speed cineradiography, laryngography, glottography, etc.) outside research laboratories.

Even if non-invasive technology for assessment and biofeedback (Fourcin, 1974; Gilbert, Potter and Hoodin, 1984; Guillemin and Nguyen, 1984), were to be standard clinical equipment, many of the procedures involved would not be feasible for use with small, multiply handicapped people. In any case, it is important to remember that, in general, isolating and examining parts of a complex whole does not yield much of clinical value and can be misleading. For instance, it is attractively straightforward to examine the infant mouth for oral reflexes in the absence of food. The significance of results is probably nil (Ingram, 1962). It is almost always possible to elicit some primitive activity, but this does not permit inferences about the availability of rooting and effective sucking during feeding. Observational analysis of the function(s) under scrutiny is inescapable, now and in the forseeable future.

Conventionally, the therapist uses assessment devices borrowed from clinical practice with acquired voice disorder, for example, examining maximum phonation time for vowels, judging frequency range and intensity (Boone, 1983; Darley, Aronson and Brown, 1975; Hardy, 1983).

Evaluating performance requires teasing out the nature and degree of contributory factors that are due to primary and secondary neurophysiological impairment: hearing loss, anxiety, pain, and so on. Further information is provided by the patient's response to intervention and (as is common in the treatment of other disorders), speech therapy assessment and treatment are intertwined. Monitoring treatment properly provides continuous ongoing assessment, increases insight of both therapist and patient into the nature of difficulties and ways to minimise them. At the same time well chosen and sensitively administered assessments are often therapeutic.

Respiration and Breathing for Speech

Disordered respiration usually coexists with laryngeal and articulatory dysfunction in individuals with cerebral palsy. If this were not the case, speakers would probably be able to compensate in the way that those with neuropathies, such as poliomyelitis, are able to do (Hixon, Putnam and Sharp, 1983).

It is probably true to say that reduced respiratory control alone does not produce speech which is 'clinically significant' (Hardy, 1983). Unfortunately, the central lesions of the cerebral palsies lead to disrupted patterns of movement, not to discrete paralysis of individual muscle groups. This fact does not preclude the possibility of different kinds of disruption being caused to different components, or subsystems of speech. However, at the moment it is not possible to translate hypotheses about regulatory control from contemporary research (Lesny, 1980; Abbs, Hunter and Barlow, 1982), to clinical fingertips.

In the present state of clinical knowledge, the symptoms identified, ways in which they are described, measured and interpreted, and selection of subsequent treatment methods, are likely to be based on a concept of hierarchical neurophysiological organisation (see p. 101) and inevitably constrained by the feasibility of investigative procedures (see p. 109). As always, therapists need to understand the patterns of movement involved and their purpose, in order to both appraise malfunction and alleviate it.

In a consideration of respiration for speech, this may entail relinquishing some myths about the importance of capacity, and concentrating instead upon (compensatory) control. Vast amounts of air are not required for phonation and attempts to obtain them by people with cerebral palsy are generally counterproductive and time-wasting; they should not be encouraged by clinicians, nor by parents (who may intuitively, but erroneously, urge children to 'take a deep breath'). The importance of inspiratory chest expansion and the way that it seems to facilitate recoil of expiratory muscles is not disputed. However controlling egressive air pressure is equally important, and probably presents the greater problem for the majority of speakers with developmental dysarthria.

In normal speech the outgoing air is obstructed by adducted vocal cords and by the organs of articulation. The sudden, rapid alterations in impedance that are caused, demand appropriate and prompt increases in subglottic air pressure. Typical problems of instability (associated with athetosis and ataxia), lack of mobility (associated with spasticity), and difficulty in obtaining graded muscular contraction, which is seen in all types, often result in breath being *pushed* out. This is done by simultaneously contracting ribcage and abdominal musculature and it works up to a point. As Cavallo and Baker (1985) point out, it is an inefficient method of increasing air pressure. Success is limited, since this mass effort cannot provide for speedy alternation between high and low pressures. The vocal symptoms produced by the strategy range from loud, uncontrolled voice at the onset of phonation, which becomes increasingly breathy and then aphonic, to delayed onset of voice and a low pitched monotone. Determined disciples of this technique may risk incurring abdominal pain or discomfort.

This is certainly experienced by some adults with athetosis. It is possibly due to the combined effects of the effort to phonate, and involuntary movement, and may be exacerbated by pain from degenerative skeletal changes.

Early intervention would aim to prevent a child acquiring the habit of forced phonation in this way. If therapy is successful, speech will still be dysarthric, but it will be less abnormal than it would otherwise have been. There will be fewer secondary handicaps associated with speech attempts, such as further disturbance of posture, balance and facial movement, fatigue and pain.

It seems unhelpful to work on respiration separately from vocalisation, except perhaps in the case of children with paradoxical breathing (see below). Facilitating automatic adjustments via careful positioning and movement, and controlling unwanted activity during voicing, seem to be more productive than attempting conscious regulation of breathing (which would be impractical anyway with young children). This, of course, represents an important digression from traditional approaches to other, acquired dysphonias. The traditional concept of therapeutic relaxation is also inappropriate. Attempts to invoke Jacobsen (1929) – style progressive relaxation, which is consciously controlled, are contraindicated. Exhortations to 'relax' or encouragement to 'try harder' are similarly doomed, at least until the child has experienced muscle tone and movement patterns which are as near to normal as possible, in other words, when treatment has facilitated 'neurophysiological relaxation' (Mysak's term).

Inspiration and expiration can both be influenced by practising prolonged vowel sounds. This might involve using an extended neutral vowel in games where the vowel represents the engine noise of a car, for instance. Feedback from successive attempts to prolong the vowel/make the car travel further, should result in increasing both intake of air and control of output. The system responds to the demand more efficiently, providing appropriate techniques have been used.

Adopting a Bobath approach, techniques might include exploiting features of extension and flexion (associated with breathing in and out, respectively) and using upright, weight-bearing positions to make use of gravity and proprioception, thereby maintaining active extension and sufficiently raised muscle tone in hypotonic children, or those with fluctuating tone. This last group of children are those most likely to show symptoms of paradoxical or reverse breathing. In this pathological pattern the downward movement of the diaphragm is not withstood by the ribcage. Instead of simultaneous intercostal contraction swinging the rib-cage upwards and outwards, the chest wall is pulled inward by the descent of the diaphragm. These children have flared lower ribs and indented thoracic walls, and sometimes the sternum is also indrawn. Treatment involves inhibiting or delaying diaphragmatic movement, so preventing inspiratory intercostal movement being overwhelmed. Merely restricting movement of the child's lower chest with your hands, often elicits visible upper chest movement, and this can be carried out in infants while on their mother's knee, easily maintaining face-to-face contact and conversation. It is, however, difficult to ascertain generalisation, or 'carry over'.

Aims in breathing for speech practice include the following.

Long Vowel Sounds

This means sustaining controlled voice for at least four seconds (personal clinical observation). Normal individuals can maintain a vowel sound for at least 15 seconds and Hirano (1981) suggests that less than 10 seconds is pathological. This exercise is considerably simpler than sustaining voice in connected speech, and unless four seconds or so can be achieved, phonation in speech seems to be extremely disrupted.

Vowel-to-Vowel Phonation

Some of the difficulties experienced by clinicians and their clients in phonation work may be associated with too quick a transfer to meaningful speech, or at least with excessive phonetic demand. Consonant/vowel combinations demand a degree of co-ordination and synchronisation, which may be beyond an individual's capability at the time they are tried. It seems sensible to aim first for graded jaw movement during sustained phonation. Initiating voice without exaggerated jaw opening is important, and a neutral vowel position helps to inhibit hyperextension.

Ideally, all the vowel sounds should probably be elicited early so that the child has a wide repertoire as soon as possible. If this can be achieved, together with some control of pitch for intonation, there is a considerable impact on the intelligibility of early communication.

Vowel-to-Consonant Combinations

Some children have less difficulty than others, so this might precede or accompany vowel-to-vowel combinations. It is often helpful to interrupt nasalised vowels with tongue movements (such as for velar sounds) and then progress forward. Some would correlate this with developmental features of early sounds. As soon as possible, the sequence should form meaningful words.

Early Inhibition of Undesirable Features

These include hyperextension of the jaw, jaw retraction and voicing on ingressive air. This last undesirable feature may be an attempt to compensate for low or fluctuating tone. Some individuals probably find that the tensor tone associated with breathing in helps to sustain voicing. However, this manoeuvre only serves to produce a grossly abnormal voice.

An appreciation of the whole pattern is required; for example, there is little benefit to be derived from attempts to manually control jaw opening, or tongue thrust without regard to the position of the upper body at least.

Timing

Phonation is rather like flying; danger points tend to be takeoff and landing, and particular attention must be paid to the initiation of voice and its cessation.

Eliciting vowel-like sounds may follow a sequence like this:
[ɜ:]; [ɑ:]; [ɜ:] [ə:]; [ɜ:] [u:]; [ɜ:] [i:]
It is important that voicing is maintained during transition to the second target sound of each pair. At first, movements are slow and sounds are prolonged (indicated by length marks). With practice, positional and acoustic changes are accomplished more quickly, although diphthongs are longer than normal: [eɪ;]; [aɪ;]; [əΩ:] [aΩ:] and eventually: [eɪ; aɪ; aΩ: aΩ:] on one expiration.

Children and Adults

Increasing age is accompanied by increases in physical and psychological demands. There is a need for more information on all aspects of behaviour, vocal function included. Typically, it seems that treatment of all kinds becomes less available with age (Thomas *et al.*, 1985). Schoolchildren should probably have more treatment to maintain and develop progress. There should be a closer overview of general physical state and follow-up of communication. This would include voice, speech and language.

Therapy of all kinds certainly becomes less available after school-leaving age. It is important to remember that while the cerebral palsies are persistent, their symptoms are not unchanging. Their natural history can be helpfully influenced by anticipating the likely deleterious effects of primary symptoms and working towards minimising them. This is a long-term operation, and criteria for success will vary from individual to individual. Sometimes treatment benefits can only be identified by listing the number of potential pitfalls that have been avoided. Sometimes pitfalls only come into view in middle age, for instance some individuals become dysphonic, probably due to the influence of worsening posture and gait, associated with degenerative changes and pain (Bleck, 1984). Again there is a need for more research.

Physical Methods for Motor Problems

Speech therapists tend to be practised in telling patients what to do: typically, we excel in using verbal direction and explanation, in treatment. Such skills alone are of little use in the treatment of developmental dysarthrias. These are sensorimotor disorders; therapists and parents have to learn ways to teach via movement and the child learns through movement. Physical contact and manipulation are required. It is a challenging, taxing business which can be frustrating beyond belief when things do not work, exciting and rewarding when they do. Some of the secret of success is to avoid continuing with techniques that are not working, while persisting with those that show signs of efficacy, despite fluctuations in performance. The delight engendered by even small successes in achieving voluntary control of laughing; calling 'Mummy', 'Daddy' or a sibling's name, producing a recognisable 'yes' or 'no', testifies to the unique significance of human voice. Attempts to reach a level of at least minimum performance should not be abandoned lightly.

Descriptions of the different philosophies and techniques employed in the physical management of cerebral palsy appear elsewhere (Mysak, 1980; Scrutton, 1984). It is important that the speech therapist is acquainted with the current principal ones (that is, those based on the work of Fay, Kabat, Rood and the Bobaths), and has a good understanding of the one employed in the treatment of children with whom she is involved. Treatment approaches used by physiotherapists, occupational therapists, speech therapists, family and, where appropriate, teachers or other care staff must be compatible. It is important to avoid 'cancelling out' the effects of treatment by injudicious mixing of different techniques founded on conflicting rationales. However, some apparent controversies would appear to be unnecessary. Given current theoretical knowledge, for instance, the dispute over the relationship between reflexive vocalisation and speech is only intellectually interesting to therapists faced with a severely dysarthrophonic child. It is not dissimilar to debating whether badminton skills assist or interfere with prowess in playing tennis. Both games involve developing skills which, although they differ, share similar orientation. Importantly, there is a common background of knowledge about anticipating movement of the ball, holding the racquet, etc. The situation of a cerebral palsied child without a normal postural background, with no experience of normal primitive (albeit reflex-based) behaviours is not dissimilar from the predicament of a candidate for Wimbledon centre court who has never held a racquet.

Conclusion

The management of dysphonia associated with neurodevelopmental spasticity or dyskinesia cannot be separated from the management of all coexisting symptoms. Consideration of vocal function must be made in the context of each individual growing child and neurological systems which have been damaged during development. Each child presents a new challenge to the clinician; therapy has little hope of success if it is not founded on careful and comprehensive assessment, and then carried out with at least a modicum of determined optimism. Optimism is more easily sustained if the clinician has developed a rationale for his/her approach based on a good understanding of current speech production and syndromes of cerebral dysfunction. A real difficulty for all members of the therapeutic team is often to achieve a balanced therapeutic diet which includes the right combination of remediation for coexisting problems, let alone engineering delivery of appropriate amounts.

References

Abbs, J., Hunter, C. and Barlow, S. 'Differential Speech Motor Subsystem: Impairment in Subjects with Suprabulbar Lesions: Neurophysiological Framework and Supporting Data', University of Wisconsin Speech Motor Control Laboratories Pre-prints (1982)

Aronson, A. E. *Clinical Voice Disorders* New York (Decker (Thieme-Stratton Inc.), New York, 1980)

Bleck, E. E. 'Where Have All the CP Children Gone? The need of adults', annotation in *Developmental Medicine and Child Neurology*, 26, 674–6 (1984)

Bobath, K. and Bobath, B. 'The Facilitation of Normal Postural Reactions and Movements in the Treatment of Cerebral Palsy', *Physiotherapy*, August (1964)

Boone, D. R. 'The Voice and Voice Therapy', in *Therapy* (Prentice-Hall Inc., New York, 1983)

Bosma, J. F. 'Anatomic and Physiologic Development of the Speech Apparatus', in Tower, D. B. (ed.) *Human Communication and its Disorders*, Vol. III. (Raven Press, New York, 1975)

Bruner, J. 'The Ontogenesis of Speech Acts', *Journal of Child Language*, 2, 1–21 (1975)

Bryan, T., Donahue, M., Pearl, R. and Herzog, A. 'Conversational Interactions between Mothers and Learning-disabled or Nondisabled Children during a Problem-solving Task', *Journal of Speech and Hearing Disorders*, 49, 64–71 (1984)

Cavallo, S. A. and Baker, R. J. 'Prephonatory Laryngeal and Chest Wall Dynamics', *Journal of Speech and Hearing Research*, 28, 79–87 (1985)

Darley, F. L., Aronson, A. E. and Brown, J. R. *Motor Speech Disorders* (W. B. Saunders, Philadelphia, 1975)

Evans-Morris, S. *Pre-Speech Assessment Scale*. (Preston Corporation, New Jersey, 1982)

Fourcin, A. J. 'Vibration'. in Wyke, B. (ed.) *Ventilatory and Phonatory Control Systems* (Oxford University Press, London, 1974)

Gilbert, H. R., Potter, C. R., and Hoodin, R. 'Laryngograph as a Measure of Vocal Fold Contact Area', *Journal of Speech and Hearing Research*, 27(2) (1984)

Gleitman, L. R., Newport, E. L. and Gleitman, H. 'The Current Status of the Motherese Hypothesis', *Journal of Child Language*, II, 43–79 (1984)

Guillemin, B. J. and Ngvyen, D. T. 'Microprocessor-based Speech Processing System Research Note', *Journal of Speech and Hearing Research*, 27, 311–17 (1984)

Hardy, J. *Cerebral Palsy* (Prentice-Hall, Inc., Englewood Cliffs, New Jersey, 1983)

Hirano, M. *Clinical Examination of Voice* (Springer Verlag, Wien, 1981)

Hixon, T. J., Putman, A. H. B. and Sharp, J. T. 'Speech Production with Flaccid Paralysis of the Rib Cage Diaphragm and Abdomen', *Journal of Speech and Hearing Disorders*, 48, 315–27 (1983)

Ingram, T. T. S. 'Clinical Significance of the Infantile Feeding Reflexes', *Developmental Medicine and Child Neurology*, 4, 159–69 (1962)

Jacobsen, E. *Progressive Relaxation* (University of Chicago Press, Chicago, 1929)

Jakobsen, R. *Child Language Aphasia and Phonological Universals* (Mouton, The Hague, 1968)

Lenneberg, E. *Biological Foundations of Language* (Wiley, New York, 1967)

Lesny, I. *The Subcortical Regulatory Motor Systems in Development and its Disorders* (Acta Universitatis Carolinae, Prague, 1980)

Mysak, E. D. 'Significance of the Neurophysiological Orientation to Cerebral Palsy Habilitation', *Journal of Speech and Hearing Disorders*, 24, 221–30 (1959)

—— *Neurospeech Therapy for the Cerebral Palsied: a Neuro-evolutional Approach*, 3rd edn (Teachers College Press, New York, 1980)

Peacher, W. G. 'Neurological Factors in the Etiology of Delayed Speech', *Journal of Speech Disorders*, 14, 147 (1949)
Scrutton, D. 'Management of the Motor Disorders of Children with Cerebral Palsy', *Clinics in Developmental Medicine No. 90*. (Spastics International Medical Publications with Blackwell Scientific Publications Ltd., London, 1984)
Stanhope, L. and Bell, R. Q. 'Parents and Families', in Kaufman, J. M. and Hallahan, D. P. (eds), *Handbook of Special Education*. (Prentice-Hall, New York, 1981)
Stark, R. E. 'Features of Infant Sounds: The Emergence of Cooing', *Journal of Child Language*, 5, 379–401 (1978)
—— Rose, S. N. and McLagen, M. 'Features of Infant Sounds in the First 8 Weeks of Life', *Journal of Child Language*, 2, 205–21 (1975)
—— Rose, S. N. and Benson, P. J. 'Classification of Infant Vocalization', *Journal of Communication Disorders*, 13, 41–7 (1978)
Thomas, A., Bax, M., Coombes, K., Goldson, E., Smyth, D. and Whitmore, K. (1985) *The Health and Social Needs of Physically Handicapped Young Adults: Are They Being Met by the Statutory Services?* (Spastics International Medical Publications and Blackwell Scientific Publications, London, 1985)
Wolff, P. H. 'The Natural History of Crying and Other Vocalizations in Early Infancy', in Foss, B. M. (ed.) *Infant Behaviour, Vol. IV*. (Methuen, London, 1969)

7 VOICE PROBLEMS IN THE DYSARTHRIC PATIENT

Sheila Scott and Brian Williams

Introduction

Speech therapy for voice disorders of neurological origin used to be considered as unrealistic and of limited value, particularly in progressive disorders (Peacher, 1949; Sarno, 1968). This attitude has gradually changed with reports of successful research and case studies (Canter, 1965 a and b; Rosenbek and La Pointe, Scott, Caird and Williams, 1984). There are a limited number of type-specific treatments available, but the same kinds of therapy can be applied to many types of dysarthria, the emphasis of treatment altering for each individual.

Earlier definitions described dysarthria as 'defective articulation of speech'. This traditional approach is frequently adopted in medical textbooks despite being imprecise and inadequate (Peacher, 1949; Darley, 1984). Yet as far back as 1911 Gutzmann (Berry, 1984) indicated that dysarthria could encompass not only defects of articulation, but also respiration, voice quality, vocal pitch and rate.

Peacher (1949) suggested that in describing those neurological speech disorders in which articulation and phonation were involved 'dysarthrophonia' was a more appropriate clinical term. Grewel (1957) proposed that this term should be extended, for accuracy, to include the defective respiratory component and coined the phrase 'dysarthropneumophonia'. The implication was that this might influence therapists to consider such voice problems holistically and encourage treatment of the 'whole problem' rather than focusing attention upon one feature to the detriment of others (Greene, 1980).

Such terms are useful as a means of clinical description and thereby in the direction of therapy but they could be taken to extremes — for example, 'dysarthropneumoreasonoprosodophonia'. Fortunately we have not reached such extremes, and today it is generally agreed that the term refers to a group of speech disorders arising from neurological causes and affecting all motor and temporal aspects of the vocal tract (Darley, 1984; Netsell, 1984). Rarely does one encounter disorders of articulation and phonation occurring in isolation in such neurological disorders (Hardy, 1967).

The problems of voice described in this chapter are classically described by Darley, Aronson and Brown (1975), as being in-

Table 7.1: Prevalence of Dysarthria in Four Neurological Disorders

	Study	Prevalence of Dysarthria
Multiple sclerosis	Darley, Brown and Goldstein (1972)	49%
Parkinson's disease	Merritt (1979)	50%
Motor neurone disease	Kurland (1977)	25–30%
Stroke disease	Kurland (1975)	8.8%

Source: Enderby, 1985, personal communication

Table 7.2: Neurological Disorders Associated with Dysarthria

Central	Upper Motor Neurone	Lower Motor Neurone	Extrapyramidal	Cerebellar
Dementia	Congenital diplegia	Disorders of cranial nerves	Parkinson's disease	Multiple sclerosis
	Stroke			
	Motor neurone disease	Bulbar palsy	Chorea	Hereditary ataxias
	Head injury	Poliomyelitis	Wilson's disease	
	Tumour	Syringobulbia		Vascular lesions
	Multiple sclerosis	Tumour		

cluded in a group of related motor-speech disorders resulting from disturbed muscular control over the speech mechanism, arising from disorders of the central or peripheral nervous systems and encompassing coexisting motor disorders of respiration, phonation, articulation, resonance and prosody. Thus the use of the term dysarthria rather than dysarthrophonia is generally accepted and strongly recommended.

Our knowledge about the prevalence and incidence of the dysarthrias is limited. Statistics published usually relate to those individuals who have sought doctors' or speech therapists' help. However, epidemiological aspects of certain diseases associated with dysarthria are well known and thus the prevalence of the speech disorder may be recorded (Table 7.1). Dysarthria may complicate a wide variety of neurological disorders (Table 7.2).

Central Disorders

Dementia

It is somewhat controversial to consider dementia as a cause of dysarthria and much research is needed before the picture is clarified. However, while dysarthria can obviously be associated with dementia, it is important that the speech disturbances characteristic of dementia are mentioned and borne in mind with therapy.

Dementia is associated with a global loss of intellectual function that is usually irreversible. It affects about one in ten of the population over the age of 65 (half of them severely) and one in five of those over 80. Both sexes are equally affected but more women survive into old age and therefore female cases predominate. Senile or non-vascular dementia of Alzheimer type accounts for most cases of dementia and most of the others have vascular of multi-infarct dementia. A small number of cases (less than 5 per cent) may, however, have a remediable cause for their dementia, such as thyroid disorders or vitamin B_{12} deficiency. In the more severe cases management problems will include a tendency to wandering, nocturnal disturbance and an inexorable deterioration in self-care in association with worsening confusion. Support for relatives is a prime consideration and full-time institutional care may be necessary. Numerous drugs have been developed in an attempt to improve intellectual function but none have shown more than minor symptomatic improvement.

Speech disturbances are characteristic of the dementias. Features of voicing difficulty are manifested as disordered rate and volume with disturbed rhythm and pitch. Difficulties in initiating and maintaining speech are also common (Critchley, 1970; Espir and Rose, 1970). One of the most significant voicing characteristics is habitual use of high-pitched vocal quality.

Improvement in vocal production may be observed following intensive reality orientation treatment procedures, particularly in mild dementia. It is an area which is currently receiving much deserved study.

Upper Motor Neurone Disorders

The articulatory muscles on both sides are innervated by both cerebral hemispheres. A unilateral corticospinal lesion (such as vascular lesion in the internal capsule) may cause temporary but not usually permanent dysarthria, although an extensive unilateral lesion involving the motor cortex may cause persistent dysarthria.

Pseudobulbar Palsy

Bilateral corticospinal lesions may be due to congenital diplegia, vascular lesions of both internal capsules, motor neurone disease or tumours of the midbrain or multiple sclerosis. This syndrome is usually associated with dysphagia and impaired voluntary control over emotional expression. The tongue is usually smaller than normal because it is spastic, but the muscles are not wasted.

One of the most distinguishing features of voice production by such patients is 'laryngeal hypervalving'. Darley, Aronson and Brown (1969a) categorised this through two perceptual dimensions of voicing, 'harshness' and strain-strangled voice quality, produced with effortful phonation. Excessive nasal resonance is present where there is palatal weakness. There has been little research into the breathing patterns of such patients but the Mayo studies observed excessively short phrasing. The lack of laryngeal control and synchrony have considerable effects upon pitch and intensity variability (Darley, Aronson and Brown, 1969b). Although Kammermeier (1969) found pitch variability to be reduced he concluded that it was not more significantly reduced in pseudobulbar palsy than in other types studied. He did note, however, that in measuring vocal frequencies the pseudobulbar palsy subjects had considerably lower fundamental frequencies which were more in keeping with the levels achieved by Mysak (1959) in a normal sample (65–70 years); yet the pseudobulbar palsy subjects were on average more than ten years younger.

Aten *et al.*, (1984) have reported the benefits of modified palatal lifts. Pseudobulbar palsy patients with dysarthria showed a minimal change in phonation time with the lift, reduced hypernasality and improved overall intelligibility.

If the harsh vocal quality occurs in conjunction with extreme tension, relaxation of the supralaryngeal musculature may prove effective. Facilitation techniques, massage or electric brush vibration in the area of genihyoid and digastric muscles may be valuable (De Jersey, 1975; Rosenbek and La Pointe, 1978).

Combining forces with the physiotherapist is invaluable in these cases. Specific respiratory stimulation through excitatory cold and respiratory resistance exercises are often found to be of benefit (Goff, 1969). However, Hardy (1968) suggested the removal of the demands on respiration, as reduced vital capacity is less crucial than we commonly imagine. Therapists should emphasise an efficient use of the exhalatory air stream, by teaching the patient to make the best use of his residual respiratory support. The pursed lip breathing techniques described later are also recommended with speech phrasing and prosody. Voice therapy must co-ordinate respiratory flow with phonation (Greene, 1980).

As with other dysarthrias, therapists should aim to improve posture for speech, swallowing, and communication techniques. The exercises described above are of no value if they are carried out in isolation.

Lower Motor Neurone Disorders

These disorders include cranial polyneuritis, progressive bulbar palsy (MND), bulbar poliomyelitis, syringobulbia and brain-stem tumours. True bulbar palsy presents with wasting, weakness and fasciculation of the tongue muscles. The labial muscles are affected first and thereafter the muscles of the tongue and soft palate, producing a nasal quality in the voice. Similar dysarthric features may present in the myopathies, for example, myasthenia gravis, polymyositis and muscular dystrophy.

The speech characteristics are well described in Darley, Aronson and Brown (1969b). There is muscle weakness, with flaccidity and atrophy of individual muscles, breathy voice quality, audible inhalation, abnormally short phrases, monotony of pitch, imprecise consonants and monoloudness. Suggestions for therapy follow in the general treatment section (p. 129).

Motor Neurone Disease (MND)

This is a disease of late middle life and usually begins between 50 and 70 years of age. Variants of the disorder include amyotrophic lateral sclerosis (ALS), progressive muscular atrophy, progressive bulbar palsy and motor system disease. Degenerative changes occur in the anterior horn cells of the spinal cord, the motor nuclei of the medulla and the corticospinal tracts. More common in the male, the condition is of unknown aetiology and clinical manifestations may include either upper motor neurone lesion signs of corticospinal degeneration, with weakness and spasticity in the legs, and lower motor neurone lesion signs of weakness and wasting of muscles, or a combination of both. The patient experiences increasing difficulty in speaking and swallowing. MND is progressive and treatment is symptomatic.

The function of all the muscles used in speech may be impaired. Vocal symptoms cover the entire spectrum from none to complete aphonia. Darley, Aronson and Brown (1975) considered that the speech gestalt of ALS consisted of grossly defective articulation of both consonants and vowels, often rendering speech unintelligible; laborious speech production; marked hypernasality; and poor adduction and abduction of the vocal cords. The inefficiency of valving results in short phrasing, but the overall effects are of breathlessness, audible inspirations and severe vocal harshness. Recent studies by Putnam and Hixon (1984) support the concept that chest wall muscle weakness and wasting curtail the inspiratory and expiratory extremes of the lung volume range; they have stressed that despite this, however, subjects may still be able to produce enough volume displacement and compression to support conversational demands.

There is little specific speech therapy treatment. In the early stages of swallowing difficulty, brushing and icing can be of some assistance. Similarly, tongue movements are reinforced by head positioning. Flexion and extension of the neck facilitate depression and elevation of the tongue. Head rotation can also stimulate lateral tongue movements.

Extrapyramidal Disorders

Parkinson's Disease

Parkinson's disease (PD) is one of the more common neurological disorders and it has a number of causes, but only those due to drugs (mainly phenothiazines) or of unknown cause are numerically important. The incidence increases with age, and at any one time approximately half of those affected are over 70 years of age. The underlying cause of PD is a degeneration and loss of neurones in the substantia nigra and elsewhere in the brain, with an associated decline in dopamine synthesis. Typical clinical features include rest tremor, muscle rigidity and bradykinesia. Effective drug treatment with dopamine agonists, such as levodopa or bromocriptine, has modified the natural history of the disease and improved the quality of life for most patients.

Not all patients with PD have speech disorders, and there is no apparent relationship between the duration of the disease and the degree of speech involvement. The parkinsonian speech disorder includes hypokinetic dysarthria, and dysphonia. Levodopa effectively improves speech intelligibility in most patients (Mawdesley and Gamsu, 1971; Wolfe *et al.*, 1975). However, despite otherwise optimal drug responses, speech difficulties may persist (Scott and Caird, 1983).

The phonatory aspects of speech are often considered to be the salient feature of hypokinesia (Darley, Aronson and Brown, 1975). The vocal levels of pitch are considered to be more characteristic of an older age group. Pitch variability is limited and often monotonous.

The respiratory function of parkinsonian speakers is restricted in keeping with the other musculature involved. De la Torre, Meyer and Boshes (1960) noted irregular and inflexible breathing patterns and a marked reduction in vital capacity.

Kim (1968) and Mueller (1971) considered that the reduction and monotony of vocal intensity were attributed to the loss of amplitude and rigidity of chest musculature. However Ewanowski

(1964) noted that parkinsonian subjects performed as well as normal controls during sustained phonation, under strictly controlled conditions, when verbal reinforcement was given to them.

The vocal quality and intensity studies of Canter (1963, 1965a and b) are well known, as is the work of Darley, Aronson and Brown (1975). However, Cisler (1927) noted that the limited closure of the glottis in Parkinson's disease, in conjunction with a loss of synchrony with articulatory movement and vocal cord movement, caused a breathy vocal quality.

Table 7.3: Traditional Methods of Speech Therapy in Parkinsonian Speech Disorder

Method	Method Aim	Technique
Chewing therapy (Froeschel, 1948)	Improving voicing Correct pitch placement	Chewing vigorously while simultaneously voicing
Eurhythmic approach (Smith, 1951)	Improving breathing Improving voicing	Relaxed total body movements in rhythmic sequences during vocalisation
Forcing exercises (Butfield, 1961)	Improving vocal fold adduction	Synchronised pushing with voicing
Syllabic speech (Andrews and Harris, 1964)	Reduce tension Improve speech rhythm	Speech is timed to a slow and regular tapped syllable
Amplification (Greene and Watson, 1968)	Reduce tension Increase voice volume mechanically	Patient's voice is amplified by a mechanical aid
Metronome therapy (Wohl, 1968)	Improve speech rhythm Improve voice onset	Syllable timed speech using a metronome aid
Group therapy (Allan, 1970)	Improve voicing, rate and clarity	Group practice of selected articulation exercises, speech phrases and conversation practice

Source: Scott, Caird and Williams (1985)

The treatment of vocal disturbance in Parkinson's disease has recently been considerably modified. In the past many methods were considered; these are summarised in Table 7.3. Perhaps the most commonly encountered method was the use of amplification as advocated by Greene and Watson (1968) which was found to increase the voice volume mechanically, thereby reducing tension. However, the patients were dependent upon a mechanical aid and, although there was some carryover in the therapeutic situation, there was often very little carryover beyond this. Syllable timed speech, with the aid of a metronome advocated by Wohl (1968), was found to improve speech rhythm and voice onset time and was also a popular method of therapy for Parkinson's disease patients. This method also relied upon a mechanical aid, however, and carryover without the aid was limited. More recent methods of therapy are summarised in Table 7.4. The prosodic method advocated by Scott, Caird and Williams (1984) highlights the necessity to focus the treatment away from the improvement of respiratory, phonatory, and articulatory components, and shifts the emphasis to suprasegmental and prosodic features of speech.

Table 7.4: Recent Approaches to Speech Therapy in Parkinsonian Speech Disorders

Method	Method Aim	Technique
Pacing board (Helm (1979), after Luria)	Reduce rate Inhibit initiation difficulties	Patient feels along a stepped board The physical barrier met by the hand is transferred into speech
Delayed auditory feedback (Downie, Low and Lindsay, 1981)	Reduce rate Overcome onset difficulties	Mechanical feedback masks the patient's speech, causing reduced rate and sound prolongation
Proprioceptive (Scott and Caird, 1981)	Improve rate rhythm, Intonation, vocal expression, vocal intensity	Exercises emphasising the affective and prosodic aspects of speech
Residential holiday therapy (Robertson and Thompson, 1983)	Social and conversational improvement	Intensive group therapy

Source: Scott, Caird and Williams (1985)

Prosodic variables make a significant contribution to the intelligibility of speech, and therapeutic efforts directed at these features improves intelligibility of speech. Clinical practice suggests that articulation also improves. For too long dysarthria therapy has focused solely on attempts to improve segmental production and, although this is important, equal emphasis should be placed on the suprasegmental and prosodic features.

Description and treatment are well documented by Rosenbek and La Pointe (1978). However Rosenbek emphasises that the goal of testing should focus on treatment and not merely label the type of dysarthria. Classification is not the primary or even a necessary goal with dysarthric patients. Treatment of dysarthria is important as it can improve the patient's life both socially and functionally.

Tests. Methods of testing are wide and variable. There are specific approaches such as that of Scott and Caird (1983) for prosodic abnormality in Parkinson's disease, or more general methods, such as one outlined by Rosenbek (personal communication 1984); see also Scott, Caird and Williams (1985). One tests non-speech and speech stimuli alone and in combination.

(1) Muscles of Respiration.

(1a) (i) Command the patient to sniff (if the patient can sniff then the diaphragmatic movement is intact).
(ii) Command the patient to pant (if co-ordination of movements of the diaphragm and the abdominal muscles are synchronised and in control then the patient can pant).

(1b) If the patient can prolong a sustained vowel such as [ah], quietly and abruptly and then louder over several repetitions, the patient has the effective use of laryngeal, diaphragmatic and abdominal musculature.

(1c) Listening to connected speech one should be examining overall loudness, the appropriateness of loudness change, and the function of the respiratory muscles in producing loudness. If any of these functions are impaired, then the first treatment target is working upon impaired respiratory mechanisms and improving respiratory function.

(2) The Larynx

(2a) Command the patient to cough and observe the patient's cough reflex spontaneously, if possible, and on command.

(2b) Listen to the quality of voice (if it has a mucosal or salival quality, then it suggests a weak larynx).

(2c) Examine pitch function to determine fundamental speaking frequency and the appropriateness of pitch change (this determines if the larynx is well used in combination with other structures).

(2d) One should always judge the quality of phonation, the presence of tremor, hoarseness, harshness, and if the patient has voiceless/voiced distinctions (is the patient dysphonic?)

(3) Examine the soft palate or velopharynx, which is instrumental in the production of correct nasal balance.

(3a) Examine drinking — does the patient get water up his nose while drinking?

(3b) (i) Listen to the speech stimuli [/u/ and /i/] while occluding the nostrils and listening to the change in resonance. When occluded, is the resonance adequate or inadequate?
(ii) One would note if there was consistent nasality or inconsistent nasality in connected speech (words such as smoke, snake, snooker are very difficult to produce if velopharyngeal competence is inadequate.)

(4) Finally one examines the tongue and the jaw, the upper airway and oral facial system, and evaluates the swallowing mechanism. Watch the movements during chewing. Is there adequate lip seal? Is there symmetrical jaw movement? One examines diadochokinetic movements, asking the patient to repeat ppp, ttt, kkk, as fast as he can. Some patients can produce these adequately at fast speeds whilst some are only intelligible at a slow speed. Some patients talk better with the jaw stabilised and some are worse. A bite block might be a means of improving consonant production and articulation in some cases. Traditional observations of articulatory production are made and then judgements of why speech has gone wrong. Is it because of consonant imprecision, weak range, velocity or directional difficulty of the articulators?

General Treatment Aims in Dysarthria

The goal in treatment is seen as maximising the level of speech function available (Schow *et al.*, 1978). Darley, Aronson and Brown (1975) summarise the aims as enabling the patient to learn to make the best of his remaining speech potential and to compensate for the impairment that has altered his lifelong speech habits.

Respiratory Function

Attempts at increasing vital capacity are rarely justified. Seldom is function so restricted that it alone limits speech production (Darley, Aronson and Brown, 1975). Rather, the limiting influence is considered to be inadequate respiratory control or inefficient valving on expiration (Hardy, 1967).

There are three classes of management according to Rosenbek and La Pointe (1978).

(1) Prosthetic
(2) Instrumental
(3) Traditional phonatory.

Prosthetic. The prosthetic means of improving respiratory structures might utilise the respiratory plunger, which is a paddle placed against the abdominal muscles acting as a surrogate belly muscle. A substitute for this is to get the patient to put a hand on the abdomen inside the waistband of the skirt or trousers and press in on the expiration with speech. This is particularly useful in the treatment of patients suffering from multiple sclerosis. It is important to note that the amount of pressure and the amount of air produced is not emphasising overbreathing. Similarly one should remember posture for breathing, and mechanical or prosthetic aids to improve posture may well improve respiratory function.

In voice therapy with dysarthrics concentration upon the controlled flow of expiration is an important therapeutic aim. Initially the assessment of the patient's posture should be made, and where necessary corrected or supported to encourage an adequate range of movement and symmetrical pose.

Position the patient in a supported sitting position with the head slightly flexed in a midline position. The patient should be relaxed and comfortable.

Bearing down through the arms, onto a table top or the arms of a chair, along the ulnar border of the hand, helps to fix the shoulder girdle and strap muscles of the neck. This simple position promotes symmetry and can alone increase vocal intensity.

When the patient is adequately positioned, facilitation of respiratory control and flowing expiration can begin against this background of increased effort.

The proprioceptive neuromuscular facilitation techniques of diaphragmatic breathing are recommended, for example, gentle resistance to the intercostal musculature during the expiratory phase is beneficial. Other techniques are described by Langley and Darvill (1979) although sternum facilitation and rib springing have been found to have little value in a speech facilitation. However, they are valuable as a dramatic means to initiate respiration in a life-saving situation.

Pursed lip breathing techniques have been found to be extremely beneficial and useful for all of the dysarthrias and particularly in Parkinson's disease (Scott, Caird and Williams, 1984, 1985).

(1) The patient is instructed to count to ten and the therapist notes the ease or difficulty involved.
(2) The patient is then instructed to blow the next breath out through pursed lips as though trying to cool the soup! Gentle blowing *not* forceful blasting or puffing as in blowing out a candle.
(3) The patient is instructed to let each subsequent breath out this way for three to four expirations.
(4) The patient is asked to count to ten again on the next breath out. If done properly respiratory flow is more relaxed, breath support stronger and vocal intensity and phrasing greater. All emphasis is removed from inspiration, the patient naturally breathes in, and following a pursed blowing out inspiration is greater as the blowing relaxes the chest musculature.

Instrumental or Biofeedback Methods. For improving respiratory function, the use of manometers is often popular with the patient. Placed in an adequate posture, and with the increased background of effort already described, the patient blows into the manometer and tries to generate at least 5 cm of water up the tube for 5 seconds. This helps the patient to recognise the degree of control associated with moving that volume of water for that length of time, and Rosenbek suggests that they then learn to transfer that control to speech. The therapist then counts how many syllables a patient's respiratory mechanism can support, helping the patient to learn to identify and produce only the number of syllables that he can support with ease.

Phonatory Techniques. In many cases brushing and icing may have a facilitatory effect upon voicing intensity. A neck wrap or the use of light pressure on various parts of the larynx may well improve voice intensity. For some patients the use of a prosthetic palate reduces the palatal dome and hence reduces the muscular movement, increasing intelligibility. Similarly, a palatal lift may also facilitate improved intelligibility of speech. A bite block or jaw sling may improve upper airway function.

Gradual voicing is co-ordinated with controlled expiration. Short phrase units are generally the end aim achieved by working through improving the glottal attack, speech sounds, rhythms and inflexions. Emphasis on well-supported easy speech groups, with inflexion, stressing and volume variation is more important than concentration on articulatory accuracy.

Netsell (1984) suggested that 'chewing' therapy may facilitate speech not least because the neuromuscular stimulation involved in chewing is similar to that of speech.

Utilising laryngeal valving as involved in lifting or exerting pressure with the arms during phonation may help hypoadduction, and 'breathy' voice onset techniques may benefit hyperadduction (Wertz, 1978).

Rood (1962) suggested that light pressure to the sides of the thyroid, moving it up and down, 'releases' the vocal cords. During this movement patients are requested to phonate.

Generally modification of respiration, resonance, prosody and articulation influence intelligibility more than exercises designed to improve phonation (Wertz, 1978).

Other methods are also mentioned in Tables 7.3 and 7.4 from Scott, Caird and Williams (1985).

The amplification methods described by Greene and Watson (1968) in the management of Parkinson's disease patients, and the use of auditory feedback, are thought to modify vocal intensity, overall rate and the stress patterns. If the patient talks better when he attempts to talk more slowly, then delayed auditory feedback (or DAF) may be a suitable method of therapy with the parkinsonian patient. However, in clinical experience, delayed auditory feedback is only useful if it is used by an experienced therapist, accompanied by extensive explanation, and it is only functional with certain patients and certain stimuli so is perhaps best used as part of a total behavioural-type therapeutic programme. Similarly the amplification device had little carryover either outside the therapeutic situation, or when the aid is not in use. The pacing board described by Helm (1979) is based on Luria's theory of motor interruption and is an artificial way of improving rate and timing. Again the authors' experience with parkinsonian patients has not found it useful (although the use of pacing board with dyspraxic patients can be most effective).

Utilising traditional methods the therapist might link gesture and speech. A simple task would be counting using finger pointing and speech, and then building up to using contrasting stress drills with a question and answer format, gradually increasing the complexity of material and finally fading gesture. Work on stress and improving prosody often improves overall intelligibility and articulatory accuracy.

Conclusion

Changes in the motor aspects of speech communication are well documented in Darley, Aronson and Brown (1969 a and b, 1975), Rosenbek and La Pointe (1978). However, too often the management of these problems is given a cursory assessment, and treatment usually consists of articulatory exercises and phonemic drill building up to longer speech unit practices. Recent studies have indicated the success speech therapy can have in the management of voice disorders of neurological origin, and that they are no longer unrealistic in their aims or of limited value in the management of progressive disorders. Therapy has come a long way from considering dysarthria as merely a defective articulation of speech, and as such the treatment should look beyond this and utilise the many varied instrumental and biofeedback techniques that are readily available to therapists nowadays. The management of dysarthria in the elderly remains limited and research opportunities, although still limited, provide an exciting and much-needed opportunity for examination.

References

Allan, C. M. 'Treatment of Non-fluent Speech Resulting from Neurological Disease — Treatment of Dysarthria', *British Journal of Disorders of Communication* 5, 1–4 (1970)

Andrews, G. and Harris, M. *The Syndrome of Stuttering* (Heinemann Medical Books, London, 1964)

Aten, J. L., McDonald, A., Simpson, M. and Gutierrez, J. 'Efficacy of Modified Palatal Lifts for Improving Resonance 231', in McNeil, T., Rosenbek, J. C. and Aronson, A. E. (eds) *The Dysarthrias: Physiology, Acoustics, Perception and Management*. (College-Hill Press, San Diego, California, 1984)

Berry, W. R. *Clinical Dysarthria* (College-Hill Press, San Diego, California, 1984)

Canter, G. J. 'Speech Characteristics of Patients with Parkinson's Disease I[2], Intensity Pitch and Duration'. *Journal of Speech and Hearing Disorders*, 28, 221–9 (1963)

—— 'Speech Characteristics of Patients with Parkinson's Disease: Physical Support for Speech II', *Journal of Speech and Hearing Disorders*, 30, 44–9 (1965a)

—— 'Articulation Diadochokinesis and Overall Speech Adequacy III', *Journal of Speech and Hearing Disorders*, 30, 217–24 (1965b)

Cisler, I. 'Sur les troubles du langage articule et de la phonation au cours de l'encephalité epidemique', *Archives of International Laryngology*, 6, 1054–7 (1927)

Critchley, M. *Aphasiology and Other Aspects of Language* (Edward Arnold, London, 1970)

Darley, F. L. 'Forward in Clinical Dysarthria', in (ed) Berry, W. R. *Clinical Dysarthria* College-Hill Press, San Diego, California (1984)

——, Aronson, A. E. and Brown, J. R. 'Differential Diagnostic Patterns of Dysarthria', *Journal of Speech and Hearing Research*, 12, 246–69 (1969a)

——, Aronson, A. E. and Brown, J. R. 'Clusters of Deviant Speech Dimensions in the Dysarthrias', *Journal of Speech and Hearing Research*, 12, 462–96 (1969b)

——, Aronson, A. E. and Brown, J. R. *Motor Speech Disorders* (Saunders, Philadelphia, 1975)

——, Brown, J. and Goldstein, A. 'Dysarthria and Multiple Sclerosis', *Journal of Speech and Hearing Research*, 15, Part 2, 229–45 (1972)

De Jersey, M. C. 'An Approach to the Problems of Oral Facial Dysfunction in the Adult', *Australian Journal of Physiotherapy* 21(1), 5–10 (1975)

Downie, A. W., Low, J. M. and Lindsay, D. O. 'Speech Disorder in Parkinsonism – Usefulness of Delayed Auditory Feedback in Selected Cases', *British Journal of Disorders of Communication* 16(2), 135–9 (1981)

Espir, M. L. E. and Rose, F. C. *Basic Neurology of Speech*, 2nd edn (Blackwell Scientific Publications, London, 1970)

Ewanowski, S. J. 'Selected Motor Speech Behaviour of Patients with Parkinsonism', PhD Dissertation, University of Wisconsin (1964)

Froeschel, E. *Twentieth Century Voice Correction*, Chapter V (Philosophical Library, New York, 1948)

Goff, B. 'Excitatory Cold', Congress Lecture, *Physiotherapy* 467–9 (1969)

Greene, M. L. C. *The Voice and its Disorders* (Pitman Medical, London, 1980) pp. 298–327

—— and Watson, B. W. 'The Value of Speech Amplification in Parkinson's Disease Patients', *Folia Phoniatrica* (*Basel*), 20, 250 (1968)

Grewel, F. 'Classification of Dysarthrias', *Acta Psychiatrica, Neurologica, Scandinavica*, 32, 325–7 (1957)

Hardy, G. C. 'Respiratory Physiology, Implications of Current Research', American Speech and Hearing Association 10, 204–5 (1968)

Hardy, J. 'Suggestions for Physiological Research in Dysarthria', *Cortex* 3, 128–56 (1967)

Helm, N. A. 'Management of Palilalia with a Pacing Board', *Journal of Speech and Hearing Disorders* 44, 350–3 (1979)

Kammermeier, M. A. 'A Comparison of Phonatory Phenomenon Among Groups of Neurologically Impaired Speakers'. PhD Dissertation, University of Minnesota (1969)

Kim, R. 'The Chronic Residual Respiratory Disorder and Post-Encephalitic Parkinsonism', *Journal of Neurology and Neurosurgery and Psychiatry*, 31, 393–8 (1968)

Kurland, L. T. 'Epidemiology of a Myotrophic Lateral Sclerosis with Emphasis on Antecedent Events from Case Control Comparisons', in Rows F. C. (ed.), *Motor Neurone Disease*, pp. 1–13 (Grune and Stratton, New York, 1977)

—— 'Long Term Care Facility Improvement Study', in *ASHA Resource Materials for Communicative Problems of Older Persons*, (Washington, DC, 1975), HRPOO14306

Langley, G. and Darvill, G. *Procedures for Facilitating Improvements in Swallow, Mastication, Speech and Facial Expression; where these have been impaired by Central or Peripheral Nerve Damage* (College of Speech Therapists, London, 1979)

Mawdsley, C. and Gamsu, C. V. 'Periodicity of Speech in Parkinsonism', *Nature*, 231, 315–16 (1971)

Merritt, H. (1979) *A Text Book of Clinical Neurology*, 6th edn (Lee and Febisher, Philadelphia, 1979)

Mueller, P. B. 'Parkinson's Disease, Motor Speech Behaviour in a Selected Group of Patients', *Folia Phoniatrica (Basel)*, 23, 333–46 (1971)

Mysak, E. D. 'Pitch and Duration Characteristics of Older Males', *Journal of Speech and Hearing Research*, 2, 46–54 (1959)

Netsell, R. 'A Neurobiologic View of the Dysarthrias', in McNeil, T., Rosenbek, J. C. and Aronson, A. E. (eds) *The Dysarthrias, Physiology, Acoustics, Perception and Management*. (College-Hill Press, San Diego, California, 1984)

Peacher, W. G. 'Aetiology and Differential Diagnosis of Dysarthria', *Journal of Speech and Hearing Disorders*, 15, 252–65 (1949)

Putnam, A. H. B. and Hixon, T. J. 'Respiratory Kinematics in Speakers with Motor Neurone Disease', in McNeil, R., Rosenbek, J. C., Aronson, A. E. and Brown, J. R. (eds) *The Dysarthrias, Physiology, Acoustics, Perception and Management*, pp. 37–68. (College-Hill Press, San Diego, California, 1984)

Robertson, S. J. and Thomson, F. 'Speech Therapy in Parkinson's Disease. A Study of the Efficacy and Long-term Effects of Intensive Speech Therapy', *British Journal of Disorders of Communication* (1983)

Rood, M. 'The Use of Sensory Receptors to Activate, Facilitate and Inhibit Motor Response, Autonomic and Somatic in Development Sequence; Approaches to Treatment of Patients with Neuromuscular Disfunction', (Brown Book Company, Des Moines, Iowa, 1962)

Rosenbek, J. C. and La Pointe, L. L. 'The Dysarthrias: Description, Diagnosis, and Treatment', in Johns, D. F. (ed.) *Clinical Management of Neurogenic Communicative Disorders*, pp. 251–310. (Little, Brown and Co, Boston, 1978)

Sarno, M. T. 'Speech Impairment and Parkinson's Disease', *Archives of Physiology, Medicine and Rehabilitation* 49, 269–75 (1968)

Schow, R. L., Christensen, G. M., Hutchinson, G. M and Nerbonne, M. A., *Communication Disorders of the Aged* (University Park Press, Baltimore, 1978)

Scott, S. and Caird, F. I. 'Speech Therapy for Patients with Parkinson's Disease', *British Medical Journal*, 283, 1008 (1981)

—— 'Speech Therapy for Parkinson's Disease', *Journal of Neurology, Neurosurgery and Psychiatry*, 46, 140–4 (1983)

—— 'The Response of the Apparent Receptive Speech Disorder of Parkinson's Disease to Speech Therapy', *Journal of Neurology, Neurosurgery and Psychiatry*, 47, 302–3 (1984)

——, Caird, F. I. and Williams, B. O. 'Evidence for an Apparent Sensory Speech Disorder in Parkinson's Disease', *Journal of Neurology, Neurosurgery and Psychiatry* 47, 840–3 (1984)

—— *Communication in Parkinson's Disease* (Croom Helm, London, 1985)

Smith, Svend 'Chest Register Versus Head Register in the Membrane Cushion Model of the Vocal Cords'. *Folia Phoniatrica* (*Basel*), 9, 32–7 (1951)

Torre de La, R., Meyer, M. and Boshes B. 'Studies in Parkinsonism IX. Evaluation of Respiratory Function, Preliminary Observations', *Quarterly Bulletin of the Northwestern Medical School* 34, 332–6 (1960)

Wertz, R. T. 'Neuropathologies of Speech and Language, An Introduction to Patient Management', in Johns, D. F. (ed.) *Clinical Management of Neurogenic Communicative Disorders*, (Little, Brown and Co., Boston, 1978)

Wohl, M. T. 'The Electronic Metronome. An Evaluation Study', *British Journal of Disorders of Communication*, 3, 89 (1968)

Wolfe, V. I., Garvin, J. S., Bacon, M. and Waldrop, W. 'Speech Changes in Parkinson's Disease during Treatment with L-dopa', *Journal of Communication Diseases* 8, 271–9 (1975)

8 VOCAL CORD PARALYSES

Malcolm Stockley

Introduction

Vocal cord paresis (weakness) and paralysis (inability to stimulate contraction of muscle) comprise a number of related neurological conditions which affect the movement of the vocal cords. Other conditions may also affect the movement of the cords, for example arthritis of the cricoarytenoid joint is uncommon, but may occur in patients with rheumatoid arthritis, or after trauma. In addition, the various myopathies such as myasthenia gravis, polymyositis, and the muscular dystrophies may cause varying degrees of wasting and hence weakness.

This chapter, however, will be mainly concerned with lesions of the vagus (Xth cranial nerve) occurring at some point between its origin in the nucleus ambiguus and the laryngeal musculature. The major division of the vagus concerned is the branch known as the recurrent laryngeal nerve (RLN) which supplies all the laryngeal muscles except the cricothyroid (Hardcastle, 1976) gives a clear description of the action of the intrinsic laryngeal muscles and their effects on the movements of the vocal cords). Any condition affecting this nerve can produce weakness or immobility of the vocal cord on the affected side (usually the left, due to its longer course) giving rise to dysphonia, or exceptionally, aphonia when both recurrent laryngeal nerves are paralysed and the vocal cords adopt a paramedian position. Lesions of the superior laryngeal nerves, which part from the vagus just below the inferior ganglion and provide the sensory innervation of the supraglottis in addition to motor supply to the cricothyroid, may also occur. Both unilateral and bilateral lesions may occur and are frequently accompanied by a recurrent laryngeal nerve paralysis. The clinical features of these conditions are described below. Cord palsies are a fairly frequent problem in ENT practice; they are usually unilateral but bilateral palsies are not uncommon.

As McKelvie states: 'No more contentious subject exists than vocal cord palsy, and positions of the cord in such states, since they can come to rest in any position between full abduction and adduction' (McKelvie, 1979). Sir Felix Semon (of St Thomas' Hospital) bequeathed 'Semon's law' at the end of the nineteenth century (Semon, 1881). This comprises a description of the positions adopted by the affected cord(s). Although the exact explanation has still not been elucidated, the gist of Semon's thesis was that an incomplete lesion of the recurrent laryngeal nerve results in an *abductor* paralysis whereas a complete recurrent laryngeal nerve lesion results in both an abductor and adductor paralysis. That is, progressive damage would result initially in an adducted cord followed with a slow migration to an intermediate position. Sir Victor Negus proposed that phylogenetically speaking, the larynx was primarily a sphincter to protect the entrance to the lower tracheobronchial tree, later acquiring an opening mechanism which remains more vulnerable to neuromuscular damage (Negus, 1931). Greene (1980) discusses the behaviour of the laryngeal muscles and concludes that 'the position of the vocal cord is not subject to any fixed neurological laws, evolutionary or otherwise, but is determined entirely by the interaction of a combination of neuropathological and anatomical factors'. These factors include: the effects of unaffected muscles, for example the cricothyroid in the case of the recurrent laryngeal nerve paralysis, and the interarytenoideus in unilateral paralysis; the angle of the cricoarytenoid joint (frequently the affected cord lies at a lower level than the contralateral cord); the balance of forces between the abductors and adductors (that is, their respective bulk); and the final amount of atrophy and fibrosis which ensues. Nevertheless, the 'puzzling fact [remains] that the abductors of the vocal folds often appear to be most susceptible to paresis after partial injuries of the recurrent laryngeal nerve' (Bowden, 1974).

With the advent of improved systems of videostroboscopy via fibreoptic laryngoscopy (for example, Wolf TV-Laryngoscope), laryngeal appearance and function can be better investigated and demonstrated to the mutual benefit of surgeon and voice therapist. The work of Williams, Farquharson and Anthony (1975) is a good example of the type of research that is needed.

Aetiology

There are many possible aetiologies but the common causes of these conditions are infranuclear and include: injury (such as road traffic accidents, surgical trauma: thyroidectomy, endotracheal intubation, and bronchoscopy); pressure or stretching due to contiguous disease (for instance, cardiovascular, and neoplastic disease); and peripheral neuritis (for example, toxic: lead poisoning, infective: influenzal and herpetic viruses, streptococcal and other bacteria).

Since malignant lesions, such as carcinoma of the bronchus, upper lobe of the lung, or mediastinal growths, may affect the recurrent laryngeal nerve particularly the left, laryngologists assume this to be the case until proved otherwise. Carcinoma of larynx, pharynx, nasopharynx, thyroid, or oesophagus and secondaries in the base of the skull, neck, or hilar lymph nodes may also give rise to palsies as may aortic aneurysms and other lesions of the heart and major blood vessels. Accidental surgical trauma, for instance during thyroid surgery, is one of the commonest causes. Around 30 per cent of cases are idiopathic (of unknown/spontaneous origin), sometimes associated with a flu-like illness or perhaps congenital and associated with birth trauma. Blau and Kapadia (1972) believe idiopathic unilateral vocal cord paralysis to be a cranial mononeuropathy in which nerve function is impaired or lost, site and aetiology of lesion unknown, and having a generally high rate of spontaneous recovery within a period of a year. Most common is the condition of unilateral and incomplete (abductor) paralysis. In the author's experience of a specialist ENT hospital in London, patients presented at a rate of approximately one each month.

Nuclear level causes include multiple sclerosis, primary or secondary brain tumours, and syphilis. The lesion more often results in a bilateral rather than a unilateral paralysis.

Recurrent Laryngeal Nerve Paralysis

The four conditions which may be distinguished are: unilateral incomplete paralysis, bilateral incomplete paralysis, unilateral complete paralysis, and bilateral complete paralysis; they are described below (Figure 8.1 a, b, c and d).

Unilateral Incomplete (Abductor) Paralysis. A common presentation of this condition is as an idiopathic mononeuritis, but it may also be a sequelae of thryoid surgery or caused by carcinoma of the left lung due to the more extensive course of the left recurrent laryngeal nerve (Figure 8.1a). Injury to the nerve during thyroid surgery may be temporary, due to oedema, typically developing within seven days postoperatively. Intubation with an endotracheal tube in which the inflated cuff lies within the larynx, rather than the trachea, is also a possible cause of this condition (Minuck, 1976). Since the affected cord remains in the midline, there may be little in the way of symptoms except slight dysphonia (worse when singing), vocal fatigue, and breathlessness, and many patients learn to compensate spontaneously. An intensive burst of

Figure 8.1: Recurrent Laryngeal Nerve Paralyses

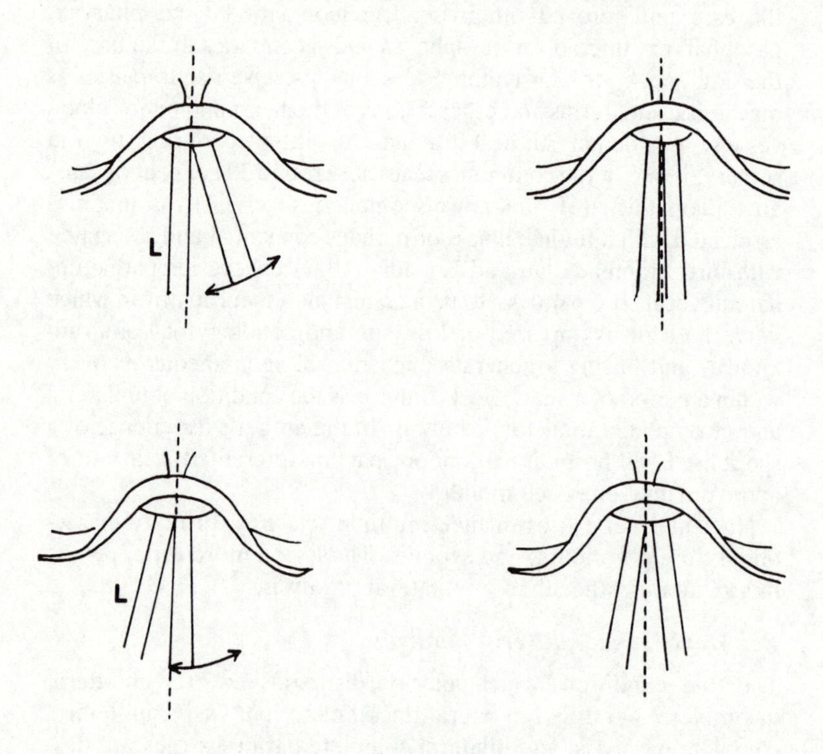

(a) Unilateral incomplete (abductor) paralysis (left cord)
(b) Bilateral incomplete (abductor) paralysis
(c) Unilateral complete paralysis (left cord)
(d) Bilateral complete paralysis

therapy is frequently efficacious in promoting better adduction of the cords and eliminating breathiness.

Bilateral Incomplete (Abductor) Paralysis. This condition, which may be an unfortunate result of thyroid surgery, is the most serious form of vocal cord paralysis (Figure 8.1b). The voice is good but patients may complain of dysponea and stridor. This is because the vocal cords adopt a position near the midline thus obstructing the airway. If the patient is not overweight and is relatively inactive it is possible to survive without surgical intervention. Exertion, or an acute upper respiratory tract infection, results in obstruction which needs to be alleviated by emergency tracheotomy. The best solution is a permanent tracheostomy, so that the patient is assured of a good airway, with a speaking valve. The usual plan seems to be to wait for about 12 months to see if any spontaneous recovery occurs. If it does not, another solution is to carry out a cordopexy, of which there are several varieties, which involve fixing one vocal cord, in a position slightly lateral to the midline, with a stainles steel suture. This solution requires intensive vocal rehabilitation since the other cord has to be trained to cross the midline to approximate with the fixed cord. Once the muscles of adduction relax, the natural elasticity of the tissues usually help the free cord to abduct slightly. The procedure is undertaken in such a manner as to create a permanent posterior glottic chink, adequate enough for normal respiration but not so large as to markedly impair the voice.

Unilateral Complete Paralysis. The left vocal cord is more commonly affected than the right due to the greater vulnerability of the left recurrent laryngeal nerve (Figure 8.1c). Damage during thyroidectomy is one of the commonest causes, despite the surgeon's attempt to preserve the nerve. The affected cord assumes the cadaveric position somewhat lateral to the midline with the result that there is a marked degree of air wastage and the voice is weak and breathy. Patients frequently complain of fatigue due to the physical effort involved in their attempts to approximate the cords. Other problems include overspill from swallowing and an ineffective cough rendering the patient liable to recurrent lung infections. If the dysphonia is resistant to voice therapy good voice may be obtained with vocal rehabilitation following Teflon paste injection (see p. 144), after allowing sufficient time for spontaneous recovery to take place.

Bilateral Complete Paralysis. Fortunately rather rare, this condition may result from the severance of *both* recurrent laryngeal nerves (during thyroid surgery), or if one nerve is damaged in the presence of an unrecognised palsy of the other nerve (Figure 8.1d). Both vocal cords assume a paramedian position initially and the patient is aphonic. Aspiration of fluids may be severe and the patient may eventually need a laryngectomy to protect the lungs; for if the condition is permanent both cords assume the more lateral 'cadaveric' position after about 6–9 months. The cadaveric position is halfway between midline and moderate abduction, and so-called because the muscles are inactive as in death. With great effort an audible whisper is possible in time as the flaccidity of the cords give way to stiffening with fibrosis and contracture.

Superior Laryngeal Nerve Paralysis

Both unilateral and bilateral paralyses may occur from lesions of the external branches, which innervate the cricothyroid muscle, although these conditions are much less frequent than recurrent laryngeal nerve paralyses due to their shorter course and 'rarely occurs without a recurrent laryngeal nerve paralysis' (Simpson *et al.*, 1967).

Unilateral Superior Nerve Paralysis. This condition results in an unequal rocking of the cricoid and thyroid cartilages. A slack, flabby cord is produced due to the failure of the backward-bracing action of the cricoarytenoideus muscle so that the arytenoid cartilage tips forward thus allowing the cords to overlap. Patients complain of vocal fatigue which results from the effort to phonate and produce sufficient intensity. The voice is quiet, lacks intonation, is breathy, and singing is impossible. There is no effective treatment for this problem. Such patients need the support of the voice therapist to explain the mechanics and implications of the pathology, to reduce general and specific musculoskeletal tension and to help obtain the optimum voice possible.

Bilateral Superior Nerve Paralysis. When the lesion (for example, carcinoma of the nasopharynx) affects the vagus at a higher level than that at which the superior laryngeal branch is given off this condition occurs together with a recurrent laryngeal nerve paralysis. The relatively wide cadaveric position of the glottis greatly exacerbates the dysphonia. The voice may be low in pitch and so restricted in range as to render singing impossible and to affect intonation. Aspiration of fluids is usually a distressing added complication. There is no effective treatment for this problem other than tracheostomy, and insertion of a speaking valve should this prove necessary to protect the patient from inhalation pneumonia.

Treatment

Surgical intervention may be necessary, such as a Woodman's procedure or a Teflon implant as described below. Vocal rehabilitation consists of so-called 'forcing' or 'pushing' exercises to encourage the active cord to compensate for the paralysed cord by crossing the midline so as to approximate with the affected cord. Voice production work should be undertaken with Teflon implant cases to ensure that full benefit is made of the surgical result. Although this aspect cannot be dealt with here, counselling is frequently of great importance: not infrequently emotional, social, and economic difficulties compound the vocal problems.

Surgical Intervention

Cordopexy. There are several types of procedure in use — the best-known being the Woodman operation (Woodman, 1946). In cases of bilateral abductor paralysis of sudden onset, due to surgical trauma, both cords are fixed in the midline causing stridor and dyspnoea, and a tracheostomy is indicated. A special cannula with a flapped valve (a speaking valve) is inserted to allow the eggressive air stream to pass through the larynx and provide a satisfactory, even good, voice. If there is no spontaneous recovery (after at least a year) cordopexy may be undertaken. This frees the patient from living permanently with a tracheostomy with its attendant restrictions and hazards, respiratory infections and water being the chief ones. However, as McKelvie points out: 'Tracheostomy remains an option for the very aged, those who have had one for many years and cope well with it, the obese and frail,. those . . . with no wish to swim, those with a brief but vital need to talk via a valved tracheostomy tube (McKelvie, 1979).

The Woodman procedure (which requires an initial tracheostomy comprises the following: arytenoidectomy with retention of the vocal process which is moved laterally and, together with fibres of the thyroarytenoid muscle, is then sutured to the inferior cornu of the thyroid cartilage. This fixes the cord in a more advantageous position of abduction. Cicatrial tissue formation during healing may change the position of the cord and voice therapy is required to achieve adequate adduction.

Teflon Injection. Teflon paste (polytetrafluoroethylene) is injected into the paralysed cord to add bulk. The increased bulk has several effects: (1) the cordal margin becomes smoother; (2) the bulk adds thickness to the cordal edge; and (3) the cord is moved slightly towards the midline, all three of which aid both adduction and vibration when the other cord moves to close the glottis and produce phonation.

As early as 1911, Brunings, a German ENT surgeon introduced a method of intracordal injection of paraffin into the affected cord. However, paraffinoma and embolisation led to its abandonment. The technique was reintroduced by Arnold in the mid-1950s using particles of cartilage in an emulsion. By the mid–1960s Teflon particles in a suspension of glycerine had become the substance of choice. This was because 'Teflon had proven to be well tolerated by human tissues' (Montgomery, 1979) and has had no carcinogenic effects.

The procedure involves direct laryngoscopy, under general anaesthesia supplied by a small lumen tube, and the use of a microlaryngoscope (see, for example, Kleinsasser, 1968) an operating microscope and a Teflon syringe. Gentle injection of approximately 1.00 cc of the paste (Teflon particles in glycerine) may be accomplished by using a motor-driven mechanism which gives a controlled dosage (for example the Lakatos' Teflon injector by Richard Wolf UK Ltd). The paste is deposited approximately 3 mm lateral to the vocal cord margin. An excellent postoperative voice may deteriorate a little as the oedema resolves and the glycerol is slowly absorbed. The technique works best with a unilateral recurrent laryngeal nerve paralysis. Bilateral injections to adduct the cords in the case of bilateral flaccid, paralysis (accompanied by a tracheostomy with speaking valve) have produced somewhat unpredictable results thus far and are not in common use. The aim of this latter technique is to prevent overspill and provide a useful voice.

Vocal Rehabilitation

Vocal assessment is indicated for all patients with a cord palsy. Most patients will also require some form of therapy; this may involve counselling and explanation, and usually some form of voice therapy to encourage optimal voice production. Although patients with an idiopathic palsy may recover spontaneously within 9–12 months, longer periods of up to three years are not unknown (McKelvie, 1979, p. 532). During this time unsupervised patients may develop poor vocal habits and even worsen their dysphonia.

The common element is habitual musculoskeletal tension which affects breathing, for example, which may become upper costal and hence shallow. The rate of breathing increases (tachypnoea) to compensate for the insufficient volume of inspired air and the air wastage through the open glottis. Some unsupervised patients even develop the habit of phonating on an ingressive air-stream mechanism. Specific tension in and around the larynx may produce all the usual signs and symptoms of vocal strain: tightness and aching in the throat, fatiguability of the laryngeal muscles (myasthenia laryngis) and disturbance of balance of resonance. The apparent paradox is that the vocal exercises used to encourage the active cord to compensate by crossing the midline to approximate with the affected cord relies on increasing laryngeal tonicity. This is certainly an area where art meets science. The aim is to exploit the natural sphincteric action of the larynx, such as occurs when fixing the chest to lift heavy weights. Thus, it is perhaps better to foster the idea of 'pushing', as first advocated by Froeschels, Kastein and Weiss (1955) and 'lifting' exercises rather than 'forcing' exercises. Depending upon the patient's age and physical condition there are a variety of ways of producing sufficient physical effort. The aim is repeated, rapid muscular tensions accompanied by attempts at vocalisation. Controlled coughing and grunts (that is, a glottal plosive followed by a vowel or nasal such as [?a:] or [?m), and a voiced glottal fricative accompanied by bilabial or alveolar closure and nasal release [hm], [hn]), should be followed by rapid muscular relaxation. No more than 60 per cent of total strength is required. Although some authorities advocate pushing against furniture etc. (Bull and Cook, 1976), it is important to bear the safety aspect in mind! Isometric exercises, such as interlocking the hands and trying to pull them apart while producing /i:/ sufficiently involves the muscles of the neck, thorax and arms to encourage compensatory adduction. This procedure also encourages better lateral expansion of the ribs and therefore greater inspiration than, say, pushing with the arms held forwards, or downwards on the arms of a chair. The vowels /u:/ and /o:/ seem to have particular value once adduction begins to improve. As soon as possible, progression from stressed syllables, to words (beginning with a stressed vowel, such as /'eg/, /'Iglu:/), phrases, reading and spontaneous conversation should follow. Not all patients require 'pushing' exercises; encouragement to use hard glottal attack on short stressed syllables may well be sufficient. Turning the head to increase tension, and digital manipulation of the thyroid cartilage have also proved useful adjuncts to the above procedures.

Relaxation exercises are frequently essential to reduce general musculoskeletal tension, and thus indirectly improve breath capacity and control, and to reduce specific neck tension following each attempt at achieving compensatory movement. The present author is an adherent of the Alexander technique (Barlow, 1973; Gelb, 1981), but recognises the difficulties of trying to *write* guidelines for students and clinicians who have had no experience, or access to a qualified teacher, of a technique which is concerned with muscular re-education in a much wider context. However, the procedures described by Mitchell (1977) can be readily understood and applied in therapy and represent an acceptable approach. To some extent the amount and type of relaxation work reflects the personal interest and therapeutic style of the clinician. Some clinicians are advocates of massage (for example, 'digital massage', see Aronson, 1980), others of music, or biofeedback (Stemple, *et al.*, 1980). Patients frequently find such work of lasting value and should be encouraged to incorporate the practice of relaxation into their lifestyle.

Conclusion

Voice pathologists find this a rewarding area in which to work as the majority of patients (who have a unilateral cord palsy) normally achieve a very satisfactory voice. Satisfaction is enhanced by close collaboration with the ENT surgeon and the use of fibreoptic endoscopes which facilitate viewing and documentation of the state of the vocal cords.

References

Aronson, A. E. *Clinical Voice Disorders* (Brian C. Decker, New York, 1980)
Barlow, W. *The Alexander Principle* (Victor Gollancz, London, 1973)
Blau, J. N. and Kapadia, R. 'Idiopathic Palsy of the Recurrent Laryngeal Nerve: A Transient Cranial Mononeuropathy', *British Medical Journal*, 4, 259–61 (1972)
Bowden, R. E. M. 'Innervation of the Intrinsic Laryngeal Muscles', in Wyke, B. (ed.) *Ventilatory and Phonatory Control Systems*, Chapter 22 (Oxford University Press, Oxford, 1974)
Brünings, W. 'Uber eine Behandlungsmethode der Rekurrenslahmung', *Verhnandlungen der Deutschen Laryngologishen Gesellshaft*, 18, 19–151 (1911)
Bull, T. R. and Cook, J. L. *Speech Therapy and ENT Surgery* (Blackwell Scientific, Oxford, 1976)
Froeschels, E., Kastein, S. and Weiss, D. A. 'A Method of Therapy for Paralytic Conditions of the Mechanisms of Phonation, Respiration and Glutination', *Journal of Speech and Hearing Disorders*, 20, 365–70 (1955)
Gelb, M. *Body Learning* (Aurum Press, London, 1981)
Greene, M. C. L. *The Voice and its Disorders*, 4th edn (Pitman Medical, Tunbridge Wells, 1980)
Hardcastle, W. J. *Physiology of Speech Production: An Introduction for Speech Scientists* (Academic Press, London, 1976)
Kleinsasser, O. *Microlaryngoscopy and Endolaryngeal Microsurgery*, translated by P. W. Hoffman (Saunders, London, 1968)
McKelvie, P. 'Neurological Affections of the Larynx and Pharynx', in Ballantyne, J. and Groves, J. (eds) *Scott-Brown's Diseases of the Ear, Nose and Throat*, 4th edn, Chapter 17 (Butterworths, London, 1979)
Minuck, M. 'Unilateral Voice Cord Paralysis Following Endotracheal Intubation', *Anaesthesiology*, 45, 448 (1976)
Mitchell, L. *Simple Relaxation: The Physiological Method for Easing Tension* (John Murray, London, 1977)
Montgomery, W. W. 'Laryngeal Paralysis Telflon Injection', *Annals of Otolaryngology*, 88, 647–657 (1979)
Negus, V. E. 'Observations on Semon's Law derived from Evidence of Comparative Anatomy and Physiology', *Journal of Laryngology*, 46, 1 (1931)
Semon, F. 'Clinical Remarks on the Proclivity of the Abductor Fibres of the Recurrent Laryngeal Nerves to Become Affected Sooner than the Adductor Fibres, or Even Exclusively in Cases of Undoubted Central or Peripheral Injury or Disease of the Roots, Trunks of the Pneumogastric, Spinal Accessory or Recurrent Nerves', *Archives of Laryngology*, 2, 197–222 (1881)
Simpson, J. F., Robin, I. G., Ballantyne, J. C. and Groves, J. *A Synopsis of Otolaryngology*, 2nd edn (John Wright, Bristol, 1967)
Stemple, J., Weiler, E., Whitehead, W. and Komray, R. 'Electromyographic Biofeedback Training with Patients Exhibiting a Hyperfunctional Voice Disorder', *Laryngoscope*, 90, 471–5 (1980)
Williams, G. T. Farquharson, I. M. and Anthony, J. (1975) 'Fibreoptic Laryngoscopy in the Assessment of Laryngeal Disorder', *Journal of Laryngology*, 89, 299 (1975)
Woodman, de Graffe 'Modification of Extralaryngeal Approach to Arytenoidectomy for Bilateral Abductor Paralysis', *Archives of Otolaryngology*, 43, 63 (1946)

9 SPASTIC DYSPHONIA: DIAGNOSIS AND MANAGEMENT

Margaret Stoicheff

Introduction

Spastic dysphonia, which has been recognised as a voice disorder for over a century, has been thrust into prominence over the past decade by Dedo's surgical management procedure (Dedo, 1976). This has made it imperative to reach some agreement on when the label of spastic dysphonia is applied. It has also highlighted the need to look carefully at the management of spastic dysphonia: possible therapy approaches, criteria for selecting a particular approach, and the changes in vocal symptoms which can be expected. In this chapter an approach to the issues of diagnosis and management is presented with the data available at this time.

When to Apply The Label 'Spastic Dysphonia'

Pathophysiology

There is unanimity in the literature that spastic dysphonia has as its basis an abnormal adductory movement or spasm of the vocal folds during phonation (Fox, 1969; Aronson and De Santo, 1983) and that this movement is involuntary, momentary and intermittent. There is also consensus that this abnormal movement may extend to the false vocal cords.

In a small percentage of patients to whom the label of spastic dysphonia has been applied, it appears that this spasmodic movement extends beyond the larynx into the hypopharynx and oropharynx (McCall, Skolnick and Brewer, 1971; Parnes, Lavorato and Myers, 1978), into the oral cavity (McCall, Skolnick and Brewer, 1971), and may even occur during respiration as well as speaking (McCall, Skolnick and Brewer, 1971; Parnes, Lavorato and Myers, 1978; Salassa, De Santo and Aronson, 1982).

The Sound of the Voice

This abnormal spasming or hyperadduction of the vocal folds is perceived by the listener as an unexpected change in voice quality – as a squeezed or strangled quality or even a choking-off of voice. This qualitative change may be very brief and widely spaced among otherwise normal phonation, or it may occur so frequently that the overall impression is of a strangled voice interrupted only occasionally by more normal voicing. The listener is also aware of the effort that the patient is putting into forcing voice through a constricted glottis. These vocal symptoms are often accompanied by visible signs of struggle such as grimaces, eye-blinking, and contraction of thoracic and abdominal musculature. Patients without exception confirm this effort and the fatigue that comes with extended speaking.

Voice tremor is found in a percentage of patients with spastic dysphonia, although it is not clear how frequently this occurs. In 1968 Aronson and his associates found that in 31 patients with spastic dysphonia, 58 per cent had a voice tremor in contextual speech, and 71 per cent had a voice tremor on prolongation of /ɑ/. A similar high percentage of voice tremor on vowel prolongation was found in a series of 33 patients on whom surgery was performed (Aronson and De Santo, 1983). Dedo and Izdebski (1983b), on the other hand, report that vocal tremor occurred in only 20–25 per cent of their 300 patients.

Onset of the Disorder

The patient typically reports that the onset of the disorder was insidious and barely noticed. Hoarseness or roughness began to appear in the voice, but there remained periods of time lasting hours or days when there were no symptoms. Usually the patient does not seek help during this period, because he does not perceive these minimal symptoms as sufficiently serious. It is only after the patient begins to experience interruptions of voicing, with some consistency, that help is usually sought some months after the initial voice symptoms. Once this stage is reached, there are no extended periods of time when the individual is free of the problem. The patient may experience greater or lesser difficulty when speaking, depending on fatigue level, emotional state and speaking situation, but he no longer experiences cessation of symptoms. The only occurrences of normal voicing are very brief and occur (for a word or phrase) in asides, during laughter, when taken off guard, sometimes when angry or shouting and when speaking at a higher pitch.

Aetiology

From 1871 to 1960 spastic dysphonia was considered by most clinicians to be a psychogenic disorder and was usually classified as a conversion reaction (Aronson *et al.*, 1968). Since Robe, Brumlik and Moore (1960) proposed that disordered function of the central nervous system was responsible for the disorder, the evidence appears to be mounting in favour of a neurological basis in at least some of these patients.

The presence of voice tremor in a high percentage of patients with spastic dysphonia and the similarity of the voice signs in spastic dysphonia to those of essential (voice) tremor, a known neurological disorder, have prompted Aronson and Hartman (1981) to conclude that 'the presence of voice tremor or rhythmic voice arrests on clinical examination, despite the absence of other neurologic signs of tremor, should arouse suspicion of essential tremor'. Aminoff, Dedo and Izdebski (1978) reported associated coexisting disorders of idiopathic torsion dystonia, blepharospasm, postural tremor and familial tremor in five out of 12 consecutive patients with spastic dysphonia evaluated clinically by a neurologist. They suggested that spastic dysphonia should be regarded as a focal dystonia of the laryngeal musculature. The appearance of abnormal laryngeal movements during breathing in three patients some months after recurrent laryngeal resection for spastic dysphonia has led Salassa, De Santo and Aronson (1982) to the conclusion that these patients had a focal, isolated form of dystonia. Schaefer *et al.*, (1983) have put their findings of VIIIth cranial nerve dysfunction in nine out of twelve spastic dysphonia patients together with literature reports such as the foregoing to hypothesise that spastic dysphonia is a disease involving multiple cranial nerves with variable presentation.

Spastic Dysphonia as a Voice Sign

Dedo and Izdebski (1983a) have indicated that a major problem with spastic dysphonia is misdiagnosis, that spastic dysphonia is confused with disorders which present similar vocal symptoms. It would appear that it may be wiser for the speech pathologist to use the term spastic dysphonia as a 'voice sign' (Salassa, De Santo and

Aronson, 1982; Aronson and De Santo, 1983) rather than as a diagnosis. This means that there is recognition that the sound of the voice may be similar in a number of disorders and that one must look beyond the label 'spastic dysphonia' to the total presenting symptomatology for a differential diagnosis.

At least the following possibilities are involved in using the label 'spastic dysphonia' in this way.

Spastic Dysphonia Associated with Psychologic Disorders of Conversion Reaction and Depression. In spite of the evidence supporting a neurological basis, there are patients with this vocal symptomatology where the basis is psychogenic (Aronson and De Santo, 1983). The patient with a psychogenic spastic dysphonia usually reports a sudden onset to the voice disorder, as well as periods of remission lasting days, weeks or months. This is not the case with neurological and idiopathic types.

In patients with psychogenic spastic dysphonia it is also possible to trigger voice free of this strained quality in the voice testing situation.

Spastic Dysphonia Associated with Hyperfunctional Voice Disorders. In the experience of this writer, some clinicians confuse hyperfunctional and ventricular dysphonias with the spastic dysphonia of neurological and idiopathic types. The main difference lies in the intermittent character of the strained or strangled component in the latter and the more continuous straining quality of a ventricular or hyperfunctional dysphonia. With close examination it may become apparent that the strained quality is a function of the muscular tension set rather than an unexpected laryngospasm. Patients in this category frequently complain of throat pain; this is not a complaint of patients with spastic dysphonia of the neurological and idiopathic types. This pain is presumably associated with the excessive muscular tension of the extrinsic muscles of the larynx in creating the necessary constriction to produce this strained quality. Trial therapy may also assist in this differentiation by demonstrating the possibility of more normal voicing with a different laryngeal set.

Spastic Dysphonia Associated with Neurological Disorders of Essential (Voice) Tremor, Spasmodic Torticollis, Blepharospasm, Pseudobulbar palsy, Dystonia. The presence of tremors in the limbs, jaw and tongue, or of involuntary movements of the head or neck, or of dysarthric involvement should alert the speech pathologist to a possible neurological condition requiring a neurological consultation. The presence of a voice tremor or of regular voice arrests without any tremor elsewhere is also a suspicious sign (Aronson and Hartman, 1981). In an organic disorder, there are no brief instances of normal voicing during laughter, asides, singing or use of a falsetto (Aronson and Hartman, 1981).

Spastic Dysphonia on an Idiopathic Basis. The use of the term spastic dysphonia has more typically been associated with this type. Aronson (1980) has summarised the characteristic features of idiopathic spastic dysphonia. These are:

(1) Presence of intermittent strained and/or strangled phonations and breaks in the voice
(2) No laryngeal lesions or paralyses
(3) No abnormal speech signs in the rest of the peripheral speech mechanism
(4) Brief periods of normal voicing during singing, laughter, shouting or anger
(5) Resistance to treatment.

The cause of the voice disorder cannot be found in this type.

Management

Discussions on management, for the most part, have made no differentiation among these four categories of spastic dysphonia. Thus it is not surprising that the literature abounds with statements such as 'Psychotherapy, speech therapy, stimulant and psychotropic drugs, hypnotism and acupuncture have all been tried as treatment without success' (Levine *et al.*, 1979). To this list might be added the most recent treatment, recurrent laryngeal nerve resection. With the term 'spastic dysphonia' being applied to differing populations, it is essential that treatment or treatments be looked at for each of these populations.

Spastic Dysphonia Associated with Psychological Disorders

Patients falling within this category respond to the type of therapy used for psychogenic disorders in which direct work on voice, reassurance and the opportunity to progress at their own rate is permitted (Aronson, Peterson and Litin, 1966). These are not patients for whom surgical treatment is advisable. There has been some suggestion in the literature that patients with very breathy voices following recurrent laryngeal nerve resection may be those whose disorder was psychogenic (Aronson and De Santo, 1983).

Spastic Dysphonia Associated with Hyperfunctional Voice Disorders

Cooper (1973) forwarded the notion that spastic dysphonia resulted from long-term vocal abuse, with physical or psychological trauma as catalysts. In this writer's experience, patients referred by laryngologists with the label of spastic dysphonia have sometimes fallen within the category of severe vocal hyperfunction with a resulting severely strained voice quality. In these patients it has been possible to trigger voice free of this excessive tension through the generally accepted methods of relaxation therapy, and more specific relaxation of the vocal tract coupled with phonation using chewing, humming, or breathy phonations. Again, these are not patients who should be treated surgically since the problem yields to conventional voice therapies.

Spastic Dysphonia Associated with Neurologic Disorders

Within this group of patients essential tremor is the most frequent disorder. According to Aronson (1980), voice therapy is not effective in reducing the vocal tremor. Likewise propanolol, although sometimes useful in reducing the tremor in essential tremor patients, has not been shown to reduce the vocal symptomatology of spastic dysphonia (Salassa, De Santo and Aronson, 1982). Surgical section of the recurrent laryngeal nerve, which reduces or eliminates the hyperadduction of the vocal folds by paralysing one vocal cord in a paramedian position, has also been used. Aronson and De Santo (1983) reported on the long-term vocal results of surgery for a group of 33 patients, 70 per cent of whom had essential (voice) tremor. By the three-year period 64 per cent of the patients had voice disorders which were at least as severe as prior to surgery. Tape recordings were used to make these judgements. The authors attributed the failed voices to a progression of the patients' original neurological condition. Dedo and Izdebski (1983a) on the other hand, using patient self-assessment questionnaires, have reported that 90 per cent of 212 patients managed surgically considered their surgery results to be satisfactory; voice tremor was present in a small percentage of these patients. It is possible, therefore, that the discrepancy in the findings between the two studies may be, in part, due to differing patient populations in the two studies. At this time, there appears to be little in the way of known treatments that is useful in alleviating the vocal arrests in patients with spastic dysphonia associated with essential (voice) tremor.

Idiopathic Spastic Dysphonia. Various forms of treatment have been applied to this group of patients.

Voice Therapy. In 1969, Fox presented some positive therapy results with a case of spastic dysphonia. Therapy consisted basically of teaching the patient to speak in a breathy voice so that the vocal folds would make minimal, if any, contact. Fox reported that the woman was able to eliminate the tremulous strained quality 75–80 per cent of the time in daily life.

This writer has used an approach which is also directed toward decreasing vocal cord contact. For two female patients, with mild to moderately severe symptomatology, therapy was directed toward a slight elevation of pitch level, reduction in vocal loudness, and easy voice onsets combined with a 'light' voice. The concepts of easy voice onset and light voice were gradually built up through work on consonant–vowel (CV) syllables in which vowels were initiated by voiceless sibilants, then voiceless fricatives and voiceless plosives. As the patients became successful at initiating vowels easily within these contexts, voiced consonant contexts were introduced with the same easy onset of voicing as the goal. The patients used the Vocal II and Visi Pitch for visual monitoring of production. They were also trained in progressive relaxation. Although neither patient had voice entirely free of spastic dysphonia, both patients expressed satisfaction with the voice results.

It is hypothesised by this clinician/writer that these successful reports may be due to the reduced expectations of the patients and clinicians. The goal was to reduce the effort and strain in the voice rather than to achieve the occasional normal voice heard briefly in their voices. It is possible that similar results are obtainable with other patients with mild to moderately severe symptomatology when expectations are more realistic.

Surgery. Since 1976 there have been many patients treated by means of surgical resection of the recurrent laryngeal nerve. In the study by Dedo and Izdebski (1983a), in which 90 per cent of the patients had improved voices on follow-up, the assumption is that a majority of them were in the idiopathic category. Since patients' self-reports were used to judge the results, it is difficult to assess the extent of the reported improvement in voice in these patients. The authors do indicate that 80 per cent of the sample found their voices to be too weak to communicate adequately in noisy surroundings and that approximately 50 per cent reported that strangers frequently commented on their unusual postoperative voices. Thus we do know that many of the patients in this sample had improved but not 'normal' voices.

In a series of ten patients who were treated surgically, Stoicheff (1983) rated the degree of spastic symptomatology on a seven-point equal-appearing intervals scale. Eight of the ten patients had idiopathic spastic dysphonia; two had spastic dysphonia of essential tremor. Seven in the former group and one in the latter group had a reduction in their spastic symptomatology on follow-up from one to six years postsurgically. The two patients whose voices were worse on follow-up did not differ from the group except in the severity of their initial symptomatology; their preoperative voice ratings indicated the mildest spastic symptoms of the group. Of those who showed improvement in spastic symptomatology, only one patient had a voice free of symptoms; three had minimal involvement with voice close to normal; the remaining four had varying degrees of involvement. However, in addition to the residual spastic symptomatology, most patients' voices were mildly hoarse, breathy or rough due to the vocal cord paralysis. Their voices also tended to be weaker than in the normal population.

Dedo and his colleagues have indicated throughout their reports that voice therapy is needed postsurgically and that this therapy should emphasise elevation of pitch, avoidance of vocal fry and of efforts to push the voice to achieve loudness. In this writer's experience, it has been necessary to provide some therapy/counselling sessions postoperatively. Patients are cautioned against attempting to produce voice more clearly through any pushing procedures and have been advised not to attempt to use voice loudly for speaking purposes. Since patients (without spastic dysphonia) who develop a vocal cord paralysis often resort to effortful styles of speaking in order to overcome the hypoadduction of the vocal folds, it would be surprising if patients with spastic dysphonia automatically avoided such compensatory practices. Until the varying reasons for recurrence have been elucidated, such as progression of disease process, compensation for vocal cord paralysis and reinnervation of the recurrent laryngeal nerve, the speech pathologist would be well advised to help prevent one of the possible reasons through counselling and therapy.

Thus management of the varying types of spastic dysphonia requires that the aetiology be examined very carefully. This means that the speech pathologist must work together with the neurologist and psychiatrist to determine the basis of the vocal symptomatology. When the basis of the symptomatology has been taken into account, vocal results vary along a continuum from excellent to no improvement. Where there is doubt of the basis, a trial period of voice therapy should be the first treatment method considered.

References

Aminoff, M. J., Dedo, H. H. and Izdebski, K. 'Clinical Aspects of Spasmodic Dysphonia', *Journal of Neurology, Neurosurgery and Psychiatry*, 41, 361–5 (1978)

Aronson, A. E. *Clinical Voice Disorders: An Interdisciplinary Approach*, pp. 157–70 (Thieme-Stratton, New York, 1980)

—— Brown, J. R., Litin, E. M. and Pearson, J. S. 'Spastic Dysphonia. I. Voice, Neurologic and Psychiatric Aspects', *Journal of Speech and Hearing Disorders*, 33, 203–18 (1968)

—— and Hartman, D. E. 'Adductor Spastic Dysphonia as a Sign of Essential (Voice) Tremor', *Journal of Speech and Hearing Disorders*, 46, 52–8 (1981)

—— and De Santo, L. W. 'Adductor Spastic Dysphonia: Three Years After Recurrent Laryngeal Nerve Section', *Laryngoscope*, 93, 1–8 (1983)

——, Peterson, H. W. Jr. and Litin, E. M. 'Psychiatric Symptomatology in Functional Dysphonia and Aphonia', *Journal of Speech and Hearing Disorders*, 31, 115–27 (1966)

Cooper, M. *Modern Techniques of Vocal Rehabilitation*, pp. 171–8 (Charles C. Thomas, Springfield, Illinois, 1973)

Dedo, H. H. 'Recurrent Laryngeal Nerve Section for Spastic Dysphonia', *Annals of Otology, Rhinology and Laryngology*, 85, 451–9 (1976)

—— and Izdebski, K. (1983a), 'Intermediate Results of 306 Recurrent Laryngeal Nerve Sections for Spastic Dysphonia', *Laryngoscope*, 93, 9–16 (1983a)

—— and Izdebski, K. 'Problems with Surgical (RLN Section) Treatment of Spastic Dysphonia', *Laryngoscope*, 93, 268–71 (1983b)

Fox, D. (1969), 'Spastic Dysphonia: A Case Presentation', *Journal of Speech and Hearing Disorders*, 34, 275–9 (1969)

Levine, H. L., Wood, B. G., Batza, E., Rusnov, M. and Tucker, H. M. 'Recurrent Laryngeal Nerve Section for Spasmodic Dysphonia', *Annals of Otology, Rhinology and Laryngology*, 88, 527–30 (1979)

McCall, G. N., Skolnick, M. I. and Brewer, D. W. 'A Preliminary Report of Some Atypical Movement Patterns in the Tongue, Palate, Hypopharynx and Larynx of Patients with Spasmodic Dysphonia', *Journal of Speech and Hearing Disorders*, 36, 466–70 (1971)

Parnes, S. M., Lavorato, A. S. and Myers, E. N. 'Study of Spastic Dysphonia Using Videofiberoptic Laryngoscopy', *Annals of Otology, Rhinology and Laryngology*, 87, 322–6 (1978)

Robe, E., Brumlik, J. and Moore, P. 'A Study of Spastic Dysphonia: Neurologic and Electroencephalographic Abnormalities', *Laryngoscope*, 70, 219–45 (1960)

Salassa, J. R., De Santo, L. W. and Aronson. A. E. (1982), 'Respiratory Distress after Recurrent Laryngeal Nerve Sectioning for Adductor Spastic Dysphonia, *Laryngoscope*, 92, 240–5 (1982)

Schaefer, S. D., Finitzo-Heiber, T., Gerling, I. J. and Freeman, F. J. 'Brainstem Conduction Abnormalities in Spasmodic Dysphonia', in Bless, D. M. and Abbs, J. H. (eds.) *Vocal Fold Physiology*, pp. 393–404 (College-Hill Press, San Diego, California, 1983)

Stoicheff, M. L. 'The Present Status of Adductor Spastic Dysphonia', *Journal of Otolaryngology*, 12, 311–14 (1983)

10 HYPERFUNCTIONAL VOICE: THE MISUSE AND ABUSE SYNDROME

Margaret Fawcus

Introduction

The term *vocal hyperfunction* appears to have been first used by Froeschels (1943) and is characterised by a tense over-adduction of the vocal folds. It is generally regarded as the most common cause of voice disorder. Boone (1977) says, 'it is at the anatomical site of the glottal opening where the vast majority of hyperfunctional voice problems begin, because of inappropriate (inadequate or excessive) vocal fold approximation'. The resulting voice may be described as harsh or strident. Whether this type of voice use becomes a problem or not will depend on the relationship between the vulnerability of the vocal folds and the degree of hyperfunction involved in voice use. Not all strident voice users experience vocal problems, but where excessive tension results in vocal fatigue, discomfort, weakness or loss of voice and actual tissue changes in the epithelium of the larynx, there is clearly a situation which demands some form of therapeutic intervention.

The physical vulnerability of the larynx varies from one individual to another: using the voice against a high intensity background noise will lead to slight, temporary hoarseness in some speakers but not in others. Jackson and Jackson (1945) observe that 'there is great variation in the amount of abuse the larynx of different speakers will stand, but every larynx has its limit. To go beyong this limit means thickening of the cords, and a thickened cord means a hoarse voice.' The laryngeal mucosa may be resistant to an habitual pattern of over-adduction for many months or even years, but an attack of acute laryngitis will often lead to the continuing condition of chronic non-specific laryngitis because the folds are now vulnerable to improper voice use.

The term *misuse and abuse* was used by Van Thal (1961) and distinguishes between the long-term habitual pattern of hyperfunctional voice use (misuse) and those situations where hyperfunction is on a situation-tied, 'one-off' basis (for example, speaking against loud ambient noise at a disco or shouting at sports events).

Excessive tension (that is, a state of muscular tonus over and above that required for efficient vocal fold movement) is a common denominator in many cases of voice disorder. In hyperfunctional voice problems it is, by definition, the central feature. Brodnitz (1959) stated that 'the vast majority of functional voice disorders begin with excessive use of muscular force'. Tension may be manifest in a harsh or strident voice, in a hard glottal attack on vowel sounds, and in high and sometimes inappropriate intensity levels. The presenting symptoms will vary, and will depend on the condition of the vocal folds. In the early stages of hyperfunctional voice use there may be no abnormal signs on examination of the larynx. In these cases, the vocal symptoms are probably intermittent and the main complaints are of vocal fatigue, episodes of vocal weakness, throat clearing or pitch breaks. There may be slight reddening of the vocal folds when these occur. Voice therapy at this stage is an important prophylactic measure, since remediation is slower and may be less successful once the tissue changes associated with chronic inflammation, vocal nodules or contact ulcers have taken place.

The causes of vocal misuse are complex, and frequently represent an interaction of endogenous and exogenous factors. Van Riper and Irwin (1958) have placed some emphasis on the personality of the speaker and regard the users of harsh voices as 'aggressive and antagonistic individuals, highly competitive and hypertense'. They commented on the difficulty of modifying such patterns of voice use because of the close affinity between voice and personality.

In addition to personality factors, the speaker's environment is a potential source of many causes of tension. At work there may be the burden of heavy responsibilities, relationships which may be strained and difficult, excessive work loads, an atmosphere which is highly competitive, and nowadays the fear of redundancy. The interpersonal dynamics in the home environment may be even more demanding and complex.

There may, of course, be familial patterns of hyperfunctional voice use. Vocal misuse may arise initially from imitation of an adult model. Piaget (1952) and Greene (1980) have written about the vocal 'contagion' which takes place in the early months of the baby's life.

The patient's age may be a significant pointer, not only as an indicator of possible physical changes and associated problems (such as the menopause), but also of crucial changes in lifestyle. Within the family network there are many possible sources of anxiety, anguish, irritation and bitterness — all potential causes of physical tension and even lack of self-care. This holds true for both the single or the married person, for the young, the middle-aged and the old. Empathy and imagination are essential qualities if the therapist is going to evaluate the effect of the various sources of stress and tension. It is important that the presence of one obvious problem (such as overwork) should not blind one to other factors, such as poor interpersonal relationships, which may have more insidious effects and ultimately be more damaging.

The possible causes of stress and tension are endless; some may appear insignificant, but it is the cumulative effect of these causes which must be considered. Suffice to say that a systematic examination of the patient's total lifestyle, at home, at work, and at leisure, may reveal clear indications (if no easy solutions) for total management.

In addition to specific remedial techniques, the management of all such cases will involve an attempt to eliminate or modify adverse environmental factors. The emphasis in the treatment programme will obviously depend on a consideration of all possible aetiological and contributory factors in each case, and on the practical problems involved in implementing change. In planning what we may describe as the 'remediation package' it is essential that we are aware of the physical and emotional stresses in the domestic environment, the work situation and leisure pursuits. Whatever can be done to reduce these demands should be discussed with the patient. The extent to which change can be achieved will obviously depend on the degree of co-operation which we can expect from those in the patient's environment. More important still is the willingness and initiative shown by the patient trying to make changes. We are not only concerned with the question of whether the deaf relative is willing to wear a hearing aid, but also whether the client is prepared to approach the relative on the subject.

In many cases, the ultimate success of treatment will depend on the extent to which adverse environmental factors can be removed or modified and in some cases this will depend on a balance being achieved between what is the ideal goal and what is practical. There are sometimes very simple solutions to vocal abuse — the purchase of a whistle, for example, may replace shouting to call the children in from the garden (and produce a more immediate response!).

The Remedial Voice Programme

In very general terms, the remedial programme will be a two-stage process: the first step is designed to modify those habits of voice production which cause the vocal strain; the second step is the development of strategies to enhance voice production.

Traditionally, the approach to remedial voice work has been based on a singing and drama teaching model, with what would seem an inappropriate emphasis on certain aspects of the training. Improved breath control, for example, has occupied a central role in such training and has come to be considered as an essential part of all remedial voice work. In this section, we shall be considering the need to develop a treatment programme to meet the specific needs of those whose voices have been misused, rather than a training regime for those who are going to make more exceptional demands on their voices. In this context, it will be seen that improved breath control is not the most important aspect of re-training. It would seem far more important that the patient first learns to monitor his vocal output, so that he can make the necessary adjustments to improve his performance.

Auditory Training

Valuable as visual feedback devices (for example, Visispeech) may be, it is essential that the patient learns to develop his own monitoring skills. Bunch (1982) comments 'machines are important tools for research, but for the purposes of performance and the teaching of singing, the human ear and associated neural mechanisms provide a superb instrument for refined detection and analysis'. The same is equally true for the speaking voice. Nonetheless, visual feedback devices are an important adjunct in treatment in enabling the patient to compare his performance with the target model presented by the therapist. It is also important, however, that such instrumentation does not obscure the need for the patient to develop reliable listening skills.

Limited auditory monitoring ability may indeed be a poor prognostic sign in the dysphonic patient. Listening is the only tangible feedback channel since, as Boone (1977) says, 'no-one has much awareness of what he is doing laryngeally whether he is approximating his folds or shortening or lengthening them'. He goes on to discuss the problems this presents in voice work since the patient 'literally does not know what he is doing when he phonates'. This is in sharp distinction to the tactile awareness one can normally rely on in articulation work. Aronson (1980) considers that auditory discrimination and feedback 'occupy a pivotal position in voice therapy . . . because tactile and proprioceptive feedback is diminished in phonation and cannot be relied on'. A study by Fishman, McGlone and Shipp (1971), in which the larynx was anaesthetised, showed that the deprivation of sensory feedback did not affect the subject's phonation. They concluded that sensory feedback from the larynx was not essential for phonation. This study underlines the importance of developing auditory feedback skills if the patient is to recognise and correct faulty voice production. The patient must become a critical and discriminating listener, and this is probably the single most important therapeutic goal. Unfortunately, concentration on breathing in the early stages of treatment — which is normally part of a more traditional approach — inevitably distracts the patient from the more important task of listening to his own voice.

Training in procedures such as the vocal profile analysis described by Laver *et al.* (1981) will give the therapist the knowledge he or she needs in order to:

(1) Detect what the patient is doing.
(2) Model what the patient is doing, providing him with an auditory 'mirror' of his own performance.
(3) Be able to alternate normal and abnormal voice production in order to heighten the patient's awareness of the voice he is producing.

Aronson's (1980) statement that 'voice is ephemeral, lacking finite acoustic boundaries' underlines one of the difficulties on working with the dysphonic patient.

Van Riper and Irwin (1958) have described the process of 'hunting' in articulation practice and a similar approach can be used in achieving target voice. It is a form of exploratory oscillation about the target – in this case the most acceptable voice produced by the patient. Good voice may be used inadvertently on occasions and this must be recognised and reinforced by the therapist immediately it occurs. During a therapy session we may expect the patient to produce a number of 'different' voices, some nearer the desired target than others. The resourceful therapist helps the patient to place these different vocalisations on a sensitive rating scale from 'poor' to 'good' voice production. Aronson (1980) observed that 'the voice rarely changes from aphonic to dysphonic to normal without first passing through several dysphonic stages'. He goes on to say, 'in the early stages improved voice will break through suddenly and momentarily, milliseconds in duration'.

It is the therapist's role to help the patient evaluate what he is doing, with the aim of working towards the target sound, with the therapist and patient making careful judgements of the voice quality achieved at each stage. The patient becomes an active and informed participant, much less dependent on the therapist's judgement of 'correctness'.

The increasing ability to make reliable judgements for himself is essential for productive practice periods and voice use beyond the confines of the clinical situation.

Elimination of Unnecessary Tension

Implicit in the term hyperfunctional is the state of hypertonus or tension in the muscles of the larynx. It is not unreasonable, therefore, to assume that such tension localised to vocal function will be an integral part of a more generalised tension. From this assumption, general relaxation became recognised as an essential and early stage in the traditional approach to treatment. Such an approach seems logical enough in the circumstances, but closer consideration reveals flaws which would seem to demand a more specific approach. In the first place, one is aware that many very tense people do not necessarily abuse or misuse their voices. Secondly, degrees of considerable tension are a normal and indeed inevitable part of our daily living. Many professional speakers who use their voices well, need the drive of adrenalin to achieve optimum performance. What is important, however, is that muscular relaxation is achieved through the ability to quite simply 'let go' in leisure activities and off-duty hours. The most effective and lasting answer to the problem of excessive bodily tension is to help the patient gain insight into the demands he is placing on his body. This lies in the realm of counselling more than relaxation, but if we are to achieve a more permanent solution in these cases, it would seem that we must address ourselves to these issues. There are a number of ways of attempting to make such changes in the person's total lifestyle:

(1) Keeping a diary – an analysis of even a day's activities may demonstrate to the patient that there is little respite from a continuous pattern of tension and activity.
(2) A personal 'brainstorming' session in which the client is asked to suggest anything which he/she thinks may result in tension. These items should be written down so that they can be discussed by client and therapist. An analysis of these situations may reveal patterns or 'groupings' which may have considerable implications for management.
(3) Non-directive counselling (Rogers, 1981) allows the patient to develop insights into sources of stress and conflict, and possible solutions to them. It is a process which facilitates change, enabling the patient to choose between the options available to him. As the name implies, this process occurs without direct advice or guidance from the therapist (who, in any case, can view the patient's problems only from her own standpoint, however empathic she may be).

The state of general bodily relaxation is very far removed from the finely balanced tonicity required in phonation. Moore (1971) views relaxation as 'a dynamic balance, in which the opposing groups of muscles exert just enough reciprocal tension upon each other to accomplish the desired movement with perfect control'. Optimum functioning demands a dynamic balance between tension and relaxation. Boone (1977) sums up the goal of relaxation by describing it as a 'realistic responsiveness to the environment with a minimum of needless energy expended'. This same viewpoint is echoed by Brodnitz (1959) when he says 'alertness of mind and body and well-adjusted muscular tonus are characteristic for the normally functioning body'.

These statements represent a more realistic approach to relaxation, and emphasise the need to work on a more relaxed bodily state through activity rather than the more static approach of supine relaxation. The aim is freedom for action, with the elimination of unnecessary tensions which may inhibit easy movement and lead to muscular fatigue and even weakness. In the clinic situation Van Riper and Irwin (1958) believe that 'the best relaxing agent we know is a good therapist' influencing the patient's mental and physical state 'by his own relaxed behaviour, by his permissiveness and competence'. This, they claim, can create 'the balanced tonicity out of which successful learning can come'. We need an active and not passive participant.

There are a number of specific approaches to general and localised relaxation which are available to the therapist and which will be mentioned here:

General Relaxation. Boone (1977) and Greene (1980) have described approaches to general relaxation with the dysphonic patient, and readers are referred to the classic text by Jacobsen (1929). A state of relaxation may be achieved by a number of strategies. Suggestion may be used in which the therapist creates a restful scene for the patient to imagine. Used skilfully this can be a very effective technique. Some therapists use a similar approach, but the suggestion is directly related to a relaxed state of each part of the body. This is basically the method advocated by Jacobsen. An alternative method aims at heightening the patient's awareness of tension and relaxation by increasing tension in one part of the body and then releasing it. It is probably worthwhile trying all three approaches in determining the most efficacious with any given subject.

The Acquisition of a Balanced Posture. Laryngeal tension can result from a muscular imbalance caused by improper head/neck posture. Such postural problems may have interesting origins, which are not always immediately obvious to the therapist and may, in any case, be related to situations outside the clinic setting. Abnormal head/neck relationships may occur in those who spend a good deal of their working time on the telephone: it is not so much the amount of talking they do, but rather the continuously asymmetrical posture involved – particularly when the telephone receiver is tucked under the chin to free the hands! Occasionally we meet speakers who habitually cock their head to one side when they speak, which tends to create unnecessary muscular tension on the contralateral side. The following case illustrates the long-term effects of an abnormal postural problem:

The woman, in her mid-30s, had earned a somewhat precarious living from painting and occasional calligraphic assignments. She had no problems with her voice until she decided that she must take a part-time teaching post at a girls' secondary school. She had not received any form of teacher training, and had no experience of classroom teaching. She found the girls difficult to control, and under the circumstances did not enjoy teaching. She began to experience vocal fatigue and periods of voice loss and was referred to the ENT department of her local hospital. There were no abnormal laryngeal signs. She was not a particularly extrovert personality, her voice was not harsh or strident, and neither did she use it excessively outside the classroom. There seemed to be a clear case here of situation-tied vocal misuse, and a treatment programme was designed to improve the audibility of her voice without recourse to forcing it at high intensity levels. In implementing the programme it became clear that she was extending her neck, which involved the tilting back of her head, causing undue tension in the muscles of the neck and larynx. In discussing this phenomenon with her, it emerged that a fellow student at art school had drawn a cartoon of her, accentuating a somewhat underdeveloped mandible, making her look 'a chinless wonder' as she put it. She had attempted to compensate for this by sticking her chin out, which had become a habitual posture. This had not presented any problem until the tension it produced was compounded by the additional tension of using voice in the classroom for several hours a week at higher intensity levels.

A balanced posture in standing, sitting and walking avoids unnecessary tension and wasteful expenditure of energy. Alexander (1932) said 'freedom of alignment allows the body to use its energy far more economically and is especially efficient because no undue tensions are present'. Gould (1971) sums up the need for attention to posture both at rest and in action: 'posture is the dynamic interrelationship between muscular and skeletal tissues. The word dynamic is important; for alignment should be stable, but never static and fixed, if it is to be the prelude to easy flowing movement.' Barlow (1952) used the term 'postural homeostasis, to denote the 'state of steady motion which underlies all voluntary movement'. He felt that such homeostasis was 'primarily dependent on the correct equilibrium of the head/neck relationship'.

Speech therapists working with disorders of voice would undoubtedly benefit from a better understanding of Alexander's ideas and the techniques which have been developed to achieve improved postural balance. In the absence of such knowledge, they must at least be aware of the need to look for poor postural alignment which is producing tension and restricting freedom of movement. Willmore (1959) developed the concept of 'vocal homeostasis' in which 'the overriding aim of all voice therapy is the reduction of misplaced effort and tension'.

Reduction of Intensity Levels. The majority of speakers probably use their voices at higher intensity levels than the situation absolutely demands. It is, of course, only the speaker who experiences vocal fatigue or dysfunction where this actually matters. Reducing the intensity level of the speaker's voice, to a level compatible with being heard by his listener, is probably the most practical way of achieving some degree of vocal economy. Aronson (1980) speaks of 'ill-advised prescription of vocal rest'. He contends that to advise a patient to whisper or remain silent for days or weeks is 'the most deleterious advice that can be given a patient with a voice disorder'. The risk of the patient adopting a forced whisper is considerable, and this can prove infinitely more damaging than quiet voice use. In addition complete voice rest can be a psychologically distressing experience, and one which it is practically difficult to implement. It is far better to advise the patient to adjust his level of intensity to meet the fairly precise needs of a given situation – to speak quietly whenever he can, with the full understanding that this takes some of the stress off the vocal folds.

Elimination of Glottal Attack. A hard, glottal attack on vowel sounds is characteristic of hyperfunctional voice use and represents a form of vocal abuse. This type of vocal attack can be heard in some singers and, if used sparingly, does no harm. Associated with general laryngeal tension, however, it is another matter, and the speaker needs to be made aware of what he is doing. Fortunately it can largely be pinpointed to vowel sounds at the beginning of sentences, which makes it rather easier to modify.

The careful use of negative practice (Dunlap, 1932) is a very effective technique in making the patient aware of a glottal attack. With fingers and thumbs resting lightly on either side of the thyroid cartilage, the patient is asked to produce a vowel sound with a tense initiation of voice. This is then followed by a soft, aspirate attack on the same vowel sound. The process is repeated, until the patient has had the opportunity of experiencing the contrast between the two approaches to vowel initiation.

This stage is followed by practice on the conscious use of aspirate attack on vowels, first on words:

arm – only – underneath – everywhere

and then on phrases:

arm in arm	every afternoon
all the afternoon	amber eyes

Appropriate reading material, which can be prepared to include a high proportion of vowel-initial sentences, can be used to ensure that the speaker can maintain a more gentle approach at the speed of normal speech.

Biofeedback Techniques. The use of biofeedback in the treatment of voice disorder has been described by Aronson (1980) Boone (1977) and Greene (1980). Aronson states that the importance of feedback cannot be overstressed because of the 'minimal tactile and proprioceptive sensation arising from the larynx during phonation'. The aim of biofeedback is to increase the patient's awareness of laryngeal tension and to give him a tangible way of controlling it. A study detailed by Prosek *et al*. (1978) investigated the use of biofeedback training and concluded that it would be most successful in those hyperfunctional voice cases where there was no permanent laryngeal damage. They found that biofeedback (electromyography) provided an accurate external monitor of laryngeal tension, thus placing fewer demands on the auditory system and freeing the patient to concentrate on developing methods of reducing such tension. Prosek considers that biofeedback techniques facilitate the vocal re-education programme but discusses some of the problems encountered in achieving reliable feedback. Undoubtedly, such an approach is a valuable adjunct to therapy in the hands of a skilful and experienced clinician.

The Chewing Approach. Detailed accounts of the chewing approach in achieving more relaxed phonation have been given by Boone (1977) and Wyatt (1977). The patient is asked to phonate whilst carrying out vigorous chewing movements. Because such phonation is not associated with abnormal patterns of habitual voice use, its advocates claim that the patient experiences a normal degree of tension while producing voice in association with a vegetative function. Aronson (1980) has suggested that the value of the chewing method may be limited because of the patient's embarrassment at carrying out the instructions.

Much will depend on the enthusiasm and skill of the therapist, and the ability to involve the equally enthusiastic co-operation of the patient. As with so many techniques employed in voice therapy, there appears to be no evaluative study of this technique.

Developing Optimum Resonance

It is reasonable to suppose that laryngeal tension in hyperfunctional voice use coexists with tension in the variable supraglottic cavities. As Bunch (1982) has observed, 'the hyperfunctional pharynx tends to be rigid and is constricted in such a way as to leave little resonating space'. Discussing the constricting effect of tension, Brodnitz (1959) said:

> hypertension at the level of the hypopharynx and the oral pharynx will produce a constriction of the muscles in the walls of the throat resonator. The tongue is thickened by contraction of its intrinsic muscles. At the same time it is pulled backward. The result is the creation of an acoustic bottleneck.

Tense, restricted jaw movement will further inhibit the optimum use of the oral cavity. The speaker may attempt to compensate for the poor carrying power of his voice by increasing the intensity of the laryngeal note, but the resulting tension is seldom justified by the increase in audibility of the voice. At the same time, the actual quality of the voice may deteriorate and the voice may sound 'constricted, strangulated and harsh' (Brodnitz, 1959).

Bunch (1982) has described the pharynx as an adjustable, mobile muscular sleeve that can 'assume many changes of shape and variations of tension in its wall. These adjustments made by the muscles of the pharynx contribute directly to different vocal qualities.' The therapist may contract the muscles of the pharyngeal walls whilst producing /a/, or on speaking, in order to give a dramatic demonstration of the effects of tense resonators of voice.

Murphy (1964) has discussed the effect of both tense and relaxed surfaces on the quality of voice, and the need to achieve a balance if tone is to be enriched rather than 'muffled', and 'bright' rather than 'metallic'.

Relatively little attention has been paid to work on developing optimum resonance in patients with hyperfunctional voice problems. This is surprising when one considers those patients who have been struggling to meet the demands of teaching, lecturing, preaching or just using their voices a great deal against adverse noise conditions. To instruct the patient to project or 'throw' their voice without a carefully structured programme is likely to do little more than result in increased tension which will be counterproductive in improving voice quality.

Zaliouk's 'tactile approach' (1963) provides a sound foundation for developing resonance, and forms the basis for the programme outlined below. The patient obtains tactile feedback from the facial bones which focuses attention on oral and nasal resonance. In practice, the production of vibrations in the facial mask seems to be incompatible with hyperfunctional voice use and gives the patient a tangible experience of relaxed resonant voice use. This has the important advantage of ensuring that the patient can make use of such feedback in practice periods outside the clinical situation. Because there has been little reference to work on achieving resonant voice production in this way, the programme will be given in some detail. While the basic idea is Zaliouk's, the steps have been developed by the present author.

Stage I. The patient sits down, with his elbows resting comfortably on the desk or table in front of him. His head rests on the palmar aspects of his hands, with fingers extended at the side of his face. He is then encouraged to produce a very quiet 'bm–bm–bm', on a continuous sung tone. He should be able to feel the vibration in the facial bones. If not, the therapist models the voice production herself, letting the patient feel the vibrations produced by the therapist. The same task can be practised by intoning 'bm' into cupped hands – this is particularly useful where the patient has some difficulty in achieving a sufficiently vivid experience of resonance. Variations on this task can be devised, providing they are carried out on a sung tone, at quiet intensity levels and with 'continuant' sounds which the patient can prolong and therefore experience adequate tactile feedback (for example: down, beam, doom, dine, barn). The patient is encouraged to imagine voice being made at the tip of the tongue (/d/ and /n/) and between the lips (/b/ and /m/), and to feel the vibration at the point of phonetic placement.

Stage II. The basic posture and approach are maintained, but the task is extended. Phrases are now practised on a sung tone, each phrase containing only voiced sounds. Again the emphasis is on careful attention to tactile feedback, both in the facial skeleton and at the point of articulation. These consonant sounds should be prolonged to facilitate clear feedback.

moonbeam	nine men
down and down	one by one
no more room	down the lane
leaning down	ring round the moon

Nicholls (1973) found that holding pitch relatively constant in voice work reduced the complexity of vocal production, 'thus permitting perceptual awareness of the postures that produce optimal pitch and quality'. This has been described as 'chanting' by both Nicholls (1973) and Boone (1977).

Stage III. Progress should now be made from a sung tone to a spoken tone, at a fairly quiet conversational level. At this point, it is even more important to concentrate on the voiced 'continuant' sounds.

Stage IV. At this stage, provided that the 'feel' for resonance is well established, voiceless sounds can be introduced:

dream time	moon shine	love song
time to go home		one more time
climbing down		sing me a tune

Stage V. There is no strict hierarchy to be observed, but at some point the variable of pitch change needs to be introduced. Intonation patterns are the first stage in this development:

Where've you been?	Who's that man?
I'm rather bored.	When are they coming?
Wait a minute.	Where are you going?

Pitch variations can also be practised on short three-note or four-note scales (for example on 'down', 'boom')

Stage VI. While still using material carefully controlled for 'resonant' sounds, longer sentences are introduced:

How lovely to lie in the warm sun.
Nearly time to go home now.
Feeling the warm sunshine on my back.
Wandering down the lonely lane.
We shall soon see them again.
Lying down on the soft sand.

By now, the hands are held at the side of the face, as if to project the voice. Emphasis continues to be placed on the voiced sounds, but the speaker also concentrates on the movements of articulation, in a light, precise way.

Stage VII. Still concentrating on light articulation and resonant sounds, work begins on more advanced material. It is important to avoid a hard attack on initial vowel sounds, encouraging a gentle, slightly aspirate initiation of phonation.

Obviously practice material must be chosen with the patient's interests in mind, but the following are two examples of suitable passages:

Rumbling in the chimneys,
Rattling at the doors,
Round the roofs and round the roads,
The rude wind roars.

Raging through the darkness,
Raving through the trees,
Then racing off again,
Across the great grey seas.

They were not all women, for there was one quiet little man in their midst, who, when not eating cake or drinking wine, was sucking the bone handle of a woman's umbrella, which he carried with him everywhere, indoors and out. He was in the custody of the largest and grimmest of ladies, whom the others called Aunt Martha.

From *The Hole in the Wall*
by Arthur Morrison
(The Folio Press, 1980)

Stage VIII. In this final stage, the feeling of resonance is developed in spontaneous speech, 'anchoring' the voice on sounds such as /m/ /n/ /w/ /r/ /l/. The hands can be used to project voice if there is a need to increase audibility. This is the stage at which work on intonation, pause and emphasis can be introduced, which will be discussed in a later section.

Filter (1980) describes a rather similar approach in which proprioceptive–tactile–kinaesthetic feedback is used in voice therapy. Emphasis is placed on the monitoring of tension, muscle tone, effort, pressure and movement, but this is extended from the laryngeal and pharyngeal focus to the thoracic and abdominal areas.

Nicholls (1973) commented that some of the most effective therapy was achieved in conjunction with resonance dynamics.

Modification of Intensity and Pitch

The question of reducing intensity levels to a more acceptable level has already been discussed in the section on eliminating unnecessary tension. Suffice to say here that the patient needs to monitor his intensity level as carefully as possible, seeing the use of a quiet voice as a sensible way of conserving vocal energy. The practice is particularly important if the patient has an essentially extrovert personality, with a tendency to use an unnecessarily loud voice. Teachers, and others whose occupations require the use of voice at high intensity levels, need to ensure that this kind of voice use does not become habitual (in situations where the level is no longer necessary or appropriate). The effect of using a quietly resonant voice can be quite dramatic, but may initially be somewhat alien to the speaker until he becomes used to the sound of a very different voice.

The role of improper pitch levels in the aetiology of dysphonia is less clearly understood. Considerable controversy exists regarding pitch, which has been summarised by Reed (1980). Cooper (1973) claimed that 90 per cent of some 2000 patients were using too low a pitch, and the remaining 10 per cent were using too high a pitch. He therefore regards low pitch as a major contributory factor in most dysphonias. It follows, therefore, that adjustment to the optimal pitch level is 'a vital part of voice therapy in almost all cases'. He further claimed that the success of his therapy was proof of the appropriateness of this approach. Many practising clinicians would challenge Cooper's findings, and would agree with Mueller (1975) that the major focus of treatment should concentrate on the elimination of vocal abuse by effortless phonation, rather than any adjustment of habitual pitch levels. He reported on a study of 25 females (mean age 37 years) with hoarseness as a distinctive feature of their voice use. The mean fundamental frequency of this sample group was 204 Hz, which was 'well within the norms for women of this age'. 'In our opinion,' Mueller went on to say, 'raising of pitch is physiologically contrary to the elimination of laryngeal hypertonicity, which is the very core of our therapeutic efforts.' Mueller considered that if there were inappropriate pitch levels, these would 'stabilise perceptually and spectrographically following correct adjustment of laryngeal tension'.

Mueller's conclusions are supported in an interesting study by Murry (1978) in which the speaking fundamental frequency was assessed in 80 male speakers: 20 patients had vocal fold paralysis, 20 had benign mass lesions, 20 had carcinoma of the larynx, and 20 had no laryngeal lesion. The subjects had a mean age of 52 years. Murry found that the speaking fundamental frequency for these organically based disorders is not lower than that found in normal voices. He concluded that 'clinical judgements of lower pitch in pathologic voices seemed to be caused by the confounding perception of voice quality rather than the perception of pitch alone'.

A more recent study by Hufnagle and Hufnagle (1984) lends still further support to the view that there is no difference between the speaking fundamental frequency of normal speakers and those with vocal cord pathologies. They commented that the entire concept of an optimum pitch becomes 'highly suspect' when dealing with vocal fold nodules, and came to the conclusion that manipulating pitch is not appropriate in the management of these cases.

If the hoarse speaker is found to be using a lower pitch, then it is probably a matter of effect rather than cause – a compensatory strategy to achieve a 'clearer' and more comfortable voice.

There may be evidence, however, that a speaker is not using his optimum pitch level, which can be described as an efficient pitch at which we produce voice of good quality and maximum intensity with the least expense of energy. There may be evidence of vocal fry (creaky voice) particularly occurring at the end of sentences on falling intonation patterns, or an habitual pitch level near the lower end of the frequency range. Fairbanks (1960) has suggested that the optimum pitch is approximately one-quarter from the bottom of the total scale, with the optimum pitch in females one or two notes lower. It is a pitch which must be compatible with the anatomy of the larynx, and a function of such variables as the length, mass and tension of the vocal folds.

Any attempt to modify pitch towards a more efficient level should rarely be a radical one. One of the most effective approaches to pitch adjustment (towards a slightly higher pitch) is to establish a 'light' pattern of articulation. This is a method described by Challoner (Chapter 13 of this volume) in helping transsexuals to achieve a higher pitch level. The idea of speech which is 'light and bright', with concentration on the voiceless, tongue tip plosive, for example, will be effective in raising pitch one or two semitones.

If pitch is too high, then this may well be a byproduct of tension. Careful work on developing optimum resonance, with its resulting reduction in laryngeal tension, will lead to an automatic lowering of pitch.

If the therapist is faced with a hoarse voice, then it will be impossible to determine optimum pitch. As Aronson (1980) comments, 'the location of optimum is impossible to find in someone who has a lesion of the vocal folds causing the latter to vibrate abnormally'.

Working on Articulation

The articulatory agility exercises recommended by some writers normally have no place in remedial voice work. There are cases, however, where improvement in articulatory precision can significantly increase the intelligibility of speech under adverse environmental conditions. This is particularly true where the speaker is coping with a background of noise or has to be heard over a considerable distance, for example in a lecture hall or theatre.

A more precise speech pattern may effectively supplement work on improving resonance. It must be stressed that in no way is one advocating an unnatural or exaggerated pattern of articulation: work is based on improving awareness, so that the speaker can feel the quick, light movements of tongue and lips, and aim for articulation that is distinct but not exaggerated. The adjustments to be made are very small – the analogy of bringing a photographic slide into focus is a useful one here – but may make a significant improvement in intelligibility.

Initially, therapist and client combine to devise phrases and sentences in which the movements of speech can be highlighted (for example: distinct articulation, intelligent participation, capital investment). Repeated practice drills are inappropriate – the purpose of the activity is to heighten awareness of light, precise but natural articulatory movement, not to strengthen or speed up the muscular activity involved.

Increased awareness of what is happening in speech can be achieved by reading a short passage aloud several times, with emphasis on a different articulatory posture at each attempt (for instance, initial emphasis on tongue tip sounds marked thus /ṭ/, back of tongue sounds /k̭/ or lip sounds /m̲/. The aim is to heighten total awareness of articulatory movement, and although the adjustments to be made are probably very slight, they make a significant improvement in intelligibility. It is the combination of improving resonance, together with a more precise pattern of articulation, that can facilitate improved audibility and help eliminate the need for effortful phonation.

At the same time, as we have indicated in a previous section, a clear resonant quality is usually incompatible with excessive tension and the concentration on light articulatory movements also tends to enhance the feeling of easy voice production.

Developing Expressive Use of Voice

To aim for optimum resonance and clear articulation is clearly not enough – the effective speaker must also use the voice expressively. This is unfortunately not just a simple matter of making the speaker aware of more appropriate and lively intonation patterns – voice is intimately tied to personality and the speaker who is shy and diffident will not find it easy to project a more dynamic image with expressive use of voice. The therapist can model the required intonation, and give the client some idea of the range of available vocal expressions and the importance of such prosodic features in enhancing meaning and sustaining interest. This area of voice production needs to be approached with sensitivity and imagination in choosing practice material.

Effective use of emphasis and pausing will further facilitate effective voice use. Again, the use of suitable material, in line with the client's interests, is very important. It is far better to work carefully on one or two short passages, than to lose concentration on a longer text. The therapist models each phrase or sentence, discussing her performance with the patient. Given clear guidelines, the client has a good notion of what is required, and more confidence to attempt the task.

Work on intonation, pausing and emphasis in spontaneous speech, needs even more ingenuity and imagination. Different emotional responses can be encouragd ('say something enthusiastic about the weather; make a sympathetic comment about someone's ill-health; congratulate someone about their promotion; be sarcastic about a colleague's late arrival').

The extent to which work is carried out on the prosodic features of speech will be determined by the end-product the client wishes to achieve. In the case of a young teacher, for example, it is important that he or she acquires a lively speech pattern which can attract and sustain the children's attention. Personality factors must be taken into account in setting goals which are acceptable to the client and in line with the demands of the situation. There are many clients where work on expressive use of voice is neither an appropriate nor necessary goal.

Breathing for Speech

The need to improve respiratory control for speech remains an area of considerable controversy in remediation work. Greene (1980) stated categorically that 'the paramount importance of correct breathing in speech and song cannot be over-estimated. Permanent improvement in the voice cannot possibly be achieved without improvement in respiration.' Aronson (1980) considers that respiration is anatomically and physiologically normal in the majority of patients. He comments that 'exactly how important attention to respiration is in voice therapy is a matter of disagreement, primarily because the extent to which faulty breathing is implicated in voice disorders is unknown'.

The rationale for the emphasis on breathing exercises as an essential and often initial part of the rehabilitation programme rests on the assumption that people misusing their voices do so because they have insufficient or a poorly controlled breath stream for phonation. In actual practice, however, relatively few patients show such problems. They may, however, when instructed by the therapist to 'take a breath', demonstrate all the worst features of clavicular breathing (raised shoulders and shallow inspiration) in their anxiety to comply with the therapist's request. Van Riper and Irwin (1958) state their point of view quite clearly when they observe 'very little breath is used in the production of tone compared to the amount of breath potentially available' but in spite of this they say 'the myth continues that if you have a voice problem you should work on respiration'. There are clearly two opposing viewpoints, but in the final analysis the indications for working on breathing for speech must depend on an assessment of the needs of the patient.

Undoubtedly there are patients who have respiratory problems associated with asthma and bronchitis, for example, or where inadequate habits of clavicular breathing developed following a unilateral recurrent laryngeal paralysis, which may have persisted despite compensatory activity of the non-affected cord. Even in cases such as these, any problems in breath control can largely be resolved by a reduction in tension and some often minimal changes in postural balance. On the whole, however, Boone (1977) says 'while an actor or singer may require respiratory training the typical voice patient does not need special training in breathing'. Brodnitz (1959) says that most people speak and sing without paying any attention to their breathing. He goes on to say 'this is as it should be and serves the purpose as long as the natural co-ordination is not disturbed and the voice is used for ordinary conversation'.

Despite views such as this, exercises for improving breath control have played a central role in remedial voice work. The emphasis on such an approach almost certainly stems from the speech and drama model, which the present author would claim is largely inappropriate in the majority of voice cases referred for therapy. Nonetheless, one must recognise that there will always be exceptions:

(1) Where the patient is demonstrating a markedly shallow, so-called 'clavicular' pattern of breathing and, as a result, is 'running out of breath' before completing his utterance. He clearly needs practice in achieving more efficient and sustained breath support for speech.
(2) There may be cases where the client consistently needs to place additional demands on his voice (such as acting, singing or public speaking), and we may then need to concentrate some attention on improving voluntary breath control in developing 'maximum *use* of vital capacity' (Greene, 1980).

(3) Some patients may have a past or current history of respiratory problems which has resulted in poor habitual patterns of breathing, sufficiently marked to affect speech.

Even in such cases, breathing *exercises* are not generally indicated; much can be achieved by aiming for a relaxed posture, so that there is the minimum of interference with respiratory movement, and an understanding on the client's part of what is actually required in terms of breath support. Concentration on breathing may actually distract the patient from the more central aims of listening to his voice and producing good phonation.

Boone (1977) has suggested that 'the ideal respiration for conversational phonation is the easy tidal breath cycle, with a slightly extended expiration to match the length of verbalisation'. He goes on to say 'the patient's easy conversational phonation, coupled with the natural breathing that goes with it, is probably the most productive respiration "training" for the typical voice patients'.

Repeated studies by the present author have shown that the majority of young to middle-aged adult speakers can produce one hundred syllables on a single breath (without any preceding practice period) and normal speakers can be expected to produce 50 syllables on a single breath. These tasks are, inevitably, carried out without the refinement of intonation, and with low intensity levels, but nevertheless demonstrate Van Riper and Irwin's point that the normal, untrained speaker does not need special training in breathing for speech.

What kind of approach is appropriate where inadequate patterns of breath control are felt to be a contributing factor in dysphonia? Most breathing exercises seem remarkably unrelated to the demands of speech. Too often, instructions to 'breathe in' result in raised shoulders and an inhibiting degree of tension. Willmore (unpublished communication, 1948) suggested that breathing should be picked up on the exhaling phase to avoid interfering with the natural rhythm of breathing. It is probably sufficient to ensure that the speaker is sitting or standing in a balanced and comfortable way. If asked to sigh heavily (as if very relieved or fed up) the patient will experience the unrestricted thoracic movement that goes with a relaxed physical state. The most realistic approach in improving breath control is to remove the postural constrictions or muscular tensions which may be incompatible with easy thoracic wall movements. To put labels on the type of breathing is unnecessary. As Brodnitz (1959) observed 'unfortunately many of these methods' (of breath control) 'defy physiologic fact, sometimes to the point of absurdity'. Aikin (1951) summed the matter up when he said 'the increased capacity of the lungs to be acquired by the singer must confine itself to the increased expansion of the lower ribs, and the proportionately increased contraction of the diaphragm, in imitation of ordinary physiological breathing, only on a larger scale'. The same holds true for an actor or public speaker, or indeed anyone who is making unusual demands on their speech, where increased breath control may need to be a focus of emphasis. A comprehensive study of normal respiration in speech and song has been given by Bunch (1982).

Considerable controversy exists (Reed, 1980) regarding poor breath control as a causative or contributory factor in voice disorders. As Reed pointed out, there is clearly a need for research here. The possibility exists, as Boone (1977) has pointed out, that disturbed patterns of respiration may be the effect of disrupted phonation rather than the cause. We have seen a parallel here in stuttering, where disturbed breathing patterns are the result of the abnormal valving behaviour of the vocal folds during the stuttering block. Breathing exercises designed to improve control for speech are as inappropriate here as they frequently are in vocal re-education. To suggest, however, that improvement in breath control is never required would be equally wrong – there are cases where poor breath support is clearly evident, creating an obvious imbalance between subglottal pressure and vocal fold tension which cannot sustain normal, easy phonation. One must ensure, however, that one interferes as little as possible with the normal, almost involuntary adjustments that are made in breathing for speech. Ideally the patient should be unaware of his breathing, leaving him free to concentrate on the far more important matter of an easy, relaxed approach to phonation.

Voice Therapy for Specific Laryngeal Conditions

In this section we shall be considering some specific approaches to conditions which arise directly from vocal misuse (such as vocal nodules and contact ulcers). There are other conditions (such as polyps) where the connection with vocal misuse is much less clear, and a question of some controversy. Finally, we shall be considering the abnormal/maladaptive compensatory behaviour which may arise not as a cause of dysphonia, but as a result of laryngeal dysfunction of some kind.

Vocal Nodules

We have already indicated that there is some difference of opinion regarding the prescription of voice rest. Total voice rest may not only be impractical, but is a psychologically traumatic experience. The best approach is undoubtedly the recommendation that voice is used at quiet intensity levels, and as sparingly as possible. Such an approach, combined with a very carefully supervised remedial voice programme, should lead to the remission of newly formed nodules. Where surgery is indicated prior to voice therapy, then it is equally important to initiate a voice rest regime post-surgically. The advice to whisper is contraindicated since this almost inevitably means the use of a forced whisper.

Aronson (1980) sums up the aims of therapy by stating that the patient 'should be taught to produce voice with less forceful stress or emphasis patterns and with easy onset of phonation rather than with a hard glottal attack'. He considers that vocal re-education is the therapy of choice and should be attempted before surgery is recommended. This is certainly an area where research is needed, since we have virtually no evidence of the efficacy of vocal therapy in the remission of vocal nodules at various stages in their development. Surgery is certainly the immediate answer to the problem, but treats the symptom and not the cause – at some stage the patient will need to learn how to use the voice in such a way as to prevent their recurrence. A remedial voice progamme has already been discussed in the previous section and will be appropriate in the case of vocal nodules, although modifications will have to be made if it is decided that the nodules are not to be removed surgically.

Contact Ulcers

The higher incidence of contact ulcers in the United States may, as Greene (1980) suggests, be a sociocultural phenomenon, in which the male cultivates a deeper voice to demonstrate his masculinity. This would suggest that attention to pitch level would be an appropriate point of departure in therapy, but if the voice is dysphonic it is impossible to determine either the patient's optimum or habitual pitch. It is generally agreed that surgical intervention is not indicated for all but the most severe cases. Boone (1977) has said that surgery may be necessary where there are large ulcers with surrounding granulations. He has emphasised that voice rest alone is only of temporary value, since vocal re-education will be needed.

Contact ulcers occur most commonly in males and rarely in trained singers and actors. Luchsinger and Arnold (1965) have described the process of 'mechanical traumatisation' and, like Aronson (1980) point to personality as a significant factor in their development. 'The evidence is clear,' says Aronson, 'that these patients are hard-driving, competitive, angry and aggressive.' He suggests that interpersonal problems and environment stress both play their part.

In therapy, particular attention is drawn to the need to correct the hard-attack which is regarded as a causative factor in contact ulcer. Von Leden and Moore (1961) described the violent clashing action of the arytenoids during phonation, viewed in high-speed cinephotography. Boone (1977) recommends both the chewing method and what he describes as the yawn–sign approach to counteract the problem of glottal attack.

He regards this second technique as an 'excellent facilitator of optimum voice' in all cases of vocal abuse. The method is based on a yawn, followed by a gentle exhalation with 'light phonation'. Boone claims that in doing this many patients experience easy phonation for the first time.

Aronson (1980) says that the quantity and intensity of voice use has to be reduced by approximately 50 per cent for one month, and that smoking and drinking must also be abandoned for a similar period. Throat clearing and coughing must also be reduced as far as possible. He also recommends the use of an easy or aspirate vocal attack on vowels, and the need to feel the difference between hard and soft glottal attack. A case study by Bloch and Gould (1974) reports on the successful elimination of contact granuloma with a programme of psychological support and vocal therapy.

Laryngeal Trauma

Under this broad and rather arbitrary heading, we will be considering the voice therapist's role in cases where vocal abuse and misuse are not the primary causes of the dysphonic condition. These conditions can include the following:

(1) External trauma to the laryngeal structure such as compression, fractures and penetrating wounds, with resulting oedema, haematoma, dislocations and lacerations, and even laryngeal paralysis.
(2) Laryngeal intubation, which can lead to mucosal ulceration and the formation of granular tissue. There may also be dislocation of the arytenoid cartilages.
(3) Post-surgical problems may occur where the cords have been stripped (in cases of severe hypertrophic laryngitis), or where polyps or other benign lesions have been removed. Stoicheff (Chapter 15 of this volume) has described the effects of radiotherapy on laryngeal tissues.

Even where misuse has not previously been present, there is a very real risk that abnormal compensatory behaviour will develop and become habitual as the patient tries to improve on his dysphonic voice production. This is a very natural reaction, and it is advisable that any patient with an impaired laryngeal mechanism should be referred for speech therapy as soon as healing has taken place.

The aim of therapy is twofold – in the first place to try and prevent maladaptive behaviour as the patient tries to come to terms with the damaged larynx; secondly, to make optimum use of the available mechanism. Normal phonation may be impossible – the therapist must work with the patient to achieve the best possible results. This may mean settling for a husky or breathy voice rather than a hoarse one – as the patient is encouraged to use less effort. The use of clear articulation will help compensate for weak phonation. A balance has to be achieved between conserving voice and preventing vocal fatigue and further laryngeal damage, and the need to make voice audible. Where the patient has to make himself audible across space or above noise, then amplification may be needed. As far as possible, the remedial voice programme should be followed. There may need to be more emphasis on breath control, more attention to clear articulation and the prosodic features of pause and emphasis. The programme will have to be adapted to the specific needs of each patient. An essentially experimental approach will need to be adopted, in which patient and therapist together try out different approaches to voice production – manipulating variables such as pitch, intensity, breath control and head-neck posture. It is essential that the therapist has an exact knowledge of the state of the vocal folds, both in terms of appearance and function.

Ventricular Phonation

There are probably two reasons why ventricular phonation develops, with the false cords adducting over the true cords lying below: in the first place, it may, as Aronson says, be the extreme end stage of hyperkinetic dysphonia. If this has continued over time, then there may be hypertrophy of the ventricular folds. Secondly, they may show compensatory activity where there is a failure of normal vocal fold adduction. This can occur, for example, where there is unilateral paralysis of the vocal cords.

Ventricular voice is characteristically low in pitch, because of the larger vibrating mass of the false cords. Complete adduction along the entire length of the ventricular folds is difficult to achieve, and so there is air waste. Pitch variation is limited, and the resulting voice is monotonous, hoarse and aperiodic. If there is hypertrophy of the folds, then the voice will be even more hoarse.

Where excessive effort is involved, then the aim will be to achieve a more relaxed phonation, although this approach alone will be unlikely to achieve normal voice. There are a number of techniques which have been reported to be successful in achieving normal vocal fold phonation. Boone (1977) and others have reported on the use of reverse or inhalation phonation. The patient is instructed to phonate on the inspiratory phase of respiration. Once this has been established, he phonates on both the inspiratiom – expiration cycle. The rather high-pitched phonation produced is not consistent with ventricular voice. Van Riper and Irwin (1958) have recommended the use of glottal fry to initiate voice. They say that there is abnormal raising of the larynx in the production of ventricular voice, and suggest that a lowering of the thyroid cartilage should be achieved.

A diplophonic voice may occur in cases where true and false vocal cord vibration occur concurrently. In such cases, the procedures described above may be used to try and eliminate the 'double' vibration. The use of a humming glide has also been successful: the patient is asked to produce a hum on the highest possible note in his repertoire (at a pitch incompatible with ventricular phonation), and is then asked to produce a phonatory glide down the scale until he reaches his optimum pitch. Once this has been carried out successfully, on a number of occasions, he is instructed to sustain the note at the end of the glide, repeating words (down–down–down, dandelion) or phrases (more and more) on a sung tone at this pitch.

It has been suggested that the use of ventricular voice might be encouraged as a compensatory mechanism in cases of permanent laryngeal damage. Unfortunately the resulting voice will tire easily and the hoarse, low-pitch and monotonous quality may not be acceptable to the patient.

Obviously, the final result – and the treatment methods employed – will depend on the patency or otherwise of the true vocal folds as a vibrating mechanism. Clinical practice suggests that the elimination of ventricular phonation is by no means easy.

Bowing of the Vocal Folds

The oval bowing of the vocal folds on phonation reflects a weakness of the thyroarytenoid muscle. The condition has been described as myasthenia laryngis or hyperkinetic phonasthenia. As the second term implies, the vocal weakness is caused by vocal strain, resulting in fatigue and weakness of the internal tensor of the vocal folds. The voice is characterised by air waste and is therefore weak and husky, lacking depth of resonance. Luchsinger and Arnold (1965) claim that the condition results from 'continuous over-exertion, particularly when tense phonation with hard attacks and poor respiratory support are at fault'.

A regime of quiet voice use, with a reduction in the amount of talking, will be needed in the initial stages of treatment. A programme of remedial voice work will follow, to encourage effortless phonation and prevent a recurrence of the condition.

Bowing may be seen as part of the ageing process, as the laryngeal muscles tend to atrophy. This is one of the several changes which result in the vocal changes associated with senescence.

The Voice of Senescence

Well-recognised changes take place in the voice during the normal process of ageing. The age at which these changes occur, and the extent to which the voice changes, will vary considerably from one person to another. The singing voice will be affected before the speaking voice, with a reduction in both power and range. In general, both the pitch range and the intensity of the voice will be reduced, and phonation may be characterised by what has been described as a senile tremulo. Luchsinger and Arnold (1965) claim that this particular feature is caused by an irregular pattern of expiration during phonation. The increased weakness of the voice is associated to some extent with a reduction in the older speaker's vital capacity, but there are a number of changes in the larynx itself which combine to produce the voice of senescence. Luchsinger and Arnold list the following factors: gradually increasing ossification of the laryngeal cartilages; a loss of elasticity in the vocal ligaments and arthritic changes in the joints; diminishing muscle tone; arteriosclerotic changes in the blood vessels supplying the larynx; reduced endocrine function and a tendency to dehydration of laryngeal tissues. It is probaby the gradual atrophic changes in the laryngeal muscles which give rise to an increase in fundamental frequency of the male speaking voice which has been noted in a number of research studies (Mysak, 1959; Hollien and Shipp, 1972; Honjo and Isshiki, 1979). Interestingly this phenomenon does not appear to occur in women. Atrophy of the muscles may also lead to bowing of the folds on adduction.

Deterioration in the intensity and quality of voice can be compounded by respiratory problems associated with bronchitis, to which the elderly seem particularly prone.

The ageing speaker may complain that talking is tiring. This may result from trying to make oneself heard to a peer group who are showing signs of increasing presbycusis. If an elderly person has to spend a good deal of time talking to a deaf friend or relative, then it is well worth discussing the possibility of a hearing aid for them (although such a prescription is not always acceptable to the elderly deaf). Increasing loss of auditory feedback may account for the sometimes inappropriately loud voice used by some old people.

It is probably rather rare for the elderly to complain about, or even be aware of, the changes taking place in their voice, unless these are causing marked communication problems. It is even less likely that they would welcome the idea of speech therapy. It would certainly not be realistic to embark on a remedial voice programme unless the speaker was genuinely concerned about his/her voice and had specifically requested help. The emphasis should be on voice conservation, using it quietly whenever possible, and complementing any weakness by speaking as clearly as possible (particularly when talking to the deaf). Attention to phrasing may help to ensure that the reduced breath support available is used more efficiently. Unnecessary effort should be discouraged, since hyperfunctional voice use can lead to only further fatigue.

The process of voice change is an inevitable one with increasing age, but to some extent compensatory strategies may be used to improve the quality of phonation if the elderly person is seriously interested in resisting the effects of ageing on the efficiency and effectiveness of their voice use.

Voice Therapy as an Effective Learning Situation

Over the past few years there has been a 'quiet revolution' in the way many therapists approach their patients, in all areas of communication disorder. We have moved increasingly from a medical model in which the patient is a passive recipient in the therapy we think best for him. This changing philosophy is mirrored in many other areas of 'treatment' in which the importance of the patient as an informed participant is being increasingly recognised, even though the process may not always be a comfortable one for the therapist, physician and surgeon. The following comment by Thruman (1973) sums up the current situation regarding our approach to the dysphonic patient:

> A brief statement of objectives at the beginning and a summary at the end of a session helps keep the client informed about what he is doing and why. If the clinician cannot provide such statements, he should examine and clarify in his mind his concept of the problem and his plan for correction. Each session, each procedure must have a specific purpose that contributes to the voice change desired. It is the client's right to understand, insofar as he can, what those purposes are and what progress is being made.

Thurman begs the question, how far can we judge what the patient is capable of understanding? Because he lacks a knowledge of our particular professional jargon, we must not underestimate his ability to understand a jargon-free explanation. The need for the therapist to explain often has the unexpected and beneficial effect of clarifying her own ideas, and as a result the therapy situation may become as much a learning situation for the therapist as for the patient.

Some of these same philosophies have been underlined and elaborated in Heinberg's (1973) systems approach to vocal behaviour modification. Heinberg has emphasised the need for what he terms 'cognitive competence' in vocal rehabilitation. He says that there must be a very clear specification of the product to be achieved. 'Once that has been accomplished,' he continues, 'alternative processes are considered for achieving that product, and each alternative is evaluated in terms of its relative productivity.' The patient must know the rules of each learning situation and the criterion of each learning system. Heinberg believes that the patient has to learn that his goal is to acquire a 'repertoire' of vocal strategies to meet the demands of different situations.

The goals must be clarified for the patient by the use of a clear rationale and, if necessary, the goal must be 'modelled' by the therapist. Furthermore, precise feedback must be provided on the patient's performance, each attempt being measured against the target voice. A precise numerical rating will help facilitate the learning process, since we are building up the patient's confidence in his auditory monitoring skills as we teach him how to listen and make judgements. It is essential that he learns to monitor his vocal performance reliably, otherwise self-supervised practice can do more harm than good. Furthermore, we are dealing with very fine differences which are not obvious to the patient until his ear has been trained to listen. The therapist's role is to 'shape' voice production towards the target goal as she reinforces the patient's more successful attempts.

Drudge and Philips (1976) give an interesting and detailed account of voice therapy in which 'the behaviour is gradually shaped using procedures such as ear-training, negative practice and feedback until carry-over into spontaneous speech in life situations is achieved'. While the therapist provided feedback in the initial stages of each therapy situation, the client was given increasing responsibility for the evaluation of his own responses. They concluded that 'appropriate self-evaluations, that is, internalised knowledge of the desired behaviour, appeared vital to the consistent accomplishment of that behaviour'. They went on to say, 'when correct self-evaluations began to occur with consistency, the responses were observed to become consistently correct'.

The approach described by Drudge and Philips is in marked contrast to the areas of emphasis of more traditional approaches, and sums up the current trend towards a more 'behaviour orientated' approach in voice therapy.

Each session should be an optimum learning experience for the patient, a process of self-discovery, with the satisfaction of experiencing and correctly evaluating his own successful achievements. In order that he can experiment with his voice, it is clearly essential to create a comfortable and permissive atmosphere. He needs to develop confidence in his ability to bring about change, and to recognise those changes when they occur.

As therapy progresses, the patient becomes increasingly responsible for his own management – drawing up a list of realistic situations in which he can practise his new voice skills, noting the situations in which he is at risk of misusing his voice, being increasingly aware of aspects of his lifestyle which create conflict and tension and being prepared to explore ways of bringing about change.

Prophylaxis

It is interesting that so little has been written on the prevention of voice disorders, particularly when so many professional voice users are at risk of misusing their voices. With the exception of the majority of actors and classical singers, very few speakers who depend on their voice professionally have received any instruction in proper voice use or conservation. This means that many lecturers, preachers and teachers have little idea of the demands they are making on their voices, and it is largely a matter of chance whether they use their voice effectively or not. Well-trained singers and actors should not experience voice problems, unless they continue singing or speaking when suffering from laryngitis. Greene (1980) reported that she had found vocal nodules only in untrained singers.

There are, undoubtedly, some singers battling against techniques learned through poor teaching methods. It is important to find out what these teaching methods were, and whether the patients' ideas about good voice production are compatible with easy phonation.

It would seem important to ensure that all those whose

occupations may make excessive demands on voice use should have guidance during their training in using their voices effectively, with the minimum of unnecessary tension. An understanding of the vocal mechanism, and of how to use it efficiently, with an appreciation of the possible effects of vocal misuse and abuse, could go a long way to preventing disorders of voice. This would seem a cost-effective process in the long term.

Conclusion

A remedial voice programme has been described, appropriate to the needs of those who show evidence of hyperfunctional voice use. The weighting given to any one part of that programme will depend on a careful assessment of all parameters of voice use. It will also depend on the demands which the patient has to make on his voice. However, auditory training, the elimination of excessive tension and the development of effortless, resonant phonation would seem to be the essential core of all vocal remediation work. The importance given to other aspects of the programme will be determined largely by the occupational needs of the patient. If the voice is dysphonic due to tissue changes in the larynx then work on developing resonance, intonation and pitch flexibility will obviously be impossible, and indeed positively contraindicated in most cases.

It has been suggested that traditional approaches to voice therapy, still very much in current use, are based on a inappropriate model derived from singing and drama teaching. Not only are some of the techniques practised irrelevant to patient's needs, but they actually serve to distract from the real cause of the problem – the hypertonicity involved in voice use.

In other chapters very specific approaches and techniques for a number of dysphonic conditions will be described. Some of the principles outlined in the present chapter may be appropriate, particularly where the patient has developed a maladaptive response to some form of functional inadequacy. Laryngeal tension, with excessive and unnecessary vocal effort, is a very common symptom in many cases of voice disorder. Nearly all dysphonic patients need to develop the ability to monitor their voices during vocal re-education, and the acquisition of vocal habits which facilitate the easiest and most effective form of voice production.

Some of the core elements described in the preceding pages will be found to be appropriate in many types of voice disorder.

References

Aikin, W.A. *The Voice — An Introduction to Practical Phonology* (Longmans, Green, London, 1951)

Alexander, F. M. *The Use of Self* (Methuen, London, 1932)

Aronson, A.E. *Clinical Voice Disorders: An Interdisciplinary Approach* (Thieme-Stratton, New York, 1980)

Barlow, W. 'Postural Homeostasis', *Annals of Physical Medicine*, 1, 3 (1952)

Bloch, C. S and Gould, W. J. 'Vocal Therapy in Lieu of Surgery for Contact Granuloma: A Case Report', *Journal of Speech and Hearing Disorders*, 39, 4 (1974)

Boone, D. R. *The Voice and Voice Therapy* (Prentice Hall, Englewood Cliffs, New Jersey, 1977)

Brodnitz, F. S. *Vocal Rehabilitation*, 4th edn (American Academy of Ophthalmology and Otolaryngology, Rochester, Minnesota, 1959)

Bunch, M. A. *Dynamics of the Singing Voice* (Springer-Verlag, New York, 1982)

Cooper, M. *Modern Techniques of Vocal Rehabilitation* (Charles C. Thomas, Springfield, Illinois, 1973)

Drudge, M. K. M. and Phillips, B. J. 'Shaping Behaviour in Voice Therapy', *Journal of Speech and Hearing Disorders*, 41, 3 (1976)

Dunlap, K. 'The Technique of Negative Practice', *American Journal of Psychology*, 55, 270 (1932)

Filter, M. D. 'Proprioceptive-tactile-kinaesthetic Approach to Voice Disorders', *Proceedings of the 18th Congress of the International Association of Logopaedics and Phoniatrics* (Washington, 1980)

Fishman, B. V. McGlone, R. E. and Shipp, T. 'The Effect of Certain Drugs on Phonation', *Journal of Speech and Hearing Research* 14, 2 (1971)

Fairbanks, G. *Voice and Articulation Handbook* (Harper, New York, 1960)

Froeschels, E. 'Hyperfunction and Hypofunction — Hygiene of the Voice', *Archives of Otolaryngology* 38 (1943)

Gould, W. J. 'Effect of Respiratory and Postural Mechanism upon Action of the Vocal Cords', *Folia Phoniatrica (Basel)*, 23 (1971)

Greene, M. C. L. *The Voice and its Disorders* (Pitman Medical, Tunbridge Wells, 1980)

Heinberg, P. 'A Systems Approach to Vocal Behaviour Modification, in Cooper, M. (ed.) *Modern Techniques of Vocal Rehabilitation* (Charles. C. Thomas, Springfield, Illinois, 1973)

Hollien, H. and Shipp, T. 'Speaking Fundamental Frequency and Chronologic Age in Males', *Journal of Speech and Hearing Research*, 15 (1972)

Honjo, I. and Isshiki, N. *Laryngoscopic and Vocal Characteristics of Aged Persons* (Kansai Medical University, Osaka, Japan, 1979)

Hufnagle, J. and Hufnagle, K. 'An Investigation of the Relationship Between Speaking Fundamental Frequency and Vocal Quality Improvement', *Journal of Communication Disorders* 17 (1984)

Jackson, C. and Jackson, C. L. *Diseases of the Nose, Throat and Ear* (Saunders, London, 1945)

Jacobsen, E. *Progressive Relaxation* (University of Chicago Press, Chicago, 1929)

Laver, J. D., Wirz, S. L., MacKenzie, J. and Miller, S. (1981) 'A Perceptual

Protocol for the Analysis of Vocal Profiles', *University of Edinburgh Work in Progress. Linguistics Department*, vol. 14 (University of Edinburgh, Edinburgh, 1981)

Luchsinger, R. and Arnold, G. E. *Voice, Speech and Language* (Constable, London, 1965)

Moore, G. P. 'Voice Disorders Organically Based', in Trevis, L. E. (ed.) *Handbook of Speech Pathology and Audiology* (Appleton-Century-Crofts, New York, 1971)

Mueller, P. B. 'Comment on Spectographic Analysis of Fundamental Frequency and Hoarseness Before and After Vocal Rehabilitation', *Journal of Speech and Hearing Disorders*, 40, 2 (1975)

Murphy, A. T. *Functional Voice Disorders* (Prentice Hall, Englewood Cliffs, New Jersey, 1964)

Murry, T. 'Speaking Fundamental Frequency Characteristics Associated with Voice Pathologies', *Journal of Speech and Hearing Disorders* 43, 3 (1978)

Mysak, E. 'Pitch and Duration Characteristics of Older Males', *Journal of Speech and Hearing Research* 2, 1 (1959)

Nicholls, A. C. 'Motivations and Manipulations in Voice Therapy', in Cooper, M. (ed.) *Modern Techniques in Vocal Rehabilitation* (Charles C. Thomas, Springfield, Illinois, 1973)

Piaget, J. *Play, Dreams and Imitation in Childhood* (Heinemann, London, 1952)

Prosek, A., Montgomery, A. A., Walden, B. E. Schwartz, D. M. EMG 'Biofeedback in the Treatment of Hyperfunctional Voice Disorders', *Journal of Speech and Hearing Disorders* 43, 3 (1978)

Reed, C. G. 'Voice Therapy: 'A Need for Research', *Journal of Speech and Hearing Disorders* 45, 2 (1980)

Rogers, C. *Client-centred Therapy* (Constable, London, 1981)

Thurman, W. L. 'Restructuring Voice Concepts and Production', in Cooper, M. (ed.) *Modern Techniques in Vocal Rehabilitation* (Charles C. Thomas, Springfield, Illinois, 1973)

Van Riper, C. and Irwin, J. V. *Voice and Articulation* (Prentice Hall, Englewood Cliffs, New Jersey, 1958)

Van Thal, J. H. 'Dysphonia', *Speech Pathology and Therapy*, 4, 1 (1961)

Von Leden, N. and Moore, P. 'The Mechanics of the Cricoarytenoid Joint', *Archives of Otolaryngology* 73, 541 (1961)

Willmore, L. 'The Role of Speech Therapy in Voice Cases', *Journal of Laryngology* 73 (1959)

Wyatt, G. L. 'The Chewing Method and the Treatment of the Speaking Voice', in Cooper, M. and Cooper, M. H. (eds) *Approaches to Vocal Rehabilitation* (Charles C. Thomas, Springfield, Illinois, 1977)

Zaliouk, A. 'The Tactile Approach to Voice Placement', *Folia Phoniatrica (Basel)*, 15, 147 (1963)

11 PSYCHOGENIC VOICE DISORDER: A MULTIFACTORIAL PROBLEM

Margaret Freeman

Introduction

There are as many different patterns of causality as there are patients having voice disorders (Murphy, 1964, p. 2)

Traditionally, it has been widely accepted that many voice disorders are caused by psychological or emotional problems. As one looks closely at definitions of psychogenesis, however, it becomes apparent that a variety of philosophies of cause have been considered. Discussions of psychogenic voice disorder includes references to psychiatric states (Aronson, 1980; Greene, 1980), reactions to life stress (Brodnitz, 1981) and concepts of the voice as an expression of personality or soul (Brodnitz, 1981; Monday, 1983). An exploration of some of these philosophical views will form one of the themes of this chapter.

Most interpretations of psychogenic aetiology have focused on two main issues. First, there is the question of how to explain a voice disorder which is not ostensibly caused by disease or structural abnormality. Secondly, there is the fact that many patients do indeed have psychosocial difficulties, tension, anxiety or similar problems which cause them to be unable to respond to speech therapy. These two elements have typically been considered as cause and effect; some known or unknown event or unconscious motivation has interfered with 'normal volitional control over phonation' (Aronson, 1980, p. 131). If we accept this, then it seems that we could consider voice therapy to be primarily a form of psychotherapy. The clinician's first goal, then, is to help the patient to identify and work through the underlying problem, rather than concentrate therapy on the mechanisms of the voice disorder; the voice disorder is secondary to this.

A number of clinicians have argued that if we place all our emphasis on the voice disorder as a symbolic problem, we are faced with attempting to define 'an unanalyzable mechanism of control over the vocal apparatus' (Weaver, 1924; cited by Moore,

1977). This has led to what Brodnitz (1965) described as a swing of the pendulum away from voice and emotion and towards the scientific description of voice as a behaviour. The result was an increase in detailed descriptions of vocal behaviour and more attention to therapeutic techniques (Boone, 1983a; Moore, 1977; Perkins, 1983).

In theory, the combination of psychological insights and increased knowledge of vocal function should provide us with the basic tools for the appraisal and management of patients with voice disorders. In practice, clinicians can be aware that there are signs and symptoms both in the patient's history and in their overall behaviour which suggest that somehow, stress and tension or some other similar problem are part of the disorder. As current theory tends to emphasise either a psychotherapeutic approach or symptom-based therapy, the clinician can still feel unsure of which aspect to treat, or even whether this patient needs speech therapy.

Part of the problem is that theories of aetiology still tend to suggest that a voice disorder which is not specifically organic in origin must be caused by 'psychological' factors. This is not a tendency which is exclusive to speech pathology; Hay (1981) has noted that it used to be concluded in most medical diagnoses that if a patient's symptoms were not shown to be related to disease, 'they were attributed to personal failure or neurotic behaviour' (p. 9). In speech pathology, it is not long ago that a number of communication disorders, including dysfluency and some speech disorders were classified as predominantly psychogenic. Detailed study of the specific characteristics of these problems has confirmed that although the speech pathologist must be aware of psychological variables, there are other more salient processes to be considered (Baker, 1977; Bloch and Goodstein, 1971).

It seems probable that further clinical research may differentiate specific types of vocal dysfunction, in the same way that particular types of spastic dysphonia have been identified (see Stoicheff, Chapter 9 of this volume). Developments in the diagnosis and management of spastic dysphonia in particular have called into question the way in which diagnostic labels of psychogenesis can be applied. Izdebski and Dedo (1981) have pointed out that the characteristic social withdrawal, facial tics and rather erratic vocal control which were previously considered to be signs of a personality disorder, may actually be *a consequence* of the problem, rather than the cause.

With the group that can be loosely described as 'functional voice disorders', the problem of discriminating between subgroups requires identification of subtle differences. Rammage, Nichol and Morrison (1983) state that:

> Diagnostic labels such as ventricular band dysphonia, bowed cords, spastic dysphonia, functional aphonia or dysphonia, hysterical aphonia, conversion reaction dysphonia or aphonia are used commonly to describe voice disorders, but by their natures are often redundant and contradictory and need specification of characteristic symptoms and signs (p. 317).

It may be that the differences between types of functional voice disorder can best be identified by attention to the physiological and mechanical detail. Already, current research has identified a range of subtle but significant changes in respiratory patterns (Gordon, Morton and Simpson, 1978; Greene, 1983), tension in skeletal muscle (Zipursky *et al.*, 1983) and in the musculature of the vocal tract (Berry *et al.*, 1982; Hirano, 1980). Whether these factors are the result of chronic or acute life stress (Aronson, 1980; Brodnitz, 1981; MacCurtain, 1983) or a discrete organic lesion (Bridger and Epstein, 1983; Ward, Hanson and Berci, 1981) is not yet clear (Zipursky *et al.*, 1983).

Recently, the suggestion that functional voice disorders may be best considered as multifactorial in origin has come from two separate sources. Kitzing (1983) describes the need to look at voice disorders at a series of levels. Rammage, Nichol and Morrison (1983) consider that many patients present with multiple aetiologies, in which physiological, organic, psychosocial and behavioural variables combine to cause the patient's voice disorder. As Murphy (1964) suggested, the probability is that each individual patient has a unique pattern of causality. The clinician's work is to combine understanding of the processes of phonation with insights into the processes of symptom development.

Multifactorial Aetiology

The recent increase in research into stress and stress-related diseases has led many workers in psychosomatics and behavioural medicine to believe that most illness is the result of a combination of circumstances (Bakal, 1980; Lipowski, 1977). Although it is known that a sudden change in life circumstances can be linked with the development of minor or more chronically disabling physical or emotional disturbances (Holmes and Rahe, 1967; Holmes and Masuda, 1974), many people cope with the stress of divorce, the death of spouse or a sudden change in employment without damaging effects. Similarly, although a demanding lifestyle, smoking, alcohol and diet all increase the risk to health, some people who are apparently at high risk of illness appear to be able to stay well (Winefield, 1981).

The conclusion of most researchers is that a certain level of stress is acceptable and perhaps even desirable (Ursin and Murison, 1983). The type of stressor, the predictability of the stress and its duration, the person's attitude, coping resources and the level of support available in other areas of life all seem to be important variables (Cooper, 1981). If the person can maintain a sense of equilibrium in life, vulnerability to physical and psychological distress is reduced. Wadsworth and Ingham (1981, p. 353) suggest that there are four general categories of factors which can increase or decrease the chances of stress-related illness:

(1) External physical agents such as infectious agents, toxic substances and nutrition;
(2) Internal physical agents, such as genetic constitution, physical fitness and immunity;
(3) Psychological factors; the individual's personal resources; and capacity for coping with threat — this interacts closely with
(4) External socioeconomic factors. Social resources include support from close confidants (see Brown, 1976) which probably affords some protection against the adverse effects of threat.

Reactions to Stress

Stress reactions can be physiological, psychological or both (Dobson, 1982; Griffiths, 1981). A sudden, novel threat tends to bring into play some of the 'flight or fight' mechanisms related to autonomic nervous system arousal (Cannon, 1932). If the individual can anticipate the threat and has developed strategies for coping with such situations, the physiological effects can be quite markedly reduced. In some cases, psychological defences such as denial, detachment or rationalisation may be employed; if these are helpful and effective, the person may use these strategies in other circumstances, to good effect (Lazarus, 1976). If the coping strategy is inadequate for, or inappropriate to the situation, and other support is unavailable, or if the situation itself cannot be changed, then the chances are that depression and anxiety or a sense of helplessness can result (Seligman, 1975).

The awareness of inability to cope or development of physical or emotional symptoms may not be a sudden effect. Hay (1981) suggests that there is an analogy with a complex machine; if it gets out of tune and nothing effective is done about it, the eventual result is a breakdown of some sort. Because the response is *adaptive*, or a coping strategy, however, it may be initially helpful in coping with stress; it is the constant effect of strain which takes its physical toll.

Stress and Psychophysiology

Some of the ways in which the body reacts under conditions of sudden threat (Cannon, 1932) and prolonged stress (Selye, 1950) have been recognised for some considerable time. Over the past few years, the detailed study of psychophysiological reactions to various types of stress have revealed that the type of response depends on the person's perception of the stimulus. Physiological responses, such as heart rate, changes in blood glucose levels and muscle tension have been shown to differ according to the demands of the situation, the complexity of the task and the person's previous experience of this and similar tasks (Dobson, 1982). Lazarus (1976) has shown that when people can develop adaptive strategies for coping with emotionally disturbing events, physiological responses tend to be less extreme.

It seems probable that few people become ill after one sudden event or circumstance; more probably, we take 'small physiological steps in the direction of full-blown illness' (Graham, 1971; see also Sheldon, 1970). Wadsworth and Ingham (1981) underline this when they ask at what stage a person becomes ill; is it when they attend the doctor, or at some stage previously, when early signs and symptoms may have been ignored or are not yet apparent? This leads on to yet another highly relevant question, why do people go to the doctor?

Why People Go to the Doctor

Most people have a range of symptoms in any given period, but comparatively few of these will cause them to consult the doctor

(Winefield, 1981). In general, it seems that an unfamiliar symptom or one that is having disruptive effects on the individual's way of life may be more likely to lead to a consultation (Wadsworth and Ingham, 1981). Mechanic (1966) suggests that a third reason for consultation is a change in circumstances; at a period of change or stress, the person may become aware of a symptom which has previously been accepted as familiar. In a sense, then, a change in circumstances may be the reason why the person notices, rather than develops the symptom.

There is some indication that for some people, going to the doctor or being ill may be a way of coping with stress. Parsons (1951) called this adopting the 'sick role'; the person requests the doctor's permission to be exempted from normal duties because he or she feels unable to cope. Mechanic (1966) suggested that this was part of 'illness behaviour'; the feeling of being unfit can be quite valid, particularly if the individual is tense and anxious. For some people, being seen as unwell and therefore unable to work may be preferable to being considered incompetent (Shuval, Antonovsky and Davies, 1973). There is some indication that social factors can be involved here; family patterns of 'illness-behaviour training' may influence how people use health care facilities (Winefield, 1981). This can also work in reverse; some people who would be readily diagnosed as physically ill may avoid seeing the doctor for fear of being placed in the sick (dependent) role, of admitting to themselves or to others that they are ill, or for economic reasons (Mechanic, 1966).

Stress, Disease and Voice Disorder

The issues raised above seem to be relevant to the understanding of voice disorder for a number of reasons. First, it seems probable that voice disorder, like most illnesses, is caused by multiple, rather than single aetiological factors. Secondly, although a voice disorder may be a sign of organic disease, there is plenty of evidence to suggest that people tend to tolerate wide variations in vocal change (Graham, 1983; Greene, 1980) unless it is having disruptive effects on their lives. In this sense, a voice disorder is similar to most symptoms which cause people to consult their physician (Wadsworth and Ingham, 1981). We know very little about the motivation for the consultation, perhaps because we are not at the front line of patient contact.

We also have very little idea of the effects of the stress incurred between the patient's initial consultation, referral to the laryngologist and first contact with the speech pathologist. It may be assumed that during this period some of our patients may be attempting some form of coping strategy or making some attempt to control or alleviate the vocal symptoms (Wadsworth and Ingham, 1981; Mechanic, 1972). If the motivation for reporting to the doctor was a coping strategy (in other words, to request exemption from normal duties), what does the referral to the laryngologist mean to the patient? Does it reinforce the 'sick role' or does it trap the patient into needing the symptoms in case they could be considered to be malingering?

Whether the patient has a subtle physiological disorder of primary organic nature (or developed as a habitual response to stress), or is 'using' the symptoms as illness behaviour, there are several other variables to be taken into account:

(1) Having a voice disorder of any sort is frustrating and limits social communication; the person's changed vocal characteristics may affect the listener in various ways, as Aronson (1980) and Izdebski and Dedo (1981) have noted — this could be a further form of stress.
(2) General medical awareness of causes of voice disorder tends to be restricted to a diagnosis of either organicity or hysteria; the chances are that the patient will be given little indication of either possibility by the general practitioner, so that the voice disorder can assume a mysterious quality.
(3) People tend to notice a symptom either when its characteristics change, so that they become aware of it, or when there is a change in circumstances; this means that there is a chance that they will not associate other relevant symptoms with the present complaint, which can affect the process of diagnosis (Mechanic, 1972). Greene (1980) and Aronson (1980) have emphasised that misdiagnosis of voice disorders can occur all too easily; the clinician must be aware of the need to investigate all possible aetiological factors thoroughly.
(4) Harris (1977) has remarked that there is rarely a direct line between the therapist's understanding of the patient's problem and the patient's change of behaviour: 'Fear of change and of the unknown can generate a strong resistance to the therapist's attempts to intervene' (p. 72); most people need help, support

and short-term goals to maintain their motivation to change; the onus must be on the health professional to encourage the patient to share in his or her own health care (Winefield, 1981).

Diagnosis: The Patterns of Causes

The Diagnostic Interview

In any diagnostic interview, the clinician needs to be able to draw on two broad areas of resources, knowledge of possible issues which may be raised and skills of communication (Griffiths, 1981). In most cases, the clinician will have at least some information about the patient's medical and voice history and a description of the state of the vocal tract, from the laryngologist's referral. Ideally, of course, it helps to be present during the laryngeal examination, as being able to see how the vocal folds are moving can make more sense of the sound of the voice (Simpson, 1971). Where this is not possible, the clinician can still make use of the information from the referring letter and available medical notes to prepare for the interview.

The interview itself is a time of mutual evaluation. From the clinician's point of view, questions such as the history, the diagnosis and the patient's ability to respond to therapy may be the dominant issues. The patient will also have some questions, which probably include some need to know exactly what speech therapy is and how it is supposed to help, as well as what has caused the voice problem. The clinician who asks for the patient's views and attempts to satisfy their expectations will gain more than additional information. Several studies have shown that when patients feel that the interviewer has taken a personal interest in their problems, they tend to be more responsive to any subsequent guidance offered by the professional person (Ley, 1977; Korsch and Negrete, 1972).

If we take the view that the patient has to be a very active partner in consultation and treatment (Stimson, 1974), the clinician's role as both communicator and persuader becomes even more important. This calls into question such issues as the type of questions used by the interviewer, the use of counselling skills and the readiness to listen and respond. The patient who has been told that there is no physical reason for the voice problem may need to air his views, as the chances are that the patient or someone else will already have suggested that the problem is 'psychological' or 'all in your head'. The patient may wish to discuss this type of comment for its relevance to his or her own case, or may seek assurance from the clinician that the symptoms are indeed valid.

There are several good models of the type of information the voice therapist needs to obtain (Aronson, 1980; Boone, 1983a; Greene, 1980; Moncur and Brackett, 1974). Aronson (1980) emphasises that the clinician should consider collection of the data and interpretation of findings as two separate issues. It is this particular point which is emphasised here. There are several possible elements which can be interpreted more than one way; if we are looking for a pattern of cause, we must be ready to challenge each part of the data, as we should not presume or infer connections which may not be valid for the individual patient.

The Patient's Concept of the Cause

A knowledge of the patient's ideas of what caused the problem is of primary importance to the speech pathologist. The history of symptom development is also vital. As few people understand medical terms or human anatomy (Boyle, 1970) or how possible symptoms are linked (Mechanic, 1972), the therapist will need to guide the discussion and seek clarification at all points. It seems that Ley's (1977) suggestion that open-ended questions yield more information is relevant here. The specific question 'what do you think caused the problem?' tends to elicit opinions; a more general request to 'tell me how you came to be referred' tends to be answered as a description of the events the patient considers relevant.

Previous History

Pointers such as previous voice and throat symptoms are important. Boone (1983b) states that the sudden onset of voice loss or change in an adult whose voice has been normal is unusual and should be a signal for further medical investigation. Many patients will have a previous history of episodes of vocal change, in which case, the possibility that some of the current episode is related to long-term compensatory behaviour or misuse should be considered. Cooper (1973) suggests that attention should be paid to sensory symptoms such as pain in the neck or shoulder region, soreness in the throat and awareness of the need to clear the throat. The typical pattern of when and how the voice can change is also relevant.

Posture and Physical Tension

It is here that two factors become closely linked. The patient's level of physical tension can be interpreted as a sign of anxiety, personality type or as a sign of chronic life stress (Aronson, 1980; Brodnitz, 1981). Although musculoskeletal tension is described as a response to life stress (Dobson, 1982), it is also possible that the person's habitual posture has been a cause of the problem; the Alexander Principle (Barlow, 1973) originated from Alexander's own observations that his habitual stance and movement caused his voice problems. Postural changes may also be influenced by attempts to control or force phonation. Certainly, this latter concept of compensatory behaviour has been suggested in relation to spastic dysphonia (Izdebski and Dedo, 1981) and in relation to some neurologically based problems (Ward, Hanson and Berci, 1981). Changes in posture and tension levels can have quite marked influences on the mechanics of phonation (Simpson, 1971; Wyke and Kirchner, 1976). The automatic assumption that physical tension is a sign of psychogenesis has been challenged by several clinicians (Boone, 1983a; Cooper, 1973).

The Influence of Other Contributing Factors

A number of conditions have been described as having a subtle effect on vocal function. Generally, such factors as allergy, menstrual hormones, postnasal drip, respiratory diseases and some medications have been considered to affect specifically the fine control of the vocal folds. It has been presumed that although singers might notice the effect, these subtle changes would be insufficient to explain voice change with normal use (Lawrence, 1983). As more is learned about the very fine control and balance required for normal speech, however (Borden, 1980; Abbs, 1981; Wyke and Kirchner, 1976; Sawashima and Hirose, 1983), it seems feasible to consider that repeated, subtle changes to the mucosa and vocal fold surfaces may lead to minor but significant changes in control of voicing. There are a number of striking similarities between the effects of alterations in sensory feedback on speech gestures and the type of factors which can affect phonation (the reader may wish to compare, for example, Borden's (1980) summary of feedback and Boone's (1983a) list of facilitating techniques).

Life Stress

The relationship between stressful life events and feelings or symptoms of being unable to cope is complex. On the one hand, the patient may attribute the onset of symptoms to a given event correctly or incorrectly; on the other hand, it may be that a connection which seems obvious to the clinician may be rejected, at least initially by the patient. It can be that issues raised by the clinician may help the patient to re-evaluate the meanings of, or associations between, certain events and their relationship to the voice disorder. In some cases, as Rammage, Nichol and Morrison (1983) and Aronson (1980) have pointed out, even when a specific event triggered the development of vocal symptoms, if the stress recedes, the patient may be left with a residual pattern of vocal misuse which may respond to direct therapy.

Does the Patient Want Speech Therapy?

The patient who has been referred after a consultation with a laryngologist may comply with the doctor's advice (Ley, 1977) and attend for one appointment, but be unwilling to accept a course of speech therapy. Before the clinician offers therapy, it is important that the patient knows something about possible expectations and the commitment of time and action which will be required of him or her. The patient has the right to refuse treatment or to question the probable benefits; the clinician should be ready to discuss this.

The Patient's Individual Pattern

By the end of the diagnostic interview, the clinician will have some information, some observations and some impressions of the patient and of the patient's vocal use. The assessment of vocal function and physiological measures, using available resources is also vital, of course. Coleman (1983) suggests that it will soon be feasible for all clinicians to use microcomputer or minicomputer- assisted instrumentation for clinical evaluation. Where this is not possible, Young's (1983) evaluation of parameters of vocal function and a subjective assessment of voice (Gordon, Morton and Simpson, 1978) can provide the clinician with some baseline assessment

The clinician's main task is to consider whether speech therapy is an appropriate form of help for the particular patient. There may be indications from the history to suggest that an organic problem is present, or a symptom may need further investigation. Similarly, if the patient's history and ability to relate to the clinician cause concern in any way, it is advisable to seek further help immediately. In fact, it is highly desirable for the speech pathologist who works regularly with patients with voice disorders to develop a good working relationship with a psychologist or psychiatrist who will be able to help the clinician to identify the influences of the psychological variables in all voice therapy and to be directly involved in diagnosis and management, when appropriate (Butcher and Elias, 1983; Rammage, Nichol and Morrison, 1983).

The Aphonic Patient

The patients who tend to cause most alarm are those who are aphonic, have a tense, strained voice or periods of aphonia which appear unpredictable. Most textbooks associate the sudden onset of aphonia with acute life stress and conversion reaction, and in general recommend that the therapist works to attempts to remove the symptoms first and then works on resolving any further or residual emotional problems, using psychotherapeutic techniques (Brodnitz, 1969; Greene, 1980). Aronson (1980) advocates open discussion with the patient of the possibility of psychogenic causality, as the first essential, whereas Boone (1983a and b) suggests symptom-based therapy, with a degree of suggestion and ongoing support. From their descriptions, it seems that most experienced clinicians agree that a patient with a conversion reaction may relinquish the symptoms readily, especially if there is some time-lag between symptom onset and an appointment with the speech pathologist. If the patient is treated firmly and with a conviction that the voice will return, then the chances are that voice will return rapidly, although the therapist may initially need to accept an approximation to 'normal voice' and be prepared to shape the patient's vocal behaviour (Aronson, 1980; Boone, 1983a).

In the past, methods such as faradism or intralaryngeal injections have been used in attempts to 'prove' to the patient that phonation is possible. These 'tactics' (Greene, 1980) are generally agreed to be inappropriate for two main reasons: first, the forced adduction of the vocal folds induces involuntary phonation, which Tarneaud (1958) suggests will be 'unable to restore the correct coordinations and synergies of the speaker's . . . voice' (cited by Cooper, 1973). Secondly, if the voice disorder is indeed considered to be 'hysterical', then to focus on symptom removal alone is unlikely to be effective (Aronson, 1980).

In contrast to conversion reaction, it must be noted that several clinicians also describe cases in which the patient appears to have lost 'the set of the voice' (Aronson, 1980, p. 150; see also Boone, 1983a; Cooper, 1973). This may occur after the vocal folds have been stripped or may follow other surgical intervention or prescribed long-term voice rest, or after a respiratory tract infection. Lawrence (1983) describes how a viral infection of the lower respiratory tract may cause damage to the mucosal surfaces of the trachea or of the bronchial mucosal lining; the resultant coughing and throat clearing 'can be ruinous to the vocal folds mucosa and the arytenoid surfaces'.

The patterns here tend to be differentiated by such factors as the medical history, the patient's affect and the response to attempts to phonate. One of the standard suggestions is that a conversion reaction may be suspected if the patient can phonate when asked to cough but not when asked to produce voice (Aronson, 1980; Brodnitz, 1965). In this author's experience, the two activities can be approached quite differently by the patient. As coughing is a gross vegetative function, and voicing for linguistic use requires far more fine control and a degree of learned behaviour, the probability that the two should be viewed as separate behaviours should be considered carefully.

Although some patients will associate the onset of their voice problem with a specific incident, the clinician may not be fully convinced that the event identified actually fits the situation. For example, there may be a long time-lag between a 'shock' and the associated voice loss. Often, another factor is the patient's apparent indifference to the disorder and its disruptive effects.

In fact, it may be that general public awareness of hysteria and hysterical dysfunction has removed the symbolic significance from the classic cases of conversion reaction (Bakal, 1979; Veith, 1965). Again, in this author's experience, many aphonic patients are anxious to be reassured that they are not considered hysterical. It can be extremely helpful to discuss the management of this type of issue with the psychiatrist or psychologist. In the sense that the patient is actually doing something physically outside the normal range of behaviours which produce voice, it is possible to state this to the patient. There is a fine line, however, between agreeing that it is possible for the patient to relinquish the behaviours and confirming the patient's conviction that the problem does not require them to take action to change.

The Duration of the Voice Problem

When a patient has a short history of voice loss, it may be that the voice may be regained quickly. For a surprising number of patients, the laryngologist's reassurance that there is no malignancy seems to release tension and facilitate the return of voice. In these cases, however, it is advisable for the clinician to offer a brief course of voice therapy, particularly focusing on relaxation, posture and breath control, as the chances are that some vocal misuse will have occurred, so that under stress the patient may be again susceptible to voice change.

One of the more confusing types of problem is when the person seems to develop almost a random pattern of vocal control, which may sometimes be associated with a specific context, such as a certain type of conversational topic, or in certain situations. One possible cause here is a hearing loss. With some patients, the clinician may use a gentle reminder to the patient when the pattern changes, to bring the need for control to the patient's attention. Some people seem to increase the likelihood of voice change by an alteration of head position or a change in relationship between the cervical spine and the jaw, in which case, relaxation and postural awareness can help. Occasionally, a patient may have specific voicing problems with certain phonetic contexts, such as voiced – voiceless contrasts or with certain vowels; it seems probable that this could be influenced by the supraglottic structures (Sawashima and Hirose, 1983) so that relaxation of the articulators may help overcome this.

Whatever the underlying cause, all patients who have a fairly long history of aphonia or dysphonia will have an acquired habitual pattern that has to be broken down. It is not unusual for quite marked tension in the suprahyoid region to be present, with slight changes to the posture of the jaw, some tongue retraction and raising of the thyroid cartilage and hyoid bone. Subtle changes in lip and facial movements may also be noted, often in the patient's non-verbal as well as speech gestures (Rammage, Nichol and Morrison, 1983). The pattern of external change can reflect similar muscle patternings, as seen by xeroradiography (MacCurtain, 1983). As this pattern is often extremely strong and well established, to break it down requires a great deal of tenacity and motivation from both clinician and patient, and considerable mutual trust and co-operation.

Approaches to Therapy

The Therapeutic Relationship

The clinician and the patient need to work in close partnership to effect the change. The clinician's work is to ensure that the patient has a reasonable target, knows how to reach it, and how often to practise. The patient's work is to attain the target behaviour and to practise. One of the factors that promotes the change is the relationship that develops between therapist and patient. The therapist who can set attainable goals, reassure the patient that change is possible and desirable, and who is empathetic and ready to listen, discuss and explain therapy techniques, can best help the patient to effect change (Baker, 1977; Harris, 1977).

The probability is high that the responsive therapist is also more likely to be trusted with information about the patient as a person. As new issues arise, it may be that the clinician feels that a direct focus on voice is no longer the main issue. Again, at this stage, discussion with a colleague may help the therapist to reconsider the goals of therapy. The clinician must address the questions: what is to be gained from the speech therapist changing the emphasis? Does the patient need voice therapy or psychotherapy? Are the therapist's counselling skills adequate to cope with the patient's problems and ideas? Is this an appropriate use of a *speech therapist*, or should a professional more skilled in understanding psychological problems be called in? All of these should be considered at this stage (Baker, 1977; Harris, 1977; Aronson, 1980).

Breaking Down the Behaviour

Relaxation and breath control exercises, followed by specific techniques to facilitate optimum phonation continue to form the core of voice therapy (MacIntyre, 1983; Moore, 1977). A number of clinicians are also paying increased attention to the mechanics of posture and body use (Barlow, 1973; Faure, 1983). All of the techniques require that the patient becomes cognitively aware of contrasts in body use, can perceive comparatively subtle changes and make appropriate and equally subtle alterations to his or her behaviour and body image.

The alteration of any established behaviour can be difficult and demanding. In therapy for dysfluency, it is well recognised that a change in habitual speech behaviour needs to be broken down into small, attainable goals; most fluency programmes utilise behaviour modification techniques on an intensive daily basis. There is a strong argument for the use of a similar approach with patients with voice disorder. MacIntyre (1983) reports that a two-week period of intensive work, which includes controlled voice rest, can help to break down old habits and reinforce new ones. This author has also used this approach to good effect with patients who had failed to respond to less frequent therapy.

Other Psychological Variables

As well as the theme of counselling and psychotherapeutic approaches, there are several other factors in therapy itself which require specific psychological insights:

Patients May Forget Instructions. Ley's (1977) studies of responses to medical instructions show that patients can fail to understand or forget what they are told quite rapidly, especially if the instructions are too complex or require any sort of anatomical knowledge. In addition, patients feel diffident about telling the health worker that they have not understood. Even when the patient has understood, the chances are that up to half of the instructions given may be forgotten within 80 minutes of the consultation. (How many speech pathologists have found that patients have reversed the instructions for breath control, in their home practise, for example?) Ley (1977) found that certain techniques improved patient's total recall:

(1) Using short sentences and simple vocabulary; this leads to an increase of up to 20 per cent in the chances of the patient recalling information.
(2) Repeating the information.
(3) Giving concrete and specific advice, in terms of how much or how often.

Failure to Learn may Reflect the Teaching. It is often stated that if the patient does not respond to therapy, this can be a sign of psychogenic aetiology. If the speech pathologist has not given the patient adequate instruction or does not work to ensure the goals of therapy and of homework are clearly established, then therapy itself is counterproductive and may be an additional form of stress.

Different Individuals Will Respond to Different Techniques. Some patients may find techniques such as relaxation difficult to master initially; use of books and tapes (Madders, 1981) or biofeedback techniques (Boone, 1983a) can be helpful, although these should not be a total substitute for the therapist and patient working together on relaxation. For some patients, the emphasis on an auditory target or on a specific type of facilitating technique (Boone, 1983a) may not be sufficient. Filter (1974, 1980) has advocated far more emphasis in proprioceptive–tactile–kinaesthetic awareness as a basis for therapy. The techniques employed include encouraging the patient to recognise, describe and monitor feelings of pressure, tension, effort and movement in abdominal, thoracic, oral, pharyngeal and laryngeal areas. Sensory awareness and relaxation techniques used are similar to those described in the Alexander Principle (Barlow, 1973) and by Jacobsen (1938; 1964).

Visual Feedback

For some patients, one of the biggest problems is to find and hold an auditory target, in which case the use of other sensory modalities can be highly effective. Visual feedback, using instrumentation, such as Visipitch, Visispeech or the laryngograph (electroglottography) can provide the patient with an appropriate change of focus. One excellent benefit of this type of instrumentation is that the clinician can give the patient guidance in facilitating techniques (Boone, 1983a) or in sensory awareness (Filter, 1974, 1980) simultaneously. As the patient can see the effects of the suggested change, the immediate effects of the therapist's directions can be appreciated and the patient may be more convinced that therapy is working!

The Patient Who Has Specific Problems

Emotional problems, underlying anxiety, depression or other unresolved psychosocial difficulties may still be part of the patient's problem. In these cases, the likelihood of speech therapy alone being effective is low. The most appropriate action is for the therapist to arrange consultation with a psychologist or psychiatrist. Descriptions of constructive results from conjoint work have been reported by Rammage, Nichol and Morrison (1983), using a psychotherapeutic approach and by Butcher and Elias (1983), using cognitive-behavioural therapy. Joint consultation has many benefits, including the fact that the patient does not feel that the problem is 'too hard' to handle, or that the speech therapist is rejecting him or her as a person.

Speech pathologists have also worked with others, using personal construct theory (Berry *et al.*, 1982), group relaxation therapy (Hayward and Simmons, 1982) and hypnosis, for deep relaxation in particular (Lucas and Levy, 1984). The decision to use a particular type of approach will depend partly on the availability and interests of the professionals involved and the suitability of a particular approach for the individual client's needs.

Finally, some people may have specific psychiatric or psychological problems which include changes in voice quality or other parameters of speech, which the speech pathologist clearly recognises as outside his or her area of expertise and knowledge (Darby, Simmons and Berger, 1981). Most of the references to changes of vocal parameters in psychopathology seem to indicate that 'voice' is used quite loosely and may actually include rate of speech and specific pitch restrictions related to affect, such as monopitch in depression. The distinction between vocal dysfunction and speech characteristics is only part of the symptom picture.

Conclusion

Speech pathologists need to draw on a range of psychological skills and insights in all of their work with patients. In voice therapy in particular, the association between stress, emotional states and voice has led to a very strong emphasis on psychodynamic theory in the explanation of the causes of some types of voice disorder.

It seems that the traditional approach which emphasises 'psychogenesis', 'personality' and 'vocal psychodynamics' actually incorporates many other psychological concepts. While we may describe everything as 'psychogenic', there is a danger that we do not recognise our own role in therapy. Much of the detail remains, as Weaver (1924) suggested, 'unanalyzable'. By looking more closely at the detail both of parameters of vocal function and of the processes in therapy, speech pathologists can identify a large number of factors which can affect the onset of a patient's voice disorder and its subsequent rehabilitation.

There is no doubt that voice therapy can be complex, but as Aronson (1980) points out, it is probably no less complex than dysphasia therapy, for example. One of the major difficulties with voice therapy is that the patient often continues his or her normal daily life throughout therapy, so that the development of new learning may be restricted by the patient's constant use of acquired, aberrant vocal habits. As well, because voice therapy focuses on a relatively automatic process, the patient may need additional support and guidance as the enormity of the task of changing one or several parts of this process *in the context of the rest of the process of normal speech* becomes apparent. It is feasible for us to consider that vocal change itself is quite stressful.

Although it is recognised that some people referred for voice therapy will have problems which are more specificially psychiatric in nature, or problems which should be more appropriately treated by a psychologist, the major thesis of this chapter is that much of what has been described as 'psychogenic' can be explained by a holistic approach, in which the individual person's pattern of lifestyle and behaviour is the main focus.

References

Abbs, J. H. 'Neuromotor Mechanisms of Speech Production', in Darby, J. K. (ed.) *Speech Evaluation in Medicine*, pp. 181–98. (Grune and Stratton, New York, 1981)

Aronson, A. E. *Clinical Voice Disorders* (Thieme-Stratton, New York, 1980)

Bakal, D. J. *Psychology and Medicine* (Tavistock, London, 1980)

Baker, J. 'Emotional Problems in Relation to Communication Disorders — An Overview', *Australian Journal of Human Communication Diseases*, 5, 79 (1977)

Barlow, W. *The Alexander Principle* (Gollancz, London, 1973)

Berry, R. J., Epstein, R., Freeman, M., MacCurtain, F. and Noscoe, N. 'an Objective Analysis of Voice Disorder: Part 2', *British Journal of Disorders in Communication*, 17, 72 (1982)

Bloch, E. L. and Goodstein, L. D. 'Functional Speech Disorders and Personality: A Decade of Research', *Journal of Speech and Hearing Disorders*, 36, 295–314 (1971)

Boone, D. R. *The Voice and Voice Therapy* (Prentice-Hall, Englewood Cliffs, New Jersey, 1983a)

——, 'Management of Voice Disorders in Adults', *Seminars in Speech and Language*, 4, 259–71 (1983b)

Borden, G. J. 'Use of Feedback in Established and Developing Speech', in Lass, N. J. (ed.) *Speech and Language: Advances in Basic Research and Practice*, vol. 3, pp. 223–42 (Academic Press, London, 1980)

Boyle, C. M. 'Difference Between Patients' and Doctors' Interpretations of Some Common Medical Terms', *British Medical Journal*, 2, 286–9 (1970)

Bridger, M. W. M. and Epstein, R. 'Functional Voice Disorders: A Review of 109 Patients', *Journal of Laryngology and Otology*, 97, 1145–8 (1983)

Brodnitz, F. S. *Vocal Rehabilitation* (American Academy of Ophthalmology and Otolaryngology, Rochester, Minnesota, 1965)

——, 'Psychological Considerations in Vocal Rehabilitation', *Journal of Speech and Hearing Disorders*, 46, 21–6 (1981)

Brown, G. W. 'Social Causes of Disease', in Tuckett, D. (ed.), *An Introduction to Medical Sociology*, pp. 291–333 (Tavistock, London, 1976)

Butcher, P. and Elias, A. 'Cognitive-behavioral Therapy with Dysphonic Patients', *Bulletin of the College of Speech Therapy*, 377, 1–3 (1983)

Cannon, W. B. *Wisdom of the Body* (Norton, New York, 1932)

Coleman, R. F. 'Instrumental Analysis of Voice Disorders', *Seminars in Speech and Language*. 4(3) 205–15 (1983)

Cooper, C. L. *The Stress Check* (Prentice-Hall, Englewood Cliffs, New Jersey, 1981)

Cooper, M. *Modern Techniques of Vocal Rehabilitation* (Charles C. Thomas, Springfield, Illinois, 1973)

Darby, J. K., Simmons, N. and Berger, P. A. 'Speech and Voice Parameters of Depression; A Pilot Study', *Journal of Communication Disorders*, 17, 75–85 (1984)

Dobson, C. B. *Stress: the Hidden Adversary* (MTP Press, Lancaster, 1982)

Faure, M-A. 'Aspects of Relationship Between States of the Spine and the Acoustic Qualities of the Voice from a Magnetoscopic and Sonagraphic Study, *Proceedings of the Congress, International Association of Logopaedics and Phoniatrics, 14–18 August 1983, Edinburgh* (1983)

Filter, M. D. 'Proprioceptive–tactile-kinaesthetic Feedback in Voice Therapy', *Language, Speech and Hearing Service in Schools*, 5, 149–51 (1974)

——, 'Proprioceptive–tactile–kinaesthetic Approach to Voice Disorders', *Proceedings of the 18th Congress, International Association of Logopaedics and Phoniatrics, 4–7 August, 1980, Washington* (1980)

Gordon, M. T. Morton, F. M. and Simpson, I. C. 'Air Flow Measurements in Diagnosis, Assessment and Treatment of Mechanical Dysphonia', *Folia Phoniatrica (Basel)*, 30, 161–74 (1978)

Graham, D. T. 'Psychophysiology and Medicine', *Psychophysiology*, 8, 121–31 (1971)

Graham, J. 'The Course of the Patient from Presentation to Diagnosis', in Edels, Y. (ed.) *Laryngectomy: Diagnosis to Rehabilitation*, pp. 1–17 (Croom Helm, London, 1983)

Greene, M. C. L. *The Voice and Its Disorders* (Churchill Livingstone, Edinburgh, 1980)

——, 'Anxiety State and the Chronic Hyperventilation Syndrome: Relevance in Speech and Voice Disorders', *Proceedings of the 19th Congress International Association of Logopaedics and Phoniatrics, 14–18 August 1983, Edinburgh* (1983)

Griffiths, D. *Psychology and Medicine* (Macmillan, London, 1981)

Harris, R. D. 'The Speech Pathologist as Counsellor', *Australian Journal of Human Disorders in Communication*, 5, 72–8 (1977)

Hay, M., Foreword, in Madders, J., (ed.) *Stress and Relaxation*, p. 9 (Martin Dunitz, London, 1981)

Hayward, A. and Simmons, R. 'Relaxation Groups with Dysphonic Patients', *Bulletin of the College of Speech Therapists*, 359 (1982)

Hirano, M. *Clinical Examination of Voice* (Springer-Verlag, Wein, 1980)

Holmes, T. H. and Masuda, M. 'Life Change and Illness Susceptibility', in Dohrenwend, B. S. and Dohrenwend, B. P. (eds.) *Stressful Life Events: Their Nature and Effects* (Wiley, New York, 1974)

—— and Rahe, R. 'Holmes–Rahe Social Readjustment Rating Scale', *Journal of Psychosomatic Research*, 2, 213 (1967)

Izdebski, K. and Dedo, H. H. 'Spastic Dysphonia', in Darby, J. K. (ed.) *Speech Evaluation in Medicine*, pp. 105–127 (Grune and Stratton, New York, 1981)

Jacobsen, E. *Progressive Relaxation* (University of Chicago Press, Chicago, 1938)

—— (1964), *Anxiety and Tension Control* (Lippincott, Philadelphia, 1964)

Kitzing, P. 'Die Behandlung von Storungen der Stimmfunktion', *Folia Phoniatrica (Basel)*, 35, 40–65 (1983)

Korsch, B. and Negrete, V. 'Doctor–Patient Communication', *Scientific American*, August, 66–74 (1972)

Lawrence, V. L. (1983), 'Vocal Problems of the Professional User of Voice', *Seminars in Speech and Language*, 4, 233–43 (1983)

Lazarus, R. S. *Patterns of Adjustment* (McGraw-Hill, New York, 1976)

Ley, P. 'Communicating with the Patient', in Coleman, J. C. (ed.) *Introductory Psychology* (Routledge and Kegan Paul, London, 1977)

Lipowski, Z. J. (1977), 'Psychosomatic medicine: Current Trends and Clinical Applications', in Lipowski, Z. J., Lipsett, D. R. and Whybrow, P. C. *Psychosomatic Medicine: Current Trends and Clinical Applications* (Oxford University Press, New York, 1977)

Lucas, H. and Levy, M. (1984), 'The Use of Hypnosis in an Unusual Voice Disorder — A Combined Clinical Psychology and Speech Therapy Approach', *Bulletin of the College of Speech Therapists* 383, 1–2 (1984)

MacCurtain, F. 'Vocal Tract Function in Psychogenic Voice Disorders', *Proceedings of the 19th Congress, International Association of Logopaedics and Phoniatrics, 14–18 August 1983, Edinburgh* (1983)

MacIntyre, J. M. 'An Evaluation of the Incidence, Causes and Types of Dysphonia Observed Over a Period of Ten Years in One District of an Industrial City', *Proceedings of the 19th Congress, International Association of Logopaedics and Phoniatrics, 14–18 August 1983, Edinburgh* (1983)

Madders, J. *Stress and Relaxation* (Martin Dunitz, London, 1981)

Mechanic, D. 'Response Factors in Illness, a Study of Illness Behaviour', *Social Psychiatry*, 1, 11–20 (1966)

——, 'Social Psychologic Factors Affecting the Presentation of Bodily Complaints', *New England Journal of Medicine*, 286, 1132–9 (1972)

Moncur, J. P. and Brackett, I. P. *Modifying Vocal Behaviour* (Harper and Row, New York, 1974)

Monday, L. A. 'Clinical Evaluation of Functional Dysphonia', *Journal of Otolaryngology*, 12(5), 307–10 (1983)

Moore, G. P. 'Have the Major Issues in Voice Disorders Been Answered by Research in Speech Science? A 50–year Retrospective', *Journal of Speech and Hearing Disorders*, 42, 152–60 (1977)

Murphy, A. T. *Functional Voice Disorders* (Prentice Hall, Englewood Cliffs, New Jersey, 1964)

Parsons, T. *The Social System* (Free Press, Glencoe, New York, 1951)

Perkins, W. H. (1983), 'Quantification of Vocal Behavior: A Foundation for Clinical Management', in Bless, D. M. and Abbs, J. H. (eds.) *Vocal Fold Physiology*, pp. 425–31 (College-Hill, San Diego, California, 1983)

Rammage, L. A., Nichol, H. and Morrison, M. D. 'The Voice Clinic: An Interdisciplinary Approach', *Journal of Otolaryngology*, 12(5) 315–18 (1983)
Sawashima, M. and Hirose, H. 'Laryngeal Gestures in Speech Production', in McNeilage, P. F. (ed.), *The Production of Speech*, pp. 11–38 (Springer-Verlag, New York, 1983)
Seligman, M. F. P. *Helplessness: On Depression, Development, and Death* (Freeman, San Francisco, 1975)
Selye, H. *Stress* (Acta, Montreal, 1950)
Sheldon, A. 'Towards a General Theory of Disease and Medical Care', in Sheldon, A., Baker, F. and McLaughlin, C. P., (eds) *Systems and Medical Care*, p. 94 (MIT, Cambridge, Massachusetts, 1970)
Shuval, J. T., Antonovsky, A. and Davies, A. M. 'Illness: A Mechanism for Coping with Failure', *Social Science and Medicine*, 7, 259–65 (1973)
Simpson, I. C. 'Dysphonia: The Organisation and Working of a Dysphonia Clinic', *British Journal of Diseases in Communication*, 6, 1, 70–85 (1971)
Stimson, G. V. 'Obeying Doctor's Orders: A View from the Other Side', *Social Science and Medicine*, 8, 97–104 (1974)
Tarneaud, J. 'The Fundamental Principles of Vocal Cultivation and Therapeutics of the Voice', *Logos*, 1, 7–10 (1958)
Ursin, H. and Murison, R. (eds) *Biological and Psychological Basis of Psychosomatic Disease* (Pergamon, Oxford, 1983)
Veith, I. *Hysteria: The History of a Disease* (University of Chicago Press, Chicago, 1965)
Wadsworth, M. and Ingham, J. 'How Society Defines Sickness: Illness Behaviour and Consultation', in Christie, M. J. and Mellett, P. G. (eds) *Foundations of Psychosomatics* (Wiley, London, 1981)
Ward, P. H., Hanson, D. G. and Berci, G. 'Observations on Central Neurologic Etiology for Laryngeal Dysfunction', *Annals of Otology*, 90, 430–41 (1981)
Weaver, A. 'Experimental Studies in Vocal Expression', *Quarterly Journal of Speech Education,* 10, 199–204 (1924)
Winefield, H. R. 'Behavioural Science in the Medical Curriculum: Why and How', in Christie, M. J. and Mellett, P. G. *Foundations of Psychosomatics* (Wiley, London, 1981)
Wyke, B. D. and Kirchner, J. A. 'Neurology of the Larynx', in Hinchcliffe, R. and Hamson, D. (eds) *Scientific Foundations of Otolaryngology*, pp. 546–66 (Heinemann, London, 1976)
Young, K. 'Evaluation of Vocal Function Without Use of Instrumentation', *Proceedings of the 19th Congress International Association of Logopaedics and Phoniatrics, 14–18 August 1983, Edinburgh* (1983)
Zipursky, M. A., Ezerzer, F., Fishbein, B. M., Epstein, S. W. and Thompson, G. 'Aerodynamic Testing in Psychogenic Voice Disorders: Respiratory and Phonatory Studies', *Human Communication*, 7, 69–73 (1983)

12 PERSISTENT PUBERPHONIA

Bob Fawcus

Introduction

. . . his awkwardness about his altered speech, which swings out of control between croaks and squeaks while an ugly lump bobs in his throat like a cork . . .'

from *Shame* by Salman Rushdie (1983)

The change from a boy's voice to that of an adult male is one of the markedly overt signs of puberty, more dramatic than the first hint of facial hair and more varied in both pattern of development and onset than any other of the classical features.

There are many possible causes for the failure to develop characteristic low-pitched phonation. Aronson (1980) provides a comprehensive account of the development of structure and function of the larynx and the factors which interfere with the normal transition from a mean fundamental frequency of a little over 250 Hz to a fundamental frequency which centres around 120 Hz.

Physical and Physiological Causes of Puberphonia

Greene (1980) outlines the range of physical and physiological causes of puberphonia suggested in the literature:

(1) Unusually early breaking of the voice, leading to self-consciousness and habitual continuation of a high-pitched voice (West, Ansberry and Carr, 1957).
(2) A desire to retain a successful soprano voice which has brought distinction (Seth and Guthrie, 1935).
(3) Fear of assuming a full share of adult responsibility. (Greene rejects the often quoted link with the Oedipus complex but comments on her frequent observation of a strong bond with

the mother and the relative prevalence of puberphonia in boys without siblings.)

(4) Hero worship of an elder boy.
(5) A natural tenor voice or small larynx.
(6) Delayed pubertal development (Luchsinger and Arnold, 1965).
(7) Severe deafness (Greene, 1961).
(8) Congenital abnormalities and asymmetries, paralysis of one fold (Arnold, 1961) or congenital web (Baker and Savetsky, 1966).

Aronson (1980) would add to the list the effect of 'general debilitating illness during puberty, which not only may delay overall growth during puberty but, because of the physical restrictions of being bedfast, may reduce the range of respiratory excursions and consequently, tidal air volumes, preventing the development of adequate infraglottal air'.

He goes on to enumerate laryngeal-respiratory postures and movements which have been noted as bases for high-pitched mutational falsetto voice.

(1) The larynx is elevated high in the neck.
(2) The body of the larynx is tilted downward, apparently having the effect of maintaining the vocal folds in a lax state.
(3) With the vocal folds in a flabby state, they are stretched thin by contraction of the cricothyroid muscles.
(4) The vocal folds are thus in a state of reduced mass and offer little resistance to infraglottal air pressure.
(5) Respiration for speech production is shallow, and on exhalation infraglottal air pressure is held to a minimum, so that only the medial edges of the vocal folds vibrate and do so at an elevated fundamental frequency.

The first of these characteristics was noted by Makuen in 1899 (cited in Luchsinger and Arnold, 1965) and is quoted in almost every work on the subject of puberphonia.

Evidence derived from simple observation of laryngeal excursions during normal phonation and falsetto suggests, however, that the reported high elevation is associated with the typical upward shift in pitch which occurs when a male speaker demonstrates the switch from true cord phonation to falsetto. This usually involves a pitch change of at least an octave. If the transfer is made at the same pitch level the elevation is much reduced.

Despite the wide range of alleged causes of puberphonia there is an alternative explanation which matches our own experience and many of the accounts which occur in the literature. These typically do not include the possibility that a pubescent male may blunder into an alternative mode of phonation during the initial period of vocal mutation and then be unable to escape voluntarily.

The fact that an individual is apparently unable to shift from one mode of phonation to another should not be at all surprising. After the successful transfer from falsetto to true cord phonation it is often just as difficult for the former puberphonic to achieve falsetto voice.

The flexibility which some individuals appear to have in control of their phonatory and articulatory behaviour is not universal. The range of skilled behaviour evident in such activities as mimicry and singing suggests that a significant proportion of those with a normal speech mechanism are unable to achieve even average performance (Fawcus, 1980). Luchsinger and Arnold (1965) comment that 'while their peripheral auditory perception is usually normal many of these [puberphonic] patients are not musical'. They also mention the influence of auditory factors reflected in the occasional occurrence of falsetto voice in profoundly deaf males.

It is of advantage to consider when falsetto phonation is employed by the normal speaker: it is a feature of war cries in many cultures, and can also be heard on British Army parade grounds in the issuing of orders during drill. More peaceful phenomena include giggling, laughing, yodelling and the singing of the countertenor.

At the London Conference of the International Association of Logopaedics and Phoniatrics in 1959, Moses traced the swings in fashion which were associated with the castrato singing voice over the previous 200 years and made the confident prediction that male singing styles were about to enter a new phase in western culture. Many in the audience found this prediction difficult to accept. With the possible exception of a single popular male alto, Alfred Deller, the overwhelming majority of male singers rarely strayed into falsetto phonation. On the popular stage as well as the concert hall, male singers exuded as strong a masculine image as possible.

For the past quarter of a century successions of highly successful popular singers have laboured consistently to lend credence to Moses' prediction. The Beatles, the Beachboys, Tiny Tim, the Jacksons, and hosts of others, have spent a major portion of their time producing falsetto phonation to the evident delight and full acceptance of their followers.

Gutzmann (1897) described the role of the crycothyroid in the production of falsetto voice in the normal larynx by means of a 'functional over-contraction'. Arnold (1961) investigated the operation of the laryngeal musculature by means of electromyography and confirmed that the external vocal cord tensor (cricothyroid) is the muscle chiefly involved in falsetto phonation. Hirano, Vennard and Chala (1970) studied the regulation of register, pitch and intensity in the larynges of a small group of singers using hooked wire electrodes.

Traditionally, falsetto voice has been considered as the main component of head register and part of the constituent pattern of the mid-register or mixed register. It is not held to be involved in the highest range, known as the whistle register, or the lowest described as chest register. The Hirano recordings show most differences occuring in the trace derived from the vocalis muscle of one of the authors (Vennard), an accomplished bass as well as a speech scientist.

In the course of two decades at both the Middlesex Hospital and Guy's Hospital, the opportunity was afforded to work with a series of young men referred with persistent puberphonia.

All were reported to have laryngeal structures within normal limits and there was no evidence of endocrine disorders. None of the young men gave cause to either the referring ENT surgeon or the speech therapist to consider the necessity for psychiatric referral. Their complaints centred on the basic acceptability of the high-pitched voice and in no case did this seriously affect social adjustment.

Treating Puberphonia

Diverse techniques as well as accounts of their success abound in the texts devoted to voice disorders. Greene (1980) suggests a number of activities, principally concerned with postural adjustments and relaxation. Gutzmann's pressure test, for example, cited in Luchsinger and Arnold (1965) is recommended by

Aronson (1980) as a successful therapeutic technique. It requires digital pressure on the thyroid cartilage during attempts at phonation.

After one has taken the necessary case history it is obviously important to investigate the patient's pitch range. The first problem encountered is that he is very likely to be able to produce falsetto voice at or near the normal adult male fundamental frequency. This is, however, clearly different from the normal male voice. It usually has a slightly breathy tone, tends to be weak and somewhat flat. Depending on how long the individual has been using falsetto, however, the stage of growth of his vocal cords, and idiosyncratic factors related to phonation patterns, it is possible that he may have achieved a reduction in breathy quality and more power than is usual for a puberphonic voice. This can be seen most clearly in the male alto who can typically achieve considerable intensity with a minimum of breathiness.

The principal test is to listen to conversation or reading aloud to determine whether or not the low pitch is maintained and whether the transition to a higher pitch is a smooth one without voice breaks.

Many individuals find singing scales difficult or embarrassing, and it is just as satisfactory to proceed in simple steps to pairs of notes up to the top of his comfortable range and then down to the lowest point. The therapist who is not a musician may find it simpler to employ a small electronic keyboard which is usually nowadays portable and inexpensive. This has many applications with other types of dysphonic patient as well as offering a broad range of opportunities in work on listening skills with young children.

A laryngograph or voiscope (Fourcin and Abberton, 1971) preferably with hard copy printout can provide the therapist with a visual display of the pattern of phonation. The puberphonic does not produce the typical sawtooth output of the normal speaker, but a wave form which closely approximates to a sine wave.

It is the absence of the characteristic bursts of laryngeal output which is responsible for the weaker almost ethereal tone of the falsetto. The tissues of the vocal folds are vibrating with reduced mass and a lower level of tension in the closed phase. They are behaving like a tuning fork or the air in a flute and the resulting voice is reminiscent of these sounds.

It is preferable not to attempt to alter the mode of phonation too quickly in the session. The abrupt change in voice which is relatively easy to achieve is usually very difficult for the patient to adjust to. It is important to determine if he has been aware of any occasional shifts into true phonation. These can occur accidentally, but it is not usually possible for the puberphonic male to reproduce them at will.

The exploration of range of falsetto may have resulted in production of 'creaky voice' particularly in the lower frequencies. It is very useful to assess how easily the patient can achieve 'creaky voice', or 'glottal fry' as it is known in the American texts on dysphonia. Of all techniques suggested the most effective with the above group of persistent puberphonic cases at the Middlesex Hospital and Guy's was the transfer from falsetto phonation first to glottal fry (creaky voice) and then into true cord phonation.

One should ask the patient to initiate 'creaky voice', and when he is comfortably producing this mode of phonation ask him to raise the pitch gradually. There is a reasonable chance that he may shift dramatically into normal phonation immediately. If this does not occur then it is necessary to attempt the task two or three times and then divert to a relaxation task; if there is repeated failure (see Greene, 1961, 1980) after an interval the technique may be repeated. Many authorities, however, report success within a few minutes of commencing the process.

Such success leads almost without exception to one of the major paradoxes in the field of speech therapy. A young man has come to the clinic, complaining that his voice is too high pitched and that he is often upset by people mistaking him for a woman when speaking on the telephone. Within a matter of minutes it is possible for him to achieve true cord phonation. The pitch drops accordingly and he has achieved exactly what he requested. The most common, initial reaction is to reject the new voice. The reasons given differ from individual to individual, but with very few exceptions this is a typical response.

This behaviour only served to confirm the views held by psychoanalysts, and those therapists who were inclined to their philosophy, that the young man actually preferred his original state and that it was the result of a process of 'symptom-choice'.

Establishing the New Voice

Although disconcerting to the therapist, even if the response is anticipated, it would be a serious mistake to interpret the rejection of the new voice as anything but a normal and temporary reaction.

It is very similar to the panic described by some stammerers when they realise for the first time that they can approach speaking situations with a low risk of stuttering (Dalton and Hardcastle, 1977). This is usually the result of a rapid response to a specific therapy procedure which can leave him feeling 'naked and vulnerable', as a stammerer once described it.

Another example is the response of the adult patient who requests therapy because he or she habitually uses a lateral /s/ or uvular /r/ and wishes to learn to speak 'normally'. In both such cases it is possible to achieve, sometimes with singular difficulty, the performance which they claimed to desire, only to find that they dislike the result.

Appropriate advice and counselling can usually overcome this very human, quite normal reaction to change. The most effective approach can be to accept the negative response as a normal reaction. It has to be remembered that if the therapist is disconcerted, the individual himself is not unaware of the paradox and is likely to feel just as uncomfortable about his protestations as he does about the quality and 'feel' of his new voice or new articulatory pattern.

In the puberphonic it is helpful to work on developing and establishing the new voice in spite of the initial protests. This entails exploring the vocal range, and encouraging the young man to experiment with the new mode of phonation. He should be encouraged to use his new voice as often as possible with strangers before he encounters his family, friends or colleagues at work. Some gain great benefit from talking on the telephone or having a face-to-face conversation with a sympathetic friend prior to approaching a situation which may be potentially threatening.

It can be emphasised that, contrary to his expectations, people in the patient's environment are not likely to notice the change. Furthermore, it should be pointed out that he himself will be much more aware of any difference as most people will tend to listen to what he says rather than how he speaks. It helps to keep the volume down at first as this aids the maintenance of stability and tends to limit the attention paid by others.

Strong reassurance can be given but this will be greatly reinforced if some assignments are attempted. These can include telephone calls to strangers, and being interviewed by a colleague of the therapist unfamiliar with the original puberphonic voice.

Sometimes the young man is more anxious about the reaction of parents and siblings than strangers.

Case History 1

KS, a young man whose family were immigrants from Pakistan had been criticised and ridiculed for up to a year by relatives, particularly his uncles. He was very concerned about their reaction to his new voice but found that they did not notice the change until he brought it to their attention.

Case History 2

TJ, a young man in his early twenties, showed a particularly distressed reaction to achieving a very serviceable male voice in the first session of therapy. 'Well as you know, I work for a construction plant hire firm, and have to deliver and demonstrate vehicles on site. I often get a bit of leg pulling about my voice but this will be terrible. Tomorrow I'm getting married and when I get back from my honeymoon, they will all fall about laughing.'

He resigned from work that day and sought a similar post in another district after his honeymoon.

Case History 3

PM was referred in his mid-forties after an ENT examination, following a period of laryngeal discomfort. His father had undergone laryngectomy a few months previously, and he was, understandably, very conscious of his own larynx.

His response to therapy employing a glottal fry initiation was rapid and effective, and he showed less concern about the change than the younger cases mentioned previously.

It was agreed that he should return after a few days to make a laryngographic recording, so that we could examine the transition from falsetto to true cord phonation and obtain a visual record.

When he returned to the clinic, he was quite unable to achieve falsetto voice, he was now as locked into the normal mode of phonation as he had been trapped into the former phonatory pattern since puberty.

In some cases of persistent puberphonia prior to therapy, and in a few instances during the course of therapy, the voice of the patient shows features of dysphonia. This may result from the individual's own effort made to achieve a more masculine voice, or during therapy from his own misapplication of techniques designed to alter the mode of phonation.

It might be suspected that dysphonia could directly result from many of the techniques suggested. These would include glottal fry, as suggested above and recommended by many authorities, but more especially those which involve increased tension, such as hard glottal attack (Aronson, 1980). It is vital to minimise and eliminate the dysphonia particularly before any attempt is made to consolidate the new voice. The principles and techniques discussed in Chapter 10 will provide the necessary guidance if required.

Similarly, most of the work required to establish and maintain the new voice will follow the same principles as those expressed in relation to hyperfunctional voice use (Chapter 10, this volume).

References

Arnold, G. E. 'Physiology and Pathology of the Cricothyroid Muscle', *Laryngoscope*, 71, 658 (1961)

Aronson, A. E. *Clinical Voice Disorders: An Interdisciplinary Approach* (Thieme-Stratton, New York, 1980)

Baker, D. C. and Savetsky, L. 'Congenital Partial Atresia of the Larynx', *Laryngoscope*, 77 (1966)

Dalton, P. and Hardcastle, W. J. *Disorders of Fluency and their Effects on Communication* (Arnold, London, 1977)

Fawcus, R. 'The Treatment of Phonological Disorders', in Jones, F. M. (ed.) *Language Disabilities in Children* (MTP Press, Lancaster, 1980)

Fourcin, A. J. and Abberton, E. 'First Applications of a New Laryngograph', *Medical and Biological Illustration* 21, 172 (1971)

Greene, M. C. L. 'Problems Involved in the Speech and Language Training of the Partially Deaf Child', *Speech Pathology and Therapy*, 4, 22 (1961)

—— *The Voice and its Disorders* (Pitman Medical, Tunbridge Wells, 1980)

Gutzmann, H. Sr. 'Ein Beitrag zur Frage der Eunuchenähnlichen Stimme'. *Medizinische Padagogische Monatsschrift*, 33 (1897)

Hirano, M., Vennard, W. and Ohala, J. 'Regulation of Register, Pitch and Intensity of Voice — An Electromyographic Investigation of Intrinsic Laryngeal Muscles', *Folia Phoniatrica (Basel)* 22 (1970)

Luchsinger, R. and Arnold, G. E. *Voice, Speech and Language* (Constable, London, 1965)

Makuen, G. H. 'Falsetto Voice in the Male', *Journal of the American Medical Association*, 32, 474 (1899)

Seth, G. and Guthrie, D. *Speech in Childhood* (Oxford University Press, Oxford, 1935)

West, R., Ansberry, M. and Carr, A. *The Rehabilitation of Speech* (Harper, New York, 1957)

13 THE VOICE OF THE TRANSSEXUAL

Judith Challoner

Introduction

It may seem a departure from the traditional view of the speech therapist's role in the treatment of voice disorders to include a chapter on voice work with transsexuals (individuals who feel they have been born into the wrong-sex body). However, it is important to realise that this type of work is increasingly becoming the responsibility of the speech therapist as part of a medical team working with these clients. Consequently there is a need for these therapists to be aware of the medical programme involved when sexual reassignment is considered, and be conversant with the transsexual condition and the many ramifications that work of this type entails – in addition to any therapy procedures that may be undertaken.

The object of this chapter, therefore, is to give speech therapists a background knowledge about transsexualism, guidelines for approaching voice work with these clients, and suggestions about general management.

Most transsexuals want to have a sex-change operation, and with a view to possibly qualifying for this very serious undertaking they must undergo rigorous screening. Part of this preoperative period may include help to make their voices sound as convincingly feminine as possible.

Much of the discussion in this chapter is based on personal experience gleaned over a number of years working with groups of these preoperative transsexual clients, during which time more than 50 individuals were referred to the programme.

The groups ran weekly for two hours in 12-week blocks with many clients attending for two blocks. The numbers in a group ranged from six to a maximum of ten. At all times a total approach was aimed at, with a beauty therapist working closely with the speech therapist. Individual voice work was coupled with general communication skills.

Final results regarding the voice work were, in general, very satisfactory at a subjective level. Approximately a quarter of these clients eventually had a sex-change operation; some are still waiting, and approximately a quarter dropped out of the programme or were encouraged to leave. It is always accepted that many individuals in a situation of this kind are simply not able to satisfy the rigid requirements imposed during this trial period.

Long-term contact has been sustained with many group members whom it was felt achieved a satisfactory voice result, and in general their own attitude to their voices is one of ease when speaking, with little attention to the mechanics involved. They feel, for the most part, that their voices are acceptable and no longer cause them personal concern. This is the compromise that the therapist hopes to achieve – a convincing sounding voice and a confident unselfconscious speaker.

The first referral of a transsexual client to a speech therapist may well present a daunting prospect. This is not surprising as it is unlikely that there will have been much reference to work of this type during training; consequently it will probably be a situation far removed from both clinical and personal experience.

In England the majority of work with transsexuals is concentrated in three London hospitals, Charing Cross, King's College and the Maudesley, and speech therapists associated with these centres, particularly at Charing Cross tend, by strength of their experience, to handle these cases. Because of the extreme confidentiality of the client's situation, and consideration for his personal feelings, there is usually little if any speech therapy student involvement.

The fact that there is increasing interest and research into more sophisticated measurements of differences between male and female voices, with precise data regarding fundamental frequency and intensity findings, as well as linguistic features, is very encouraging to those exploring this area of work. This will be discussed below in this chapter. It is hoped that any therapist who feels that he or she has a client who is a suitable subject for self-monitoring work with instrumentation techniques, or if the precise progress needs to be recorded, will realise the possibilities in this area.

This discussion, however, is largely a basic and practical guide based on empirical observation to be expanded by individual therapists as their own knowledge and expertise increases, and to suit each particular situation.

The Transsexual Condition

The term transsexual was coined by an American psychiatrist, Harry Benjamin (1966), who reported on a number of cases and became one of the prime initiators to stimulate study of the subject.

In her study on bisexuality, Charlotte Wolff (1979) defines transsexuals as people who believe that their mind is trapped in the wrong-sex body. As she explains, some are satisfied with hormone therapy, but many insist on surgery. There is a violent clash between their sexual and gender identity. It is the sense of belonging to the opposite sex that disturbs them rather than the qualities of 'masculinity' or 'femininity'.

Benjamin believed that there were a number of causes for the condition (far more common in men than women) and that some were biological and some psychological. There are many other psychiatrics with a variety of theories, but no clearcut consensus has evolved. It is clear, however, that there is not a chromosomal abnormality in these individuals.

Whatever the aetiology, these people feel overwhelmingly that they are in the wrong-gender body. This conviction has been with them their entire life and has been the dominant feature of existence. Mentally and emotionally they completely identify with the opposite sex, and feel that their body is a tragic mistake.

In their study on gender identity, Money and Ehrhardt (1972) explain that the transsexual is driven by a compulsion to have the appearance, body and social status of the opposite sex.

Most transsexual clients referred to a speech therapist would be candidates for a gender reassignment operation. They would be having psychiatric consultations, and if necessary seeing the psychiatric social worker who might be helping with the practical difficulties involved when a change of lifestyle such as this is being organised. The social worker may also be involved in family counselling of the client's partner, children or parents.

Although, of course, transsexuals can be of either sex this discussion deals exclusively with the male-to-female situation.

The sex change operation is where the male sex organs are removed or modified to create an artificial vagina. The patient is in hospital for about ten days and requires at least six weeks recuperation – usually considerably longer. For most patients the elation at finally having 'the operation' seems to transcend the very considerable discomfort immediately following the surgery.

At a later date some transsexuals also elect to have breast implantation surgery. Although hormone therapy is usually part of the preoperative treatment, and is carried on afterwards, the resulting breast development is only moderate and often not sufficient to satisfy the desire for a totally feminine figure.

There is often confusion about transvestism (the act of cross-dressing, usually in connection with sexual arousal, without the desire to actually have the identity of the opposite sex), homosexuality and certain sexual fetishes, in connection with transsexualism. One should be aware that there may perhaps have been some overlap into these areas at times, and that many transsexuals have had a variety of sexual experimentation. However, the true transsexual wants above all to appear and be accepted as the opposite sex; all other sexual considerations are very much secondary to this.

The progress of most of these clients follows a certain pattern. In early adulthood they try to conform to accepted social expectations and fit into their gender role. Many have deliberately taken on a very masculine job in hopes that it might help resolve their conflicting feelings. Quite a number of transsexuals say they have joined a branch of the armed forces for this reason.

A continuation of this pattern is that many transsexuals marry and have children, but in most cases they say that sexual relations were conducted as a duty, and that they had little interest in that aspect of the relationship. The rapport with their wives is often warm and loving; there is frequently a feeling of guilt in later years that their obsessional feeling has destroyed the marriage and caused the partner pain and distress. Many wives remain ignorant of the situation for years while others are aware of the problem, but try to live with it.

It is surprising that in this sexually enlightened age it is not uncommon for a transsexual to reach middle age and be unaware that his sexual dilemma is not unique. These people are generally those who read little and have been unwilling or unable to discuss their personal feelings and voice their fears to others. Although nearly all transsexuals have had experiences of cross-dressing (wearing clothing of the opposite sex) even as children, this may have continued as an entirely secret pastime into adulthood.

Case History 1

John is a 60-year-old civil servant in a provincial city. His entire early life was led against a background of emotional unfulfilment, and a feeling of anxiety that he was going insane because he had the persistent feeling that he should have been a woman. The fact that he is an extremely masculine appearing individual with heavy facial hair growth made his predicament seem, to him, compounded. He had a successful army career as a young man, and his married life was happy in spite of his disinterest in sex. There were two children and he was outwardly conforming to a routine pattern of life, although cross-dressing whenever he was alone in the house. It was reading an excerpt from the book *Conundrum* by the journalist Jan Morris (1974) which changed John's life. The book, which was serialised in a Sunday newspaper, was an account of Jan's life as James until she was over 40, and her struggle with her sexual identity, subsequent sex-change operation and adjustment to a new way of life.

John realised that his feelings were not unique, and once told the group of the feeling of joy and relief that this realisation made, even if nothing was resolved by it immediately. He was at that time recently widowed and sought medical advice from his doctor who referred him to the Gender Identity Clinic at Charing Cross Hospital in London. From there he was given counselling and included in a group of ten other transsexual clients.

After living full-time as a woman, and being medically retired from his job he was referred to the surgeon. His case ended unsatisfactorily for him as the surgeon refused to operate because he felt that in spite of a stable personality and passable voice, his appearance was too masculine, even if assisted with all possible camouflage techniques to enable him to pass successfully as a woman.

John continues to live in the female role with great support from his daughter, but no longer has contact with his son who refused to accept the situation.

One must remember the great responsibility that falls to the psychiatrist and surgeon when taking a decision to irrevocably alter another human being's life in this way. The long and often difficult 'trial period' is necessary for this reason as well as being in the client's long-term interest. It is interesting to note that not all psychiatrists view surgery as the answer. Benjamin (1966), for example, viewed it as a last resort – to be considered only if the patient was felt to be suicidal. He felt that more conservative therapy was often the appropriate course.

The majority of transsexuals seek help earlier than John. However, the age span of the group members was not particularly young, between 26 and 65 years, the main spread being between 34 and 45.

The average procedure for the client is that the psychiatrist will combine hormone therapy with counselling. The hormones produce some secondary sex characteristics such as modest breast growth, some surface fat, some reduction of beard growth and skin softening. If a client is not suitable for hormone therapy for some medical reason, such as history of thrombosis, the refusal of these drugs can cause depression and panic. Much reassurance will be needed that this therapy is not absolutely necessary.

Before referral to a surgeon the client must live full time and be able to support himself as a woman for at least a year. This latter stipulation is vital because the question of employment is often very difficult for the transsexual to resolve. It is not uncommon for an individual to live and work as a man by day and conduct his domestic and social life as a woman, sometimes for many years. It is difficult to give up a secure job for something new, particularly when there are many other pressures as well. Some clients are lucky enough and have sufficient confidence to make the transition quickly and openly.

Case History 2

Simon, 42, is a highly paid scientific officer with a large company where his expertise is very much valued. He lived a double life for years until, with the support of his wife, he approached the firm with his problem, and was allowed to continue in the same firm as a woman. He continues to live in the same house with his former wife and daughter and has now had the operation.

A further condition for surgery is that the transsexual must be divorced if married and have provided for any dependants. He must satisfy the psychiatrist that he is mentally stable before referral to the surgeon who has the ultimate decision.

Not all transsexuals, even those considered suitable for surgery, elect to have it. One extremely convincing-looking (and sounding) client who satisfied all the criteria and had, in fact, lived many years as a woman never wanted referral for the operation. He explained that counselling had enabled him to come to terms with the situation and help with voice and grooming had boosted confidence. However, he felt the operation would be an act of mutilation that would not, in his case, change his lifestyle. He continues to live, apparently successfully, as a woman.

Physical appearance has not any real bearing on the transsexualism of an individual. Often very masculine-looking men feel inwardly feminine. Appearance seems to act neither as a deterrent nor an impetus towards wanting a sex change.

Acoustic and Linguistic Considerations in Transsexual Treatment by Speech Therapists

It is appropriate at this point to discuss research work done in this area. Oates and Dacakis (1983) give a very full review of the rather scattered and inconclusive literature on communication problems of transsexuals. They understandably give considerable emphasis to research in Australia (where their own clinical work was carried out) and on published American work. Much of the information is based on results with individual patients.

As these authors emphasise, 'the validity and efficacy of management procedures remains limited, until a more comprehensive data base on sex markers in speech is delineated'. In this connection they discuss the important distinction between male and female 'speech markers' (on which there is little valid published data) and 'speech stereotypes'. The former are those features of speech both segmental and non-segmental, which constitute the clues by which we consciously or unconsciously assign gender to a speaker when other (for example visual) indicators are lacking or ambiguous.

The 'speech stereotypes' are the subjective expectations of the average person as to what they expect the speech of one or other sex to be. For the purist the speech markers are the important attributes of which we need to know more. These are ill-defined. What makes us identify an unknown voice on the radio as male or female? Even those who have carefully researched such 'markers' produce inconclusive results. Of course fundamental frequency is the most obvious of these markers. Oates and Dacakis (1983) summarise the findings of studies into fundamental frequency of adult speech as follows: adult males from 20 to 29 years have an appropriate mean of 138 Hz with a range of 60–260 Hz. Females of the same age have a mean of 227 Hz with a range of 128 to

520 Hz. They conclude, 'thus although female voices average 1.7 times higher in fundamental frequency than do those of males, the ranges for males and females overlap considerably'. It is also mentioned that in older age there is a considerable reduction in the difference between the fundamental frequencies of male and female speakers although no figures are given.

Perhaps 'stereotypes' are more important to the fulfilment of the transsexual's expectations than the fundamental speech markers. As Oates and Dacakis (1983) record 'the client's goals often arise largely from stereotypical beliefs'. In other words it is perhaps more important that the client thinks he is creating the expected image than that they are actually reproducing the precise idiosyncrasy of the intended voice.

In summary, the help that a speech therapist can give to the transsexual is still based on empirical observations. Until more fundamental research on absolute speech markers has been carried out the therapist will be guided by subjective criteria.

Responsibility of the Speech Therapist

Voice Work

The therapist gives help and practical advice on voice modification to give as plausible and acceptable results as possible to the receiver.

Encouraging General Communication Skills

There cannot be too much emphasis on developing a confident manner coupled with as convincing an appearance as possible. Expectation in the listener of hearing a female-sounding voice, because the speaker appears at ease and looks female, is often enough to defy the critical ear.

Referral to Other Agencies

This entails referral to the appropriate source for additional help if it is indicated. Advice is often sought regarding grooming, clothes or make-up. Obvious basic suggestions can be made, but referral to a beauty therapist is more satisfactory.

Information about the formalities of changing names by deed poll and queries about legal documents, and other matters of a legal nature, should be referred to the psychiatric social worker, whose responsibility it will be to talk to employers and to do any family counselling.

Nearly all male transsexuals have several years of electrolysis once or twice a week. This is very expensive and time-consuming. Many beauty clinics run evening sessions for men only, as for example the Tao Clinic.

The Albany Trust (24 Chester Square, London SW1) was set up 25 years ago to provide an information and counselling service for members of sexual minorities. This society can give a client the telephone number of a self-help transsexual group which is often able to supply useful addresses and other support facilities. The Trust can also put the client in touch with the Beaumont Society. This was originally founded for transvestites, but transsexuals are also welcome and it provides a social base; wives are also free to attend and many have found it very supportive. Some transsexuals dislike association with the Beaumont Society, but it can be a useful link since it also publishes a newsletter which includes sources for wigs, clothes, large-sized women's shoes and other items sometimes difficult to find or embarrassing to ask for in shops.

Refraining from Personal Involvement

This should be mentioned because it may be a temptation to try to undertake more in the way of counselling – often at the request of the client – than one is qualified to give. Transsexual referrals are unique in speech therapy work. One must be aware that some of the clients may be under more stress than is immediately apparent, and require specialised guidance.

Voice Work

It is assumed that anyone attempting voice work with these clients will be completely familiar with the mechanics of the normal voice and have had experience of working with adult voice patients. The anatomical differences of the voice-producing apparatus of the male and female, such as size of larynx, and length and mass of vocal tract, will be well-known.

The rationale, therefore, behind any techniques suggested will be self-evident, so it is expedient to outline the therapy programme in terms one would use in explanation to a client. All the following procedures have been practised without creating problems of vocal strain.

The only case of hoarseness among the group members started when a client was about to have the operation and it persisted to such a degree that she was seen postoperatively by an ENT surgeon. It was found to be an entirely functional problem and gradually resolved itself in a few months. This man had had a long period of caring for a dying wife, in addition to many personal problems, as well as the prospect of this major operation.

It might be argued that as this is essentially an exercise in acting it might be more expedient to send transsexuals to a drama coach. After all, the only 'disorder' of the voice is that the client views it as a hindrance to his ability to function successfully as a woman. However, these are not professional actors but troubled individuals who need the help of someone used to dealing with people under stress where there is medical back-up available.

This reference to acting may seem obvious, but it is not always easy for these clients to accept this idea. It has been my experience that much as a transsexual may wish to produce a convincing female voice naturally, he often dislikes the idea of having to deliberately work on achieving it. To concentrate on how the voice sounds and thinking about altering its production is sometimes, understandably, felt to inhibit thought and conversation.

It is the dislike of feeling they must 'put on an act' that worries the transsexual. This feeling does not extend to wearing female dress or make-up, because this is the natural taste and inclination. Clothes are simply part of the female image that he wants to project to the world and himself. To achieve concentrated effort on voice training it may be necessary to discuss the fact that although one may understandably dislike the mechanics involved, good results are possible, and with practice it will be easier and more automatic to produce an acceptable voice.

It is convenient to divide the plan for voice work into the following categories and for these to be interweaved as appropriate:

(1) Assessment.
(2) Relaxation.
(3) Voice experimentation.
(4) Breathing for speech.
(5) Pitch establishment.
(6) Elimination of chest resonance.
(7) Intonation, peaking and lilt.
(8) Role playing and self-expression practice.
(9) Non-verbal communication.
(10) Personality projection and communication skills.

Assessment

As assessment is our tool for drawing up a plan for treatment, the following outline is suggested as a useful guide. We assume that the client will present at the initial interview dressed as a woman and using his 'female voice' if he has one.

(1) Is the voice convincing enough to pass as feminine?
(2) Does it need only minor adjustments?
(3) Is it a light-sounding male voice?
(4) Is it unmistakeably masculine?

This impression will be influenced (as it should be) by how well the client presents and how much at ease he is with his voice and his ability to communicate as a woman. Many clients have been playing this role successfully for years. There can be every permutation of looks and voice with no absolute categories.

The following should be noted:

(1) Quality of voice.
(2) Impression of the degree of chest resonance.
(3) Pitch.
(4) Method of delivery.
(5) Manner of articulation.
(6) Type of breathing used for speech.
(7) Manner of speech. Is it flat and unemotional? Is there a regional accent? Has an attempt been made to make it sound feminine by being overly affected in speech?
(8) Physical impression. One needs to record how he presents as a person, how intelligent he appears to be, his size, age, and appropriateness of his clothes and make-up. One must also

> note habits that detract from his appearing to be a relaxed speaker, or communicator in general, as for example poor eye contact, rigidity of face, an over-anxious manner, covering his mouth or Adam's apple, and similar traits.

All these aspects of the speaker and his voice will give a profile, and one can draw up a list of priorities to work through, eliminating certain aspects, modifying others or capitalising on them.

In general, as was mentioned earlier, one will naturally expect the pitch to be lower. There will also probably be too much chest resonance for a female-sounding voice. It sounds very simplistic to state the following, but what one is attempting to do is to instruct the speaker in ways to modify his own speech production. The plan set out has been a useful flexible checklist to follow.

It is interesting to note that one of the most convincing speakers in any of the groups was a small frail-looking South American man with an elegant manner, and at 43 an excellent dress choice appropriate to his size and age. His gentle contralto voice, speaking English with a strong Portuguese accent, was totally feminine. I was interested that he refused to speak in his native tongue during the eight months I knew him, although I often asked him to, so I could compare the effect of speaking his second language rather slowly and deliberately, with his more fluent speech.

The glaring problem that Carlo had was complete lack of any animation, and a rigidity of face and manner that called attention to him unfavourably, and detracted from his ability to establish rapport with others no matter how good an image he created.

In this particular case we spent a great deal of time doing role-play exercises and relaxation therapy, as well as talking about the problem, of which he was well aware. He became far more animated and began to relate much more normally with others, but still had somewhat of a 'wax dummy' image that drew the eye. Too much perfection perhaps is not totally feminine. In any case he went on to have the operation and one would feel this was a total success story, but I felt far less satisfied with Carlo's ability to cope with a new lifestyle, than some who seemed more 'human' in spite of their imperfections. One must always be aware of the total person.

Relaxation

Whatever the feeling about the use of relaxation as part of voice therapy, it is a useful aid in getting an individual to feel in control of his own body. Progressive relaxation is effective and it is important to suggest that the client concentrate on feeling the state of relaxation in order to try to return to it at times of alarm or great tension. In her book on voice disorders, Greene (1975) summarises many of the various relaxation techniques.

Vocal Experimentation

Most individuals have no idea of the variety and range of sounds that the voice is capable of producing. It is often reassuring for someone to realise that it is possible to free his voice from rigid vocal habits even if he feels initially embarrassed attempting it. To accomplish this, suggest that imitation is made of sounds that have no direct connection with speech and require no intellectual effort, such as copying musical instruments, birds, sounds of nature and even animal noises. This type of exercise is very disinhibiting and encourages further voice experimentation.

Breathing for Speech

Instruction in diaphragmatic breathing, with exercises to increase the efficiency of breath control is extremely important. The procedure then explained to the client is that instead of pushing the surge of air needed for articulation into the mouth in a powerful stream, he employs another method. This 'other' method involves taking gentle 'tucks' of air into the mouth from the reservoir created by efficient diaphragmatic breathing, and then articulating. This will have the effect, if combined with light articulation, of adding a very slightly breathy quality. This breathy sound will need careful monitoring to be sure that it is not overly noticeable, but if it is done properly the softening result can be very effective.

Pitch Establishment

There is often the thought that for a man to make his voice sound more feminine he should raise the pitch to falsetto. In reality, of course, all that this accomplishes is to make the voice sound like a man speaking in a falsetto voice! In addition, even if it were effective, it would be a very difficult type of speech for most people to sustain.

As was mentioned there is considerable overlap between the pitch ranges of male and female voices. Often in the middle-aged speaker the pitch needs to be raised only slightly. It is the resonant quality that makes the voice sound more 'male' than the actual pitch. The pitch level which is finally deemed as appropriate to try to adopt will be decided both by what the therapist thinks is suitable to the individual and by a realistic appraisal of the client's abilities.

Practice and ear training are necessary, and the system many clients find satisfactory is to identify the starting pitch they wish to achieve with a note on the scale. Even the very unmusical will have done some rudimentary singing and will understand this method.

Reading aloud, first at sentence level and later expanding into poetry or prose that required some expression, is a useful method of practice in maintaining pitch level. In all stages of therapy choosing suitable reading material is important. Most of the group found it helpful to make their own tapes at home which would then be brought to the classes for discussion and comment.

Elimination of Chest Resonance

This is one of the most vital areas of this work. Using material with many /m/ phrases, have the client read them aloud in his male voice feeling the hum at the top of the chest with his hand as he reads. He can then practise humming only and gradually 'push' the sound up until the shift of vibration can be physically felt to move into the face, and then practise reading the same material as before making as little vibration as possible in the chest region. This will be done, of course, partly in connection with the work on breathing and on pitch, but it is often less confusing for the client to concentrate on one area at a time.

Articulation Techniques

Emphasis should be on 'light' articulation with suggestions that the client thinks deliberately of making delicate contact with lips, tongue and teeth as he reads a prepared passage. He should focus speech forward in the face as much as possible, in other words he should *push* the voice forward. It was mentioned earlier that suitable choice of practice material is helpful particularly if a client can identify with it and feel 'feminine' when reading it.

Peaking, Intonation and Lilt

Peaking is a term used to explain the method of raising the pitch of the voice at intervals on certain syllables to add variety and keep up the pitch level. This can be practised using a marked passage with an arbitrary marking of syllables. I have noticed that in general the female voice tends to have more pitch variation, and I have tried to mark passages accordingly.

Role Playing, Non-verbal Communication and Personality Projection

These last three items are areas that are combined together and are very much interlinked. One must always be aware that the client is a communicating individual as well as a 'voice case'. Most therapists will have had the experience of using this type of therapy in other areas of work.

Role play was used a great deal in the group situation and proved an excellent means of practising techniques learned. When emotive or controversial subjects were discussed, many clients found it difficult, initially, to maintain the voice standard they achieved in a simple clinical situation. One of the reasons that some individuals came for so many months was the chance for long-term practise.

Male mannerisms and habits need to be called to the client's attention and eliminated. These will be self-evident when the situation arises. Another point worth noting is that the circumstances of their lives have often made some transsexuals so self-absorbed that they find it hard to communicate whether as a man or a woman. Awareness of the barriers that have been built up is a step to breaking them down.

Vocal Cord Surgery

The rationale behind performing surgery on the transsexual's vocal cords was that if the cords were reduced in length (by pulling the cords through the arytenoids and fastening them) the pitch would be raised. In reality most speech therapists dealing with these patients postoperatively find little change. There does, however, tend to be some reduction in the laryngeal prominence, although not dramatically. Oddly enough, even with the knowledge of these results this is still a much-requested operation by transsexuals, regardless of the unavoidable discomfort involved.

Summary

Most transsexuals can achieve an adequately unisex voice to enable them to be absorbed into the world as females provided they are intelligent enough to understand what is expected of them. Far more important, however, than the vocal mechanics is the building of a confident manner and a feeling of self-worth in the individual. Not all transsexuals are going to completely blend into society as women, although many do and those are the ones that we do not notice. Life for some will eventually have to be a great compromise. But even this compromise can often bring a greater degree of happiness and peace of mind than has ever been experienced before. Research is going on to enable us to measure more accurately the differences between the voices of the sexes. It may be that even when there is fuller theoretical understanding of male/female discriminators this will not materially affect the present empirical pattern of therapy adopted in these cases.

References

Benjamin, H. *The Transsexual Phenomenon* (New York, 1966)

Greene, M. *The Voice and its Disorders* (Pitman Medical, London, 1975)

Morris, J. *Conundrum* (Faber, London, 1974)

Money, J. and Erhardt, A. *Man and Woman — Boy and Girl* (The Johns Hopkins University Press, Baltimore and London, 1972)

Oates, J. M. and Dacakis, G. 'Speech Pathology Considerations in the Management of Transsexualism — A Review', *British Journal of Disorders of Communication*, 18(3), 139–51 (1983)

Wolff, C. *Bisexuality, A Study* (Quartet Books, London, 1977)

14 THE VOICE OF THE DEAF

Sheila Wirz

Introduction

The speaker characteristics of hearing-impaired people are different from those of speakers who are able to use their auditory sense to monitor their production of speech. This book is concerned with voice and it is the vocal characteristics of hearing-impaired people that are discussed here. Vocal characteristics are discussed in two ways, first by a review of the literature about 'deaf voice' and secondly with illustration from a study applying the Vocal Profiles Analysis scheme (VPA) to the description of 'deaf voice'.

There are of course a whole range of reasons why and how the voice of a hearing-impaired person may be aberrant, reasons such as the degree and type of hearing loss; the age at which the person became deaf; the type and appropriateness of the auditory amplification prescribed; the educational regime which the speaker followed; and the amount of speech therapy which the speaker has had, etc.

This however, is a book about voice, not deafness and the aim of this chapter is to describe the voice of hearing-impaired speakers, not to replicate descriptions of the effects of hearing loss upon spoken language. Comprehensive reviews of these effects are included in Sims, Walters and Whitehead (1982) and in Hochberg, Levitt and Osberger (1983).

There is of course an enormous difference between the speach characteristics of a hearing-impaired speaker who has had a period of normal hearing (and normal auditory feedback) and another who has never heard. The hearing-impaired population themselves refer only to the latter, the congenitally deaf, as deaf. This chapter is primarily concerned with the voice of congenitally deaf speakers. A thorough review of the speech and voice characteristics of speakers with acquired hearing loss is given by Parker (1983). She outlines the difficulties of speech production which occur after the onset of hearing impairment. She divides these into changes in speech production which affect the 'naturalness' of speech production and those which affect intelligibility.

She refers specifically to problems which may arise in the breathing patterns of deafened adults, related or unrelated to increased tension and the effects which this can have upon phonation.

Parker also points out that a loss of the facility to control smooth and appropriate pitch changes is common among deafened speakers with marked effect upon their intonation patterns. Difficulties in controlling volume and rhythm may also occur. These speech parameters if disrupted will affect the speaking characteristics of the deafened speaker but they are unlikely to grossly affect intelligibility.

Deafened adults, Parker notes, may also have disruption at a phonetic level of speech production. Changes of the phonological structure are unlikely among speakers who have learned the rules of speech before the onset of their hearing impairment.

In this chapter, the definition of voice which will be followed is one which includes those parameters at laryngeal, supralaryngeal and subglottal levels, which interact to affect a speakers voice.

Deaf speakers have abnormal voices. Received wisdom and casual observation support this view, and the invitation to contribute this chapter to a collection such as this seems to lend confirmation to it. Yet the literature is confused and confusing in its descriptions of deaf voices. It is often difficult to establish whether a writer is referring to a disturbance at a laryngeal level, or uses the term 'voice' or 'voice quality' to refer to the over all product of a deaf speakers vocal apparatus.

In this review the relevant literature has been divided for convenience into three sections.

(1) A review of that literature which refers to the laryngeal performance of hearing-impaired speakers;
(2) A review of those studies referring to the velopharyngeal incompetence disturbing the resonance characteristics of deaf speakers.
(3) And finally a consideration of those studies which have looked at other prosodic aspects of deaf speakers.

There is, of course, considerable overlap between the various parameters of deaf speech which can be disturbed, and any division of the literature in an arbitary way like this leads to problems of classification. For example, does one classify loudness as a comment on the laryngeal performance of a deaf speaker or as a reflection of his disturbed prosody? 'Over fortis' is frequently cited (but seldom defined!) in the literature as a feature of deaf speech. Is 'over fortis' synonymous with loudness or is it an articulatory feature?

Laryngeal Features of Deaf Speech

The inability of hearing-impaired speakers to control their laryngeal performance results in different voice quality and poorly controlled pitch and intonation. These factors are commonly cited in the literature. Jones (1967) in his study lists the attributes of voice quality which are most commonly cited as: 'tense', 'flat', 'breathy' 'harsh', 'throaty', 'monotone', 'lack of rhythm', 'poor resonance' and 'poor carrying power'. Calvert (1962) also noted that none of the adjectives used by teachers of the deaf to describe the voice of deaf speakers suggested pleasing quality – all were unpleasant.

Poor laryngeal control is often attributed in the early literature to abnormal breathing patterns. Rawlings (1935) found that the speech of deaf people is 'breathy and accompanied by excessive breathing movements'. Hudgins (1937) at a similar time also noted that the deaf expended more breath on each 'unit of speech' (he appears to mean syllable) than did hearing speakers. Peterson (1953) investigated the co-ordination of breathing and articulatory timing by hearing-impaired speakers, and suggested that it was the difference in transitions which led to the perception of their voice quality as being different from that of hearing speakers. Calvert (1962) looked at harsh and breathy voices of deaf speakers and compared these with simulated voices of hearing speakers. He concluded that deaf voice quality was identified not only by fundamental frequency and subsequent harmonies but by information from the articulatory timing of deaf speech.

Stark (1972) studied the vocalisations of young (preverbal) deaf children and one of her observations was that young deaf children did not acquire control over voicing or pitch and intensity variation as did hearing children.

A variety of terms, then, such as hoarse, breathy, weak, harsh, husky or strident have been used to describe the voice quality of the deaf. (Fairbanks, 1960; Zemlin, 1968; Nickerson, 1975). While there appears to be some general agreement as to what these terms mean, there have been very few efforts to study how these perceptual features can be related to acoustic aspects or to the actual respiratory and phonatory dynamics responsible for the quality.

In attempts to describe voice quality in deaf speakers many studies have used perceptual ratings but few have gone on to demonstrate that the use of such ratings is replicable and can be used with considerable interjudge reliability. Markides (1983) asked 30 teachers of the deaf and 36 lay people to rate the voice quality of 85 hearing-impaired children. But in this study one does not know if the teachers were similarly using terms such as 'deep', 'throaty', 'hoarse' or 'soft', 'fairly normal', 'deep', or whether they were using different terms to describe the same phenomenon.

However, there are studies which demonstrate that valid reliable judgements of voice quality can be obtained using perceptual rating scales (Yanagihara, 1967; Whitehead and Emanuel, 1974; Whitehead and Subtelny, 1976). Monsen (1978) compared listeners' evaluations of the same word tokens on different occasions.

One of the qualities commonly cited as characteristic of deaf speakers is a tense/harsh voice quality. At the National Technical Institute for the Deaf (NTID) between 10 and 12 per cent of students entering college education have tense/harsh voice quality. This term is used in the voice classification scheme employed by the speech pathologists at NTID where there is high reliability of perceptual judgements by experienced judges (Subtelny, 1975). Wirz, Subtelny and Whitehead (1979) attempted to isolate the acoustic features which allowed this high interjudge reliability. An examination of the spectrographic features of deaf speakers' production showed that generally tense phonations of the vowels of hearing-impaired speakers were significantly different from those phonations perceived to be relaxed. The difference was characterised by increased distribution of higher amplitudes of sound energy in the higher frequencies of the spectrum.

It is clear that there continues to be lack of agreement in the published literature about voice quality in hearing-impaired speakers, even when care is taken in the research design to ensure objectivity with perceptual ratings. It is possible to specify reasons for this lack of agreement. Firstly, the speech item in the sample may affect the perceived quality (Rees, 1958). Secondly, a variety of spectral features contribute to a perceived quality, and although there are discernible general spectral features among deaf speakers there is also considerable individual voice variation (Wirz and Anthony 1979; Whitehead and Emanuel, 1974). Thirdly, if the aberrant quality is associated with laryngeal tension there may be accompanying supralaryngeal tension (Spector *et al.*, 1979) which affects other speech parameters.

Commonly the literature refers impressionistically to 'high pitch' among deaf speakers (see, for example, Boone, 1966; Miller, 1968; Martony, 1966; Levitt, 1971) without attempting to define more closely the pitch level. Rather than apply impressionistic labels other writers have described the laryngeal performance of deaf speakers by looking at the pitch and intonation. One of the earliest attempts to look at pitch parameters among hearing-impaired speakers through instrumentation is that of Voelker (1935). He used stroboscopic techniques to describe both mean pitch and pitch range in a group of 28 deaf children and compared them with a group of matched controls. He found that 'the average pitch of the deaf voice was identical with the average normal voice' (Voelker, 1935). However, when he investigated pitch range, he found that the deaf used a narrower range than their hearing peers — '80 per cent of the deaf have less average pitch change than the normals'. He goes on to stress that deaf speakers *do* use pitch movement although in a more restricted way and with more 'perseverated pitch patterns' than do hearing speakers.

Gilbert and Campbell (1980) studied the fundamental frequency characteristics of deaf and hearing children and found in a subject intragroup analysis of variance, there was no significant difference between the deaf and the hearing individuals. His work suggests that there is a trend for some hearing-impaired speakers to have a higher pitch than their hearing peers, but that this is not always the case. In Gilbert's study the fundamental frequency of young adult females who were hearing-impaired was approximately 30 Hz higher than the data reported by Michel, Hollien and Moore (1966) for hearing young female speakers. Similarly the fundamental frequency of the young adult deaf male group was approximately 20 Hz higher than that of hearing young men reported by Hollien and Shipp (1972).

Not only is the fundamental frequency of hearing-impaired speakers reported to be different, and usually thought to be higher, but also the frequency range is reported to be narrower. Angelloci (1962) in a spectrographic analysis of deaf speech found that hearing-impaired speakers had a wider range of distribution of the mean fundamental frequencies but that the speech of the hearing-impaired speakers was monotonous. Monsen (1978) noted that there is no correlation between the speech intelligibility of hearing-impaired adolescents and either mean fundamental frequency or mean change of fundamental frequency. Thus, while noting that it is 'commonplace that poor control of fundamental frequency detracts from the speech intelligibility of the hearing impaired, it is not entirely clear how the pitch control of hearing impaired differs from normal in ways that affect voice quality' (Monsen, 1978).

Velopharyngeal Features

Nasal voice quality is frequently cited as one of the characteristics of deaf speakers.

Hudgins (1934) in his classic study was the first to describe 'excessive nasal resonance' as a feature of deaf speech. However, it is always difficult to establish the features which influence the perception of 'nasality'. Spriesterbach (1955) has demonstrated with cleft palate speakers that the perceived quality of 'nasality' is affected by features such as misarticulation and pitch variation. We can infer that this is probably the case with the speech of the hearing-impaired, and that many of the references to nasality in deaf speech refer to either misarticulation of nasals, or lack of oral/nasal distinctions, or to pitch variation, or any combination of these parameters! In addition some writers may also be referring to the actual feature of nasal resonance.

Colton and Cooker (1968) in an attempt to minimise the confounding influence of misarticulation, pitch variation etc. used backwards playback as a technique to investigate whether naive listeners perceived deaf speakers as being 'more nasal'. They found that hearing students consistently rated the deaf subjects as being 'more nasal' than the hearing even in the group where the hearing subjects read in a 'word by word' manner (attempting to simulate deaf rhythm) (Colton and Cooker, 1968). They did not find a statistically significant difference between the profoundly deaf and the less deaf, as both groups were perceived to be more nasal than the control group.

This search for a relationship between degree of hearing loss and degree of perceived nasality is followed by Seaver, Andrews and Granata (1980). They investigated the velopharyngeal characteristics of 19 hearing-impaired subjects who exhibited nasality. One of their results was a non-significant relationship between degree of perceived nasality and degree of hearing loss. They also investigated the velopharyngeal positioning of these hearing-impaired speakers by the use of lateral x-rays taken during the production of /i/ and /Θ/. Surprisingly they found that in all but one case the velopharyngeal contact observed on these x-rays was very similar to that which one would see in patient's with normal speech. This finding seems to be in direct contrast to the suggestion by Nickerson (1975) that deaf speakers have difficulty in velopharyngeal control! Seaver, Andrews and Granata (1980) conclude that 'in terms of anatomical physiological attributes, the hypernasality observed in the speech of many hearing-impaired speakers is not analogous to the hypernasality observed in the craniofacial cleft population' (p. 246). Thus, although the nasal resonance features of the deaf may be perceived to be similar to those of the velopharyngeal insufficient population they are of a different origin. Boone (1966) raises the question of how deaf speakers achieve their characteristic quality and suggests that the deaf use 'cul-de-sac' resonance by using pharyngeal tension and lowering the body of the tongue.

Other Prosodic Aspects

Other suprasegmental parameters which affect the vocal characteristics of deaf speakers include intensity, intonation and frequency. Frequency disturbances affecting pitch have been reviewed above in the discussion of laryngeal parameters.

Stoker and Lape (1980) posed the question 'is it possible to determine a (hearing-impaired) child's competence in speech with measures other than articulation?' Among the parameters they examined in their sample of 42 hearing-impaired children were breath duration and suprasegmental competence. 'Pitch', 'loudness modulation' and 'duration modulation' were rated by four speech pathologists. Only items with an interjudge reliability coefficient of 0.05 level of confidence or better were included in their study. In this respect the methodology of this study was much more rigorous than many others using ratings.

Stoker and Lape (1980) found that 'pitch modulation', and 'loudness modulation' correlated with hearing loss and intelligibility at an 0.001 level of significance, and breath control and duration modulation correlated at an 0.05 level of significance. Interestingly none of these four suprasegmental features had a significant correlation with hearing aid use, or age, or sex.

Voelker (1935) examined the pitch and timing characteristics of hearing-impaired speakers. He looked at the rhythmic quality of the speech of his 28 hearing-impaired subjects. He comments on the fact that deaf speakers commonly have an interval of 1.0 to 2.1 seconds between adjacent segments. Such intervals among the hearing control group rarely exceeded 0.5 seconds. Rhythm also was disrupted – 'the deaf group used on average 3 times as many phonations to say a sentence as the normals' (Voelker, 1935).

Martony (1966) suggests that the reduction of vowel transitions and the increased holding of vowel postures disrupts rhythm and contributes to a lack of intelligibility.

Levitt (1971) comments on the excessive effort which deaf children use in speech. This excessive effort he refers to as an 'over fortis' of breathing and phonation which is manifest as poor pitch control and rhythm.

Penn (1955) conducted a large-scale study of the vocal characteristics of 100 conductive and 100 nerve deaf speakers in the United States armed services. In her study of suprasegmental features she found that 35 per cent of the nerve deaf subjects 'manifest a loudness that exceeded a level reasonably appropriate to the distance from the listener and to environmental noise while only 9 per cent of conductives revealed this deviation'.

It can be seen from the above review that there is a wide variation in the aspects of deaf voice which have been studied, and the methodologies used to examine these different parameters. What all these studies have in common is that they study one or, in some cases, a few parameters of deaf voice, frequently drawing comparisons with hearing speakers. These studies do not attempt to be assessment procedures but very definitely pinpoint areas where assessment of deaf voice would be advisable.

A range of assessment techniques exist but it is tempting to suggest that many of them fall into the category described by Butterworth (1980) who suggests that a common research strategy for investigating speech is for the investigator to formulate a hypothesis, hypothesise factors affecting this process, then collect data which meets the needs of his hypothesis. One feels that the assessment of voice and phonation is rather like this. A researcher or clinician lists parameters which are often disturbed in the vocal characteristics of a given group of speakers. The assessment then consists of fitting the speaker to this list of parameters.

One of the problems of a review of existing assessment procedures or an evaluation of descriptions used is that there is a lack of common agreement as to what constitutes voice. As Monsen (1978) says, voice quality is a rather ill-defined term.

> For the phonetician 'voice quality' is a technical term and refers to perceptual attributes pertaining to the way the vocal folds vibrate for example, to laryngeal gestures. In this technical sense it is separate from qualities of speech which derives from articulation. However, while it may be true that the phonetician can listen to a word and separate the poorly executed gestures of the larynx from those of the other speech articulators most listeners probably cannot!

Here Monsen is probably expressing a concern felt by many listeners and going some way to explaining the inefficiency of some of the perceptual assessment procedures reviewed above.

The Vocal Profile Analysis (VPA) Scheme

One of the problems leading to these confusions, is that phonetic theory has provided us with few tools with which to attempt the task of describing parameters (or groups of parameters) such as voice quality. Laver (1968, 1980, Laver *et al.*, 1981) is one of the few phoneticians who has addressed this question. He says:

> if it is the legitimate business of general phonetic theory to take on the task of describing phonetic realizations not only of phonological elements but also of paraphonological attitudinal signals and of the learnable features of voice quality that signal membership of a given community, then a more comprehensive scheme for accounting for phonatory quality has to be available than that at present utilized in linguistic description (Laver, 1980).

Laver (1980) provided such a phonetic description of voice quality by specifying laryngeal and supralaryngeal parameters of voice quality. Laver *et al.* (1981) devised an assessment procedure, the Vocal Profile Analysis (VPA) scheme, which can be applied to both normal and non-normal speakers. The Vocal Profile Analysis scheme is a system which allows description of those parameters at laryngeal and supralaryngeal levels that affect voice and which cannot be readily described using traditional phonetics.

The Vocal Profile Analysis scheme is based on the fact that a speaker's voice quality is derived from those laryngeal and supralaryngeal features which are idiosyncratic to him. Such idiosyncrasy is the product of both the anatomical make-up of the individual and his learned phonetic settings. The anatomy of a speaker's vocal tract will affect his vocal characteristics. These differences in anatomy may be at a supralaryngeal level — for example, a speaker with a class 3 orthodontic bite will have different oral resonance characteristics from a speaker with a class 1 bite. Or, more obviously, a speaker with an inadequate velopharyngeal sphincter will have a different oral/nasal resonance balance from a speaker who is able to achieve adequate velopharyngeal closure.

At a laryngeal level too, anatomical differences will affect phonation. An extreme difference will be the way the increased length and bulk of the vocal folds of an adult male speaker produces a very different phonation from the shorter, less massive folds of a woman or child. Similarly, the change in mass of slightly inflamed oedematous folds will change the phonation characteristics of a speaker.

As well as these skeletal differences which lead to marked differences in voice, the way in which a speaker habitually uses his vocal tract will also affect his voice quality. A speaker who has learned and habitually uses a forward tongue body posture will have a different oral resonance from a similar speaker who has a habitual back posture of tongue body.

Thus a speaker's voice quality can be said to be affected by learned muscular bias and by his anatomical make-up. The VPA identifies those supralaryngeal and laryngeal features which are affected by either long-term muscular bias or by skeletal idiosyncrasy.

These features are muscular bias or skeletal differences at the lips, the jaw, the tongue tip, the tongue body, the velopharynx, and the larynx. As well as identifying the posture of those articulators, the VPA also notes the range of movements of lips, jaw and tongue, the efficacy of phonation and the degree of muscular tension.

The degree of habitual supralaryngeal and laryngeal tension will affect the long-term muscular tension at laryngeal and supralaryngeal levels, and thus voice quality.

The phonetic theory developed by Laver (1979) suggests that by specifying a neutral point for each of these supralaryngeal and laryngeal features, and tension characteristics it is possible to measure displacement from these specified neutral points. Measurements from neutral can be made acoustically or physiologically and they can, of course, also be perceived.

Table 14.1: Parameters Included in a Vocal Profile

Supralaryngeal features	Labial features	Rounded or spread
		Labiodentalised
		Extensive or minimised range
	Jaw features	Close or open
		Protruded
		Extensive or minimised range
	Tongue tip	Advanced or retracted
	Tongue body	Fronted or backed
		Raised or lowered
		Extensive or minimised range
	Velopharyngeal	Nasal or denasal
		Audible nasal escape
Tension features	Pharyngeal tension	
	Supralaryngeal tension	Tense or lax
	Laryngeal tension	Tense or lax
	Larynx position	Raised or lowered
Phonation type		harsh
		whisper
		creak
		falsetto or modal
Prosodic features	Pitch mean	High or low
	Pitch range	Wide or narrow
	Pitch variability	High or low
	Tremor	
	Loudness mean	High or low
	Loudness range	Wide or narrow
	Loudness variability	High or low

The VPA scheme, then, provides a perceptual rating scheme based on neutral settings of supralaryngeal and laryngeal parameters and allows measurement and perceptual rating of a speaker's deviations from the neutral points. The resulting profile of these deviations from neutral is a specification of the characteristics of a speakers voice.

Table 14.1 shows the parameters included in a VPA. A trained user listening to a speaker makes a first judgement as to whether the speaker deviates from neutral for each of the supralaryngeal, laryngeal or prosodic parameters. If there is a deviation from neutral the listener judges whether this is a deviation within or outside the normal range. Having made that judgement the listener then identifies the precise nature of the deviation on a six-point rating scale. The scheme is described much more fully in a forthcoming book.

The application of the VPA can be illustrated by describing its application to the vocal characteristics of hearing-impaired speakers; 40 profoundly hearing-impaired young adults, aged between 18 and 23 years old, in tertiary education, and with an average hearing loss (over the speech frequencies in their better ear of 85 dB) were recorded reading the Rainbow Passage from Fairbanks (1960). Three trained listeners then rated these recordings using the VPA, and had an interjudge reliability of 80 per cent over the 287 scalar degrees of the VPA. They also listened to recordings of 40 hearing speakers. The results of these analyses are presented in Table 14.2.

Difference between Vocal Profiles of Deaf and Hearing Groups

It can be seen from these data that the differences between the vocal profiles of the deaf and hearing groups can be divided broadly into four groups.

(1) Ratings relating to the range of movements.
(2) Ratings relating to pitch and loudness.
(3) Ratings relating to tension.
(4) Ratings relating to laryngeal factors.

Range of Movements

The deaf speakers were markedly different from the hearing speakers in terms of the range of articulatory movements.

Table 14.2: Percentages of Hearing and Hearing-impaired Speakers exhibiting Non-neutral Supralaryngeal, Laryngeal, or Prosodic Features, Using the Vocal Profile Analysis Scheme

	Control Group % Speakers Exhibitiing the Parameter	Deaf Group % Speakers Exhibiting the Parameter
Lip rounding	45	55
Lip spreading	5	15
Labiodentalised	0	2.5
Extensive lip range	5	25*
Minimum lip range	7.5	55 ***
Close jaw	37.5	15
Open jaw	10	40
Protruded jaw	5	17.5
Extensive jaw movement	2.5	20*
Minimum jaw movement	12.5	60***
Advanced tongue tip	45	25
Retracted tongue tip	12.5	48
Fronted tongue body	37.5	20
Backed tongue body	52.5	65
Raised tongue body	42.5	40
Lowered tongue body	15	27.5
Extensive tongue range	0	0
Minimum tongue range	5	97.5***
Nasal	100	95
Audible nasal escape	0	12.5
Denasal	0	5
Pharyngeal constriction	47.5	87.5***
Supralaryngeal tension	57.5	85.0
Supralaryngeal lax	2.5	7.5
Laryngeal tense	72.5	95.0*
Laryngeal lax	0	5.0*
Raised laryngeal	17.5	55.0**
Lowered laryngeal	30.0	27.5
Harsh	25.0	72.5***
Whisper	97.5	92.5
Creak	77.5	67.5
Falsetto	0	20.0***
Modal	100.0	97.5
High pitch mean	30.0	40.0
Low pitch mean	42.5	40.0
Wide pitch range	0	7.5
Narrow pitch range	27.5	90.0***
High pitch variation	0	5.0
Low pitch variation	7.5	87.5***
Tremor	25.0	25.0
High loudness mean	17.5	10.0
Low loudness mean	2.5	47.5
Wide loudness range	2.5	2.5
Narrow loudness range	5.0	90.0***
High loudness variability	0	0
Low loudness variability	5.0	90.0***

*** $p = 0.001$
** $p = 0.01$
* $p = 0.05$

97.5 per cent of deaf speakers had *minimised tongue movement* compared with 5 per cent of hearing speakers;
60 per cent of deaf speakers had *minimised jaw movement* compared with 12.5 per cent of hearing speakers;
55 per cent of deaf speakers had *minimised lip movement* compared with 7.5 per cent of hearing speakers.

In direct contrast to this are the significant differences between the occurrence of extensive ranges of lip and jaw movements among the deaf.

25 per cent of the deaf speakers had an *extensive range of lip movements* compared with 5 per cent of hearing speakers;
20 per cent of the deaf speakers had an *extensive range of jaw movements* compared with 2.5 per cent of hearing speakers.

Pitch and Loudness

In these parameters too there is a highly significant difference between the pitch and loudness characteristics of deaf and hearing subjects.

90 per cent of deaf speakers showed *narrow pitch range* compared with 27.5 per cent of hearing speakers;
87.5 per cent of deaf speakers showed *low pitch variability* compared with 7.5 per cent of hearing speakers;
47.5 per cent of deaf speakers showed *low loudness mean* compared with 2.5 per cent of hearing speakers;
90 per cent of deaf speakers showed *narrow loudness range* compared with 5 per cent of hearing speakers;
90 per cent of deaf speakers showed *low loudness variability* compared with 5 per cent of hearing speakers.

Surprisingly the pitch means of the deaf and hearing groups were not significantly different even at $p = 0.05$ level.

Tension

Here the following results were noted: 87.5 per cent of the deaf speakers were characterised by *pharyngeal constriction* compared with 47.5 per cent of hearing subjects;
95 per cent of the deaf speakers showed *laryngeal tension* compared with 72 per cent of hearing speakers;

5 per cent of the deaf speakers showed *laryngeal laxness* but no hearing speakers showed this characteristic.

These figures are difficult to interpret. We can see that nearly all deaf speakers show *laryngeal tenseness* but so do a large number of the hearing speakers. However, the difference between the deaf and hearing groups is significant. No hearing person shows *laryngeal laxness*, but all the deaf speakers who did not show *laryngeal tenseness* show *laxness*. The difference in the incidence of the laxness too is significant.

Finally, a highly significant group of deaf speakers showed a non-neutral degree of pharyngeal constriction.

Laryngeal Factors

Of the deaf speakers 72.5 per cent show *harshness* compared with 25 per cent of hearing speakers, this is probably interrelated with the high incidence of *laryngeal tension*. Of the deaf speakers 20 per cent used *falsetto* while none of the hearing speakers did. Both *harshness* and *falsetto* are highly kinaesthetic laryngeal performances, and it is possible that the high incidence among deaf speakers is related to this fact. Of the deaf speakers 55 per cent had *raised larynx position* compared with 17.5 per cent of normals. The reported results showing the percentage of deaf and hearing speakers who exhibited a non-neutral setting of a parameter goes some way towards indicating whether a feature is common among deaf speakers, when compared with hearing speakers. Where the occurrence is greater for the deaf group than for the hearing there is some justification for calling such parameters 'typifying features' of deaf voice. In the results reported above it can be seen that there are several features in the vocal balance of these 40 deaf speakers that were significantly different from those of the 40 hearing speakers.

Visual Display Systems

This review has attempted to show that there are features which distinguish the voice quality of hearing-impaired speakers. However, because voice is seldom clearly defined, it is difficult to make cross comparisons from the literature as to precisely which are these distinguishing features. The vocal profile analysis scheme

(Laver *et al*. 1981) provides a comprehensive labelling procedure for the supralaryngeal and laryngeal components of voice, and appears to provide a very useful tool for identifying those features which typify deaf voice.

Remedial intervention to improve the vocal features of hearing-impaired speakers is a concern of teachers and therapists. This intervention may be directed towards improving inadequate laryngeal performance, resonance disturbances or prosodic difficulties. It was cited earlier in this chapter that common laryngeal difficulties of hearing-impaired speakers are in the maintenance of regular phonation, appropriate pitch range and pitch variability.

The aim of the teacher/therapist in improving the laryngeal performance of a hearing-impaired speaker, is to develop his self-perceptual skills. This is greatly aided by the use of visual display. There are a range of visual display systems which exhibit different laryngeal features. Maki (1984) reviews some of these. Abberton *et al*. (1984) describe their therapy regime with post-lingually deaf subjects as 'speech production feedback therapy' using the Voiscope display. Their term succinctly describes the two-fold nature of vocal therapy using visual display on the one hand to develop the speaker's speech production, and on the other the speaker's self-feedback mechanisms. Teaching/therapy techniques with the hearing-impaired which use visual display only as an aid to production but pay no attention to the development of self-feedback will yield poor results.

Spector *et al*. (1979) describes the use of another visual display system, the Simultaneous Spectrographic Display (SSD) in improving the voice quality of congenitally deaf young adults. Specifically Spector *et al*. used the SSD to reduce the laryngeal tension habitually used by a group of profoundly deaf young speakers.

Wirz and Anthony (1979) also describe the use of visual display, in their case the voiscope, as an agent in improving voice quality with hearing-impaired school children. Parker (1974) describe the use of the laryngograph in teaching intonation to profoundly deaf children.

The common feature of all these studies is the emphasis on visual display as a way of improving the self-perceptual skills and subsequently the self-monitory skills of hearing-impaired people. Visual display is seen as a teaching aid to heighten the hearing-impaired speaker's awareness of a speech parameter and, subsequent to this awareness, to help that speaker develop intrinsic self-perceptual skills which he could use when there is no visual display providing an extrinsic aid.

There are of course remedial objectives which can be achieved in voice therapy with hearing-impaired speakers without the use of visual display. A hard glottal attack (the 'over fortis' mentioned above) is common in hearing-impaired speakers. Therapy directed towards a reduction of this hard attack can greatly impove a speaker's voice quality. It is often a revelation to hearing-impaired speakers to recognise how little physical effort is required in order to produce easy phonation. The teacher/therapist can encourage the hearing-impaired speaker to produce different phonations and reinforce those relaxed phonations which occur in his random productions, until the hearing-impaired speaker becomes able to produce easy relaxed phonation to request and later as his habitual phonation.

Amplification

Many hearing-impaired speakers also exhibit poor laryngeal control through their habitual use of an inappropriate loudness level. If the teacher/therapist finds it difficult to encourage the hearing impaired speaker to use a lower loudness level it may be helpful to use a sound level meter as an aid to help the hearing-impaired speaker to appreciate how loudly he is speaking. If the speaker uses habitual amplification, it may be helpful to increase the level of amplification within the relatively quiet setting of the therapy session, if there is any probability of the hearing-impaired speaker being able to associate the increased volume which he uses with his proprioception of his voice production. He can then be helped to reduce his volume and learn to monitor this more acceptable intensity level.

Poor Pitch Control

A further vocal disturbance common among hearing-impaired speakers and amenable to therapy is poor pitch control. As cited above various writers (Parker, 1974; Maki, 1980) have shown how visual display can help the teacher/therapist to teach the hearing-impaired speaker to control his pitch level or variability. Without visual display too the teacher/therapist can help the speaker to appreciate the concept of pitch level by analagous use of hand positions, or by feeling the position of the larynx in the neck, or by relaxation of the musculature of the neck, or by reducing the degree of pharyngeal tension. By using procedures proven and familiar to the teacher/therapist the hearing-impaired speaker can be helped to appreciate the difference between his habitual pitch level and that of the desired objective.

Summary

The communication of hearing-impaired speakers is impaired. The degree of impairment of language is obviously the primary difficulty for most hearing-impaired children, and not unreasonably becomes the primary teaching objective for teachers and therapists of young hearing-impaired children. However, the effects which poor voice quality can have upon the listening 'set' of a naive listener to a hearing-impaired person should not be underestimated. If the teacher/therapist can encourage easy relaxed phonation among young hearing-impaired children voice problems should not develop (Ling, 1976). However, there will be many hearing-impaired speakers who do develop aberrant voice patterns where specific voice therapy will be applicable.

References

Abberton, E. *et al*. 'Speech Perceptual and Productive Rehabilitation in Electrocochlear Stimulation'. *Tenth Anniversary Conference on Cochlear Implants Proceedings*. (Raven Press, New York, 1984)

Angelloci, A. 'Some Observations on the Speech of the Deaf'. *Volta Review*, 64, 403–5 (1962)

Boone, D. 'Modification of the Voices of Deaf Children'. *Volta Review*, 68, 686–92 (1966)

Butterworth, B. *Language Production I*. (Academic Press, London, 1980)

Calvert, D. R. 'Deaf Voice Quality — a Preliminary Investigation'. *Volta Review*, 62, 402–3 (1962)

—— 'Some Acoustic Characteristics of the Speech of Profoundly Deaf Individuals'. Doctoral dissertation, Stanford (1961)

Colton, R. H. and Cooker, H. S. 'Perceived Nasality in the Speech of the Deaf'. *Journal of Speech and Hearing Research*, 11, 553–9 (1968)

Fairbanks, G. *Voice and Articulation Drillbook*. (Harper and Row, New York, 1960)

Gilbert, H. and Campbell, M. 'Speaking Fundamental Frequency in Three Groups of Hearing Impaired Individuals'. *Journal of Communication Disorders*, 13, 195–205 (1980)

Hochberg, I., Levitt, H. and Osberger, M. *Speech of the Hearing Impaired* (University Park Press, Baltimore, 1983)

Hollien, H. and Shipp, T. 'Speaking Fundamental Frequency and Chronological Age in Males'. *Journal of Speech and Hearing Research*, 15, 155–9 (1972)

Hudgins, C. V. 'Voice Production and Breath Control in the Speech of the Deaf'. *American Annals of the Deaf*, 82, 338–63 (1937)

—— 'A Comparative study of the Speech Co-ordination of Deaf and Normal Subjects'. *Journal of Genetic Psychology*, 44, 1–34 (1934)

Jones, C. 'Deaf Voice' — A Description Derived from a Survey of the Literature. *Volta Rview*, 69, 507–8, 39–40 (1967)

Laver, J. D. 'Voice Quality and Indexical Information'. *British Journal of Disorders of Communication*, 3, 43–54 (1968)

—— *A Phonetic Description of Voice Quality*. (Cambridge University Press, Cambridge, 1980)

——, Wirz, S. L., Mackenzie, J. and Miller, S. 'A Perceptual Protocol for the Analysis of Vocal Profiles'. University of Edinburgh Work in Progress, Linguistics Department, 14 (1981)

Levitt, H. 'Speech Production and the Deaf Child', in Conner, L. E. (ed.) *Speech of the Deaf Child* (Alex Graham Bell, Washington, 1971)

Ling, D. *Speech and the Hearing Impaired Child* (Alex Graham Bell, Washington, 1976)

Maki, J. 'Visual Feedback as an Aid to Speech Therapy' in Subtelny, J. (ed.) *Speech Assessment for Hearing Impaired* (Alex Graham Bell, Washington, 1980)

Markides, A. *The Speech of Hearing Impaired Children* (Manchester University Press, Manchester, 1983)

Martony, J. 'Studies on the Speech of the Deaf'. Progress Report Speech Transmission Lab Royal Institute of Technology, Stockholm (1966)

Michel, J., Hollien, H., and Moore, P. 'Speaking Fundamental Frequency Characteristics of 15, 16, 17 Year Old Girls'. *Language and Speech*, 9, 46–51 (1966)

Miller, M. A. 'Speech and Voice Patterns Association with Hearing Impairment'. *Audecibel*, 17, 162–7 (1968)

Monsen, R. 'Towards Measuring How Well Hearing Impaired Children Speak'. *Journal of Speech and Hearing Research*, 21, 197–219 (1978)

Nickerson, R. S. 'Characteristics of the Speech of Deaf Persons'. *Volta Review*, 77, 342–62 (1975)

Parker, A. 'Voice and Intonation Training for Deaf Children using Laryngographic Display'. *Proceedings of VIII International Congress on Acoustics*, (Chapman and Hall, London, 1974)

—— 'Speech Conversation', in Watts W. (ed.) *Rehabilitation and Acquired Deafness* (Croom Helm, London, 1983)

Penn, J. P. 'Voice and Speech Patterns in the Hard of Hearing'. *Acta Otolaryngology*, Supplement no. 124 (1955)

Peterson, G. E. 'Acoustical Gestures in the Speech of Deaf Children'. *Volta Review*, 55, 23 (1953)

Rawlings, C. G. 'A Comparative Study of the Movements and Breathing Muscles in Speech of Deaf and Normal Subjects', *American Annals of the Deaf*, 80, 136–50 (1935)

Rees, M. 'Some Variables Affecting Perceived Harshness'. *Journal of Speech and Hearing Research*, 1, 155–68 (1958)

Seaver, E. G., Andrews, J. R. and Granata, J. J. 'A Radiographic Investigation of Velar Positions in Hearing Impaired Young Adults'. *Journal of Communication Disorders*, 3, 239–47 (1980)

Spector, P., Subtelny, J., Whitehead, R. and Wirz, S. 'Description and Evaluation of a Training Programme to Reduce Vocal Tension in Adult Deaf Speakers'. *Volta Review*., 81, 81–90 (1979)

Sims, D., Walters, F., and Whitehead, R. *Deafness and Communication* (Williams and Wilkins, Baltimore, 1982)
Spriesterbach, D. 'Assessing Nasal Quality in Cleft Palate Speech of Children', *Journal of Speech and Hearing Disorders*, 20, 266–70 (1955)
Stark, R. 'Some Features of the Vocalizations of Young Deaf Children', in Jones, F. Bosma (ed.) *Third Symposium on Oral Sensation and Perception*. (Charles C. Thomas, Springfield, Illinois, 1972)
Stoker, R. G. and Lape, W. N. 'Analysis of Some Non-articulatory Aspects of the Speech of Hearing Impaired Children'. *Volta Review*, 82, 137–48 (1980)
Subtelny, J. 'Speech Assessment of the Deaf Adult'. *Journal of the Academy of Rehabilitation Audiology*, 8, 110–18 (1975)
Voelker, C. H. 'A Preliminary Stroboscopic Study of the Speech of the Deaf'. *American Annals of the Deaf*, 80, 243–59 (1935)
Whitehead, R. and Emanuel, F. W. 1974. 'Some Spectrographic and Perceptual Features of Vocal Fry'. *Journal of Communication Disorders*, 7, 305–19 (1974)
—— and Subtelny, J. 'The Development and Evaluation of Training Materials to Improve Speech and Voice Diagnosis in Impaired Adults'. Paper presented at the American Speech and Hearing Association, Houston, Texas 1976.
—— and Anthony, J. 'The Use of Voiscope in Improving the Speech of Hearing Impaired Children. *British Journal of Disorders of Communication*, 14, 132–52 (1979)
——, Subtelny, J. and Whitehead, R. 'A Perceptual and Spectrographic Study of Tense Voice in Normal Hearing and Deaf Speakers'. *Folia Phoniatrica, (Basel)*, 33, 23–36 (1979)
Yanagihara, N. 'Significance of Harmonic Changes and Noise Components in Hoarseness'. *Journal of Speach and Hearing Research,* 10, 531–41 (1967)
Zemlin, W. R. *Speech and Hearing Science* (Prentice Hall, Englewood Cliffs, New Jersey, 1968)

15 POST-RADIOTHERAPY VOICE

Margaret Stoicheff

Introduction

Preservation of the larynx in patients with glottic carcinoma by means of radiotherapy is a relatively recent development. In 1955 at a leading cancer treatment centre, 90 per cent of glottic cancer patients were being treated surgically and only a few by radiation therapy (Hawkins, 1975). Since then, the policy at this centre and elsewhere increasingly has become that of conserving the larynx wherever possible while minimising morbidity. With early glottic cancer, radiation therapy has become the initial treatment choice with surgery being reserved for radiation failure (Hawkins, 1975; Harwood and Tierei, 1979; Dickens *et al.*, 1983). Hawkins (1975) reported that complications arising in 673 patients treated by radiation for cure were low; transient dysphagia and an increase in huskiness during and immediately after treatments was usual; laryngeal oedema, the most troublesome feature, usually subsided but occasionally persisted, particularly following the successful treatment of extensive tumours.

It has been implicit in the medical literature that the voices of patients following radiotherapy are superior to those of patients following varying degrees of medical extirpation of the larynx, although objective studies detailing this are not available. In the medical literature the vocal results of patients treated successfully by means of radiation therapy are reported to be normal to near normal. Fletcher and Klein (1964) reported that 80 per cent had essentially normal voice after irradiation. Woodhouse *et al.* (1981) reported that voice results were good to excellent in 63 per cent and fair in 32 per cent of patients following radiotherapy. A few vocal problems have been mentioned, such as huskiness associated with persistent oedema in a few patients (Marks, Fitz-Hugh and Constable, 1971), tiring of the voice after excessive use and in the evening in most patients (Morrison, 1971; Vermund, 1970), and a deeper sounding voice (Vermund, 1970).

Quantifying Voice Changes

There are two reports, both single-case studies, which have employed objective measures to quantify changes in voice before, during and following radiotherapy. Werner-Kukuk, Von Leden and Yanagihara (1968) collected cinematographic, aerodynamic and acoustic measures for a 77-year-old male who received 6170 rads over a period of 46 days. They found that changes in the vibratory function of the vocal cords were reflected in the voice measures. One of the measures, Yanagihara's spectrographic classification of hoarseness, demonstrated a change from a type IV hoarseness before radiotherapy to a type I three months after the completion of treatments. Murry, Bone and von Essen (1974) examined the changes in phonational range, most comfortable fundamental frequency level, airflow rate and intraoral pressure for a 49-year-old male who received 5800 rads over 39 days. All measures indicated improved vocal function eight weeks after the end of treatments (the last measurement period), although the patient was still hoarse and the vocal folds were slightly reddened. The measures showed least efficient vocal function late in the treatment period when the patient exhibited second-degree mucositis and complained of difficulty in talking.

Zegger (1983) looked at longitudinal changes in voice in 12 subjects from immediately after treatments to five years following treatments. Judges rated when best and most deviant voices occurred. Ratings of most deviant voice were most frequently given immediately following the completion of treatments. The best voice ratings were distributed over a wider range of time periods with the most concentration in the eight to nine month period.

Patients who have been treated by radiotherapy for cure report satisfaction with their voices. In a questionnaire study of 227 out of 235 glottic cancer patients successfully irradiated from 1960 through 1971, Stoicheff (1975) found that 83 per cent reported that their voices were normal to near normal. However, the majority of them (80 per cent) indicated one or more of the following persisting difficulties: fatiguing of voice with much usage, reduced loudness, decreased clarity of voice, and inability to shout. It is of interest that almost one-half of the patients who were employed prior to treatments continued to work *during* the time that they were receiving radiation therapy and that most of the remainder returned to work within a 12-week period. The voice necessitated some minor changes in employment for nine patients and major changes for four patients.

Post-radiotherapy and Normal Voices

Few studies are available comparing post-radiotherapy voice with the voice of normal controls. Colton *et al.* (1978), using the technique of long-term spectral analysis, compared the spectral levels of five patients with T_1 laryngeal cancer subjected to radiation therapy with those of normals matched for age. They found that at one year post-treatment, the patients exhibited spectral levels within normal limits. Stoicheff *et al.* (1983) had listeners rate the voices of 46 male patients and control males matched for age. They found that the mean dysphonia ratings of the patients at one year post-treatment were significantly different from those of the control subjects. However, 35.3 per cent of the patients and 84.1 per cent of the controls received ratings of one or two (on a seven-point equal-appearing intervals scale) indicating that some irradiated patients' voices fell well within normal limits. In this study the listeners were also asked to indicate the predominant voice quality using the descriptions 'normal', 'breathy', 'hoarse', 'rough', and 'strained'. The qualitative classifications of the patients' voices before and after radiotherapy indicated that the characteristic quality moved closer to that of the control group following radiotherapy, with 53.5 per cent of the post-treatment voices (and only 18.5 per cent pretreatment) rated as normal or rough compared with 72.5 per cent of the control group voices. Stoicheff *et al.* (1983) concluded that these perceptual judgements tended to provide some limited support for subjective reports in the literature that voice tends to sound normal or near normal following radiotherapy. Stoicheff (1984) compared the mean speaking fundamental frequency of patients in the preceeding study with that of the control subjects and found no statistically significant difference.

Surprisingly little attention has been paid to post-radiotherapy voice by researchers. This may be partially due to the fact that these patients do not tend to be concerned about voice nor to seek assistance for it. The lack of research may also be a function of the relatively recent general acceptance of initial radiation therapy rather than surgery for early glottic carcinoma.

References

Colton, R. H., Sagerman, R. H., Chung, E. T., Yu, Y. W. and Reed, G. F. 'Voice Change after Radiotherapy', *Radiology*, 127, 821–4 (1978)

Dickens, W. J., Cassisi, N. J., Million, R. R. and Bova, F. J. 'Treatment of Early Vocal Cord Carcinoma: A Comparison of Apples and Apples', *Laryngoscope*, 93, 216–19 (1983)

Fletcher, G. H. and Klein, R. 'Dose–Time–Volume Relationship in Squamous Cell Carcinoma of the Larynx', *Radiology*, 82, 1032–42 (1964)

Harwood, A. R. and Tierei, A. 'Radiotherapy of Early Glottic CancerII', *International Journal of Radiation, Oncology, Biology and Physics*, 5, 477–82 (1979)

Hawkins, N. V. 'The Treatment of Glottic Carcinoma: An Analysis of 800 Cases', *Laryngoscope*, 85, 1485–93 (1975)

Marks, R. D., Fitz-Hugh, G. S. and Constable, W. C. 'Fourteen Years' Experience with Cobalt 60 Radiation Therapy in the Treatment of Early Cancer of the True Vocal Cords', *Cancer*, 28, 571–6 (1971)

Morrison, R. 'Review Article — Radiation Therapy in Diseases of the Larynx', *British Journal of Radiology*, 44, 489–504 (1971)

Murry, T., Bone, R. C. and von Essen, C. 'Changes in Voice Production During Radiotherapy for Laryngeal Cancer', *Journal of Speech and Hearing Disorders*, 39, 194–201 (1974)

Stoicheff, M. L. 'Voice Following Radiotherapy', *Laryngoscope*, 85, 608–18 (1975)

——, Ciampi, A., Passi, J. and Fredrickson, J. M. 'The Irradiated Larynx and Voice: A Perceptual Study', *Journal of Speech and Hearing Research*, 26, 482–5 (1983)

Vermund, H. 'Role of Radiotherapy in Cancer of the Larynx as Related to the TNM System of Staging. A Review', *Cancer*, 25, 571–6 (1970)

Werner-Kukuk, E., von Leden, H. and Yanagihara, N. 'The Effects of Radiation Therapy on Laryngeal Function', *Journal of Laryngology and Otolaryngology*, 82, 1–15 (1968)

Woodhouse, R. J., Quivey, J. M., Fu, K. K., Sien, P. S. and Phillips, T. L. 'Treatment of Carcinoma of the Vocal Cord: A Review of 20 Years Experience', *Laryngoscope*, 91, 1155–62 (1981)

Zegger, T. J. (1983), 'The Improvement of Voice Following Radiotherapy for Glottic Cancer', University of Toronto, Department of Speech Pathology (1983)

16 VOICE FOLLOWING LARYNGECTOMY

Bob Fawcus

Introduction

The proposal that surgery should be performed on the larynx or related structures inevitably causes great anxiety in patients and their families. Few people can face the prospect of any major surgery with equanimity but the risk of losing the ability to communicate through speech adds significantly to the apprehension prior to the operation.

The prime reason for major laryngeal surgery is the extirpation of carcinoma. In most cases this also involves a programme of radiotherapy, and for the past decade there has been a growing tendency in the United Kingdom to perform laryngectomy only upon those patients who have failed to respond to radiotherapy. These issues are discussed comprehensively by Berry (1983); see also Stoicheff, Chapter 15 of this volume.

One of the significant changes affecting the management of the laryngectomised patient, brought about by the change in radiotherapy practice, lies in the altered expectation of achievement of oesophageal voice. This affects the whole approach to the patient and his family, from the initial interview with the speech therapist to his final discharge (Edels, 1983).

Twenty years ago the picture was very different. The majority of patients tended to make a more rapid recovery from surgery with fewer complications. Some patients had not been given radiotherapy prior to the operation and the majority had been exposed to much lower levels of radiation than such patients today.

It was not uncommon for the patient to be buoyed along on a gentle tide of enthusiasm from the surgeon, who was grateful for something positive to offer, from nursing staff who had seen previous evidence of success, the speech therapist who evidently enjoyed exercising a specialised skill and a band of supporting players in the role of successful former patients.

As radiotherapy practice and policy changed, it often seemed hardest for the surgeon to accept that it was now less likely that the patient who had undergone extensive radiotherapy prior to surgery would achieve adequate pseudophonation. There were also a number of speech therapists who found it difficult to acknowledge the change.

Technological developments lagged disappointingly. The patient who was unable to learn oesophageal speech might be shown one of the few available transcervical vibrators, but there was often strong prejudice against their introduction. It is interesting to note that pneumatic prostheses were developed by Czermak as long ago as 1859 (see also Luchsinger and Arnold, 1965). The original design remained in use for at least a century until the development of plastic versions in Holland and Japan, and the proliferation of both transcervical and intraoral electronic prostheses (Salmon, 1979). A new generation of speech therapists (Murrills, 1983; Edels, 1983) and others were cognisant of the changes which were occurring and began to seek new answers. Some of these were derived from developments in the United States, particularly the training courses at the Mayo Clinic associated with Keith and Darley (1979) and Shanks and Duguay (1974). Other influences were derived from processes and practices which were already well established at some centres in the United Kingdom. Swallow (quoted in Damsté, 1959) had worked closely with Negus (1949) in his studies of the structure and function of the larynx and had developed a soundly based approach to the teaching of oesophageal voice. Her approach was founded on principles of 'injection', and this had influenced Moolenar-Bjil (1952, 1953) when they collaborated in London during the Second World War. Swallow continued to work with Ranger (1964) at the Middlesex Hospital until the early 1960s and their partnership laid the foundations for the subsequent publication by Edels (1983) which provided the most substantial contribution to British literature on the problems and management of the communicative sequelae of laryngectomy.

Initial Contact

When the patient who is about to undergo a laryngectomy first meets the speech therapist who is to be responsible for his management and treatment, both are afforded an opportunity that rarely occurs in the field of disorders of communication. The therapist is enabled to obtain a brief but relatively complete picture of the individual's personality and speech characteristics prior to morbidity. In the vast majority of acquired disorders referral occurs after the trauma and the therapist is wholly dependent upon the views and opinions of others.

The patient himself is afforded the rare chance to probe and examine the therapist far more effectively than will be possible for some time after the operation. The free mutual flow of information between patient and therapist provides a precious opportunity for each to get to know the other. This initial visit can, however, tragically be missed if the co-operation with medical and nursing staff is not such that the therapist is made immediately aware of the impending laryngectomy operation.

Because of the complex interaction of anatomical, physiological and psychological factors it is impossible to predict with any confidence that a patient will either succeed or fail in his first attempts to achieve oesophageal phonation. Most therapists working in the field will have encountered the individual who has undergone relatively straightforward surgery, without obvious negative reactions to radiotherapy or blatant psychological complications, who is, however, apparently unable to achieve useful audible phonation. This stands in sharp contrast to the individual at the opposite end of the continuum who produces adequate voice from the most unpromising structures.

One very unfortunate patient had a 'stomach pull-up' performed which proved unsuccessful leaving her, after a major gastrotomy, with no mechanism for the ingestion of food or drink and no possibility of achieving pseudophonation. Having survived in this condition for a matter of months it was decided, at her own insistence, that a colon transplant be performed. Within four weeks of the operation she began to achieve audible pseudophonation, and after six months was confidently using the telephone in her new role as secretary to a club for laryngectomees.

The most satisfactory approach with any patient who has undergone extensive surgery involving the larynx and related structures is a tentative, experimental progression with minimal demands in the early stages. Establishing a relationship in which the patient and therapist together explore the possibilities for voice, whether by means of the individual's own resources or with the aid of an electronic or pneumatic prosthesis, is less damaging in the long run than a confident 'hard sell' which can so often result in an exacerbation of failure.

Respiratory Control

Control of respiratory outflow is as essential for the individual attempting to achieve phonation without a larynx as it is for virtually any other type of dysphonic patient. Too often in the past this has been presented in a didactic manner by therapists more involved in running off a routine procedure than carrying out a careful appraisal of the true respiratory requirements of the paitent, and the extent to which he is capable of achieving them.

> 'Your problem is that you can't breathe', announced an earnest speech-training teacher to a young Indian acquaintance.
> 'Madam, I will have you know that I have been breathing perfectly for the past twenty seven years!' was his cheerful response.

Such a reply could as easily be offered to many a speech therapist who has embarked enthusiastically upon a programme of breathing exercises more suited to the training of a coloratura soprano than a shop assistant. Careful observation of the patient will provide essential basic information on his customary patterns of respiration, his response to physical and emotional stress, and any changes in the pattern of his respiratory behaviour when he attempts to communicate. As Gordon points out (Chapter 2 of this volume), a facility such as pneumotachography will provide hard data on a patient's performance. At the present time such equipment is rarely seen outside special research units, but the advent of the low cost microcomputer means that measurement of important acoustic and physiological parameters is rapidly coming within the reach of any interested therapist.

With virtually any postlaryngectomy patient it is as well to commence with a regime which includes learning to observe his own respiratory state and pattern of activity. This should include sitting at rest during attempts at speaking and in such activities as climbing a flight of stairs. The therapist may wish to postpone developing the patient's own awareness of the process to allow for a brief period of observation which is not complicated by the patient's attempts to control his respiration.

The advantage of starting with work on respiration is that it is an activity in which all individuals are perforce obliged to engage. Few people are unable to achieve at least a minimal marginal improvement in performance, and it may be the only activity in the early sessions in which the patient can gain any success. A similar argument may be put forward for the early introduction of a device such as the Cooper Rand intraoral artificial larynx (Geene, 1980). Not only can such an aid facilitate communication in the post-surgery period, it can serve to reduce tension and provide a much-needed source of practical success.

Control of Muscular Tension

Control and observation of respiration leads step by step to a mutual cognisance of the emotional state of the individual. In the majority of cases the level of tension is likely to be high because so much is dependent upon the achievement of audible phonation. Some therapists expressly state that relaxation procedures should be introduced either before or after surgery, or during both periods.

Prior to the operation the patient is not likely to be in a receptive state. He is usually preoccupied with the implications and possible effects of surgery and will find it difficult to concentrate on anything like a formal programme. Even after the operation such procedures are not always necessary. It is essential that the patient is as relaxed as possible but this can be achieved in a number of different ways. Humour is probably the best relaxant available, but it is difficult to introduce into a formal relaxation procedure.

How far can a therapist expect a patient to be relaxed if it appears to him that his whole future depends on the ability to attain oesophageal or similar phonation? Would one expect a tennis champion to be 'relaxed' before a crucial match, or a singer before an important début?

In teaching oesophageal phonation it is obviously essential that the patient is as relaxed as possible. The most important muscle system which must be in a relaxed state is the cricopharyngeal sphincter, or pharyngo-oesophageal segment as Diedreich and

Youngstrom (1966) describe it. Individuals who have undergone more extensive surgery may have either a pharyngogastric segment or a similar junction between the base of the pharynx, and a transplanted section of the colon or other tissues.

The overwhelming majority of patients have little appreciation of the function of the sphincteric mechanism and even less idea of how to make it relax. In attempting to teach several hundreds of speech therapy students to achieve oesophageal phonation the exercise could only be described as a dismal failure. All of them were intimately aware of the structure and function of their pharyngo-oesophageal segment and all had received some prior training in relaxation. Probably of greater significance was the fact that there was virtually no pressure on them to achieve success. Fewer than 5 per cent ever achieved sufficient control to enable them to produce oesophageal phonation.

It is considerably easier for most laryngectomees to produce oesophageal phonation than it is for the normal speaker. A small number of patients with a pharyngocolonic or pharyngogastric sphincter are left with a system in which the structure and function of the tissues are such that they actually facilitate the production of pseudophonation. This is because they have lost the capacity to contract the muscles of the segment excessively, which tends to occur whenever a normal speaker or the novice laryngectomee attempts to transfer air from the pharynx into the oesophagus.

As Damsté (1958) emphasised, the process of deliberately introducing air into the oesophagus is counter to the physiological operation of the sphincter. A small quantity of air inevitably passes into the oesophagus during the process of deglutition but the pattern of closure of the larynx in normal subjects is specifically delayed to minimise the ingestion of air into the stomach (Ardran and Kemp, 1967). This explains the common complaint of the laryngectomee that he feels an excess of air in the stomach. In fact, this is rarely due to attempts to produce oesophageal speech, but many patients are convinced that this is the cause.

Teaching Oesophageal Phonation

The three principal methods of achieving phonation by means of transferring air into the oesophagus are well documented and have been fully explained by Damsté (1958). It is noteworthy perhaps, that despite the fact that his findings were quoted extensively in major US texts including Snidecor (1962) and Diedreich and Youngstrom (1966), the implications for teaching oesophageal speech were not apparently appreciated. Both texts continued to advocate a technical approach which was based on insufflation, a procedure shown by both Damsté and by Diedreich and Youngstrom to be used by only the minority of groups of accomplished speakers in both Holland and the United States.

Swallowing Method

The technique most commonly quoted in texts on physiology and laryngology is in fact the least effective. It is generally described as the 'swallowing method' and is still not without its advocates in the field of speech pathology. It is in fact relatively easy for the laryngectomised patient to swallow air. Every time he swallows saliva, beverages or solid food he takes in more air into the oesophagus than the individual with the normally functioning larynx. Air which enters the oesophagus during the act of swallowing, with or without accompanying fluids or solids, is treated as a bolus and is automatically passed down to the stomach by peristaltic action.

It is, however, almost impossible to reverse this process voluntarily. One patient of ours, an elderly general practitioner, was able to drive excess air from his stomach with digital pressure just below the sternum, but most patients have to wait until the air pressure in the stomach reaches such a level that a bolus returns in a reverse direction up the oesophagus. Woe betide the laryngectomee who dared to allow this to occur within sight or sound of Amy Swallow without making an attempt to say something. 'Use it, use it!' she would urge.

The long delay in return of air from the stomach, and the crucial lack of voluntary control, makes this procedure totally inadequate as a means of communication. Those who claim to teach it, or use it effectively, are probably using another method without realising it. The value of experiencing oesophageal phonation via this method, particularly induced by the intake of effervescent beverages, is somewhat exaggerated. The presence of alcohol in some of the beverages favoured for this approach may well have beneficial psychological effects, but not directly linked to the transfer of gases in and out of the oesophagus.

Inhalation Method

Inhalation, also known as insufflation, was the training method of choice until the early 1960s in most centres in the United States and the United Kingdom. The process of intake of air is closely related to normal breathing for speech and it tends to be the easiest technique for normal speakers to achieve, whether for small boys wishing to discomfort their parents in formal surroundings, or guests at a Middle Eastern banquet wishing to display their appreciation.

Early attempts to view the process cineradiographically gave the false impression that inhalation was a universal technique amongst successful oesophageal speakers and should be encouraged. The radiographic image was restricted in size and could give little idea of the operation of the full system. The films which were made only served to bolster an innaccurate interpretation of the method. It was only when Damsté (1958) made measurements of the air pressures within the pharynx and oesophagus that the process was clearly revealed.

In order to teach the inhalation method the first requirement is that the patient should be sitting in a relaxed state. He is then asked to take in a sharp breath. Some authorities recommend that the patient keep his mouth open but this, in fact, is unnecessary as air can enter the nose. Other therapists demand that the patient should gasp, gulp or sniff air. This is neither essential nor advisable as it can lead to accessory movements of the face, mandible or head which become habitual and later may prove difficult to eliminate.

If the patient's pharyngo-oesophageal inlet is sufficiently relaxed, air can be induced from the pharynx into the oesophagus because of the pressure difference between the atmosphere and the thorax. It is this process which, during respiration, draws air into the lungs of the normal speaker via the oral or nasal route and into the tracheostoma of the laryngectomised patient. The induction of air into the oesophagus in the 'inhalation' process is parallel to the intake of respiratory air via the stoma. It cannot occur if the musculature at the entrance to the oesophagus is too tightly contracted. The intake of breath has to be sufficiently rapid and deliberate to achieve the simultaneous transfer of air into the oesophagus. The inhalation method is not identical to the normal process of inspiration. If the process occurred in the course of normal respiration the laryngectomee would be continually moving air in and out of his oesophagus with unmistakeable acoustic results. In practice the transfer only takes place when the patient chooses to speak.

The inhalation method possesses certain advantages but also inherent problems which lead many therapists to use the third principal technique, namely 'injection' (see below). The sharp intake of breath inevitably implies that the patient must release the excess air that he has drawn in and this usually occurs during the production of speech. This can mean that an individual is forced to phonate at a greater intensity level to counteract the audible emission from the tracheostoma. As our hearing for the low frequency output from the oesophagus (around 40–80 Hz) is considerably poorer than our detection of the broad band width noise emitted from the stoma, it is a high priority to attempt to reduce this source of interference in the process of spoken communication.

The principal advantage of the inhalation technique is that it is somewhat easier to teach in the initial stages. It involves few departures from the normal mechanisms of speech and is particularly well suited to the production of vowels and semi-vowels. Claims that it facilitates fluency are greatly exaggerated. It is very doubtful that a speaker using inhalation can achieve more than three syllables on a single intake, and very likely that accounts of individuals producing many more syllables are based on speakers employing a mixture of inhalation and injection.

Injection Method

Despite the very strong support for the inhalation technique evident in the literature of the 1940s and 1950s some authorities had described an alternative approach. Schlosshauer and Möckel (1954; 1958) outlined the process of air injection which they had observed by means of cineradiography. The contribution of Damsté (1958) was, however, crucial in our understanding of the whole process and in particular the implications for teaching oesophageal voice. In addition to making cineradiographic films of 24 accomplished Dutch oesophageal speakers, he analysed their speech output spectrographically. Two pressure transducers were inserted via the nasal cavity in order to obtain simultaneous recordings of the pressures set up in the oropharynx and the oesophagus during the production of oesophageal voice. (Figure 16.1)

Figure 16.1: Simultaneous Recordings of the Pressure in the Pharynx (P), the Pressure in the Oesophagus (O) and the Sound Pressure (S). Time signal (T) indicates 0.02 sec. All four recordings (a) to (d) show pronunciation of the syllable [pa:]. (a) and (d): injection method; (b) and (c): suction method

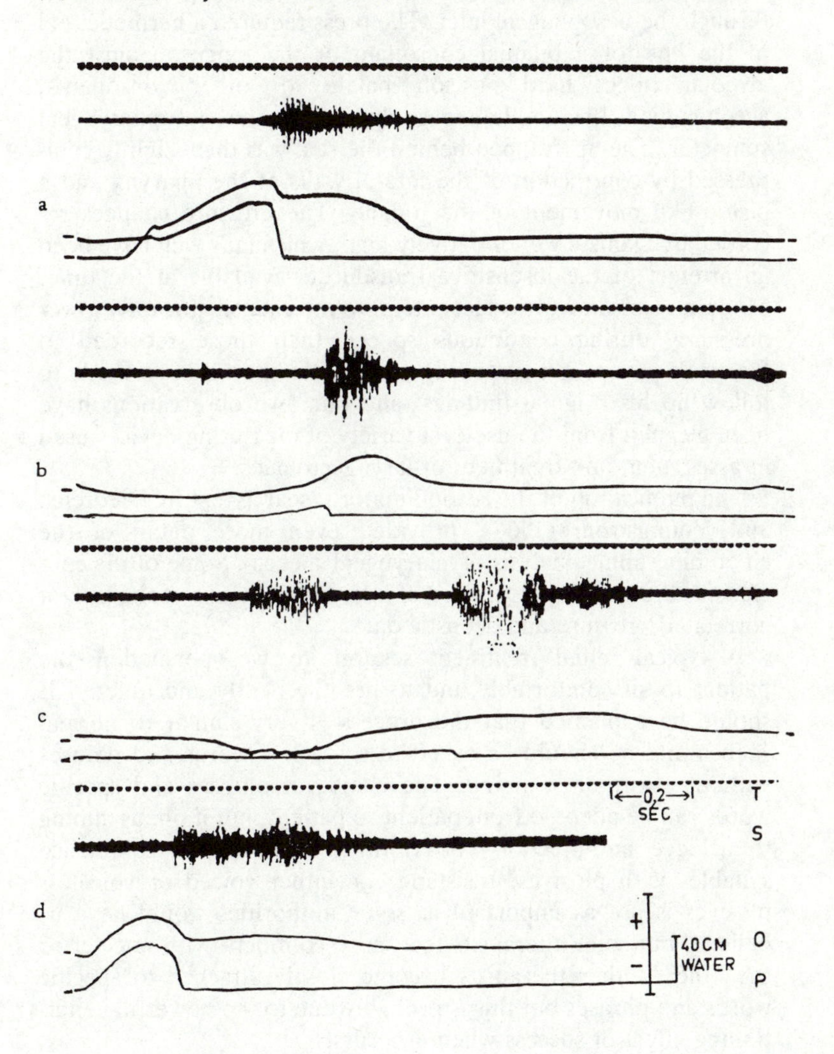

Source: Damsté (1958)

He was able to show that 23 of the subjects were employing a process which he termed 'injection', even those who had originally been taught by the inhalation method. He found evidence that the process which he described as a 'glossopharyngeal press' involved the active pumping of air from the oral cavity and pharynx down through the oesophageal inlet. The press required a hermetic seal of the lips for a bilabial consonant or the tongue against the alveolar ridge, hard or soft palate for other consonants, accompanied by simultaneous closure of the nasopharyngeal sphincter. The air trapped behind the seal was then slightly compressed by contraction of the lateral walls of the pharynx and a piston-like movement of the tongue. The pressure changes recorded by Damsté were relatively high, which may well have been an artefact of the insensitive transducers available at the time. Modern electronic transducers tend to indicate significantly lower pressures during continuous speech than those recorded in Damsté's group, but surprisingly little attempt has been made to follow up his original findings, and our own observations have been gleaned from the use of a variety of measuring devices used in assessment and treatment of laryngectomees.

The publication of the second major research text by Diedreich and Youngstrom (1966), provided even more detail of the cineradiographic analysis of 'alaryngeal speech'. Some of the conclusions drawn, however, were of less value because of the lack of correlated pressure and acoustic data.

A typical initial treatment session involves persuading the patient to sit comfortably and to breathe gently and quietly. It should be explained that the process is very similar to normal speech and he should be asked to say a few words and phrases without effort or straining. The choice of phrases and specific words can be adapted from patient to patient, but if one is aiming to achieve an injection pattern it is necessary to commence syllables with plosives. Insistence on either voiced or voiceless plosives is not as important as some authorities would have us believe, but some therapists feel more confident with one set or the other. Other therapists become closely attached to specific words and phrases but this is probably due to the powerful conditioning effect of success when it occurs.

Bilabial plosives appear to lead to a relatively high success rate. This is likely to be due to the lack of lingual involvement which can so easily lead to tension in the pharyngo-oesophageal segment.

Figure 16.2: Two Frames from a Computer Program: 'Teaching Oesophageal Speech'

(a)

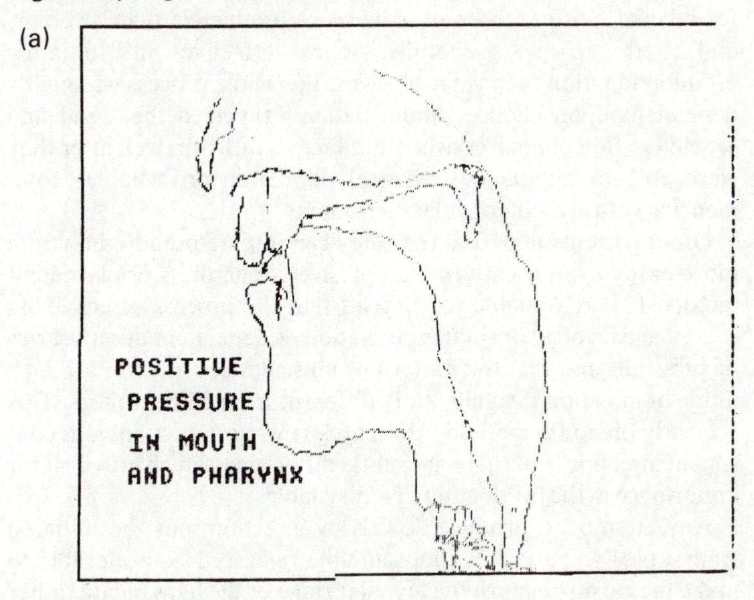

(b)

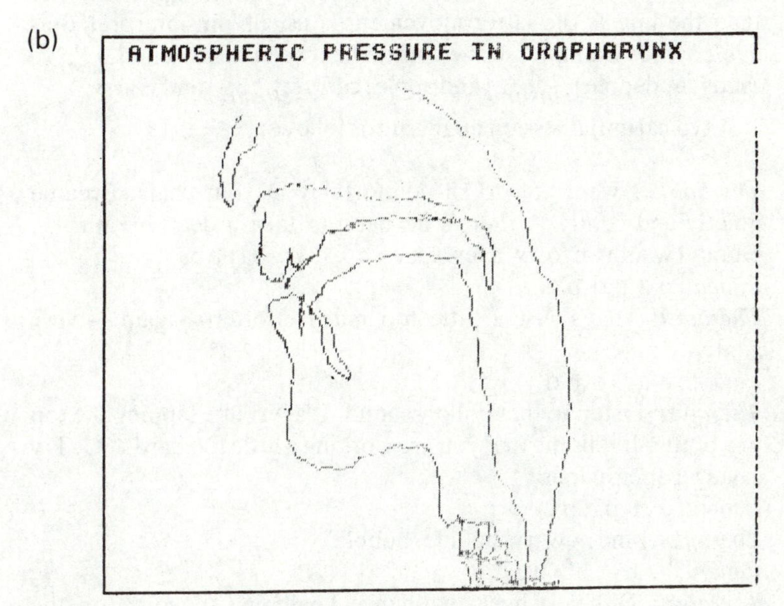

Source: Clinical Communication Studies, The City University

Observation of a long series of patients at both the Middlesex Hospital and at Guy's suggested that although there was a tendency for bilabial plosives to be initially more productive than alveolar, and both to be generally more effective in initiating pseudophonation than velar plosives, the whole process was highly dependent upon chance. Some patients reversed the trend and seemed to find bilabial consonant injection difficult, well after they were able to initiate oesophageal phonation on syllables commencing with alveolar or velar consonants.

Other patients may find that they can initiate pseudophonation more easily from fricatives than plosives, regardless of placement factors. It is reasonable to contend that the process of achieving oesophageal voice, or similar phonation, is dependent upon a series of sub-skills and that the pattern of muscular contraction for each mode of injection is significantly different from all the others. This is clearly obvious when one compares vowel production with consonant injection, but there are subtle differences which are of major importance in the production of any syllable.

Any attempt to produce vowels by injection must be initiated from a plosive pattern without audible release. It is preferable to make the closure against the alveolar ridge or the hard palate rather than the lips as the latter movement is usually misinterpreted as a /b/, as, for example, in the contrast between dandy and $[^{\ d}_{closure}]$ Andy, or dapple $[^{\ d}_{closure}]$ and apple; carry $[^{\ k}_{closure}]$ and Harry.

A typical initial session might run as follows:

Therapist: I want you to sit comfortably in your chair. Breathe quietly and gently — there's no need to take a deep breath . . . Good, I want you to say a few easy words. Try ba ba ba. . . .
Patient: p'ɑ̊ p'ɑ̊ p'ɑ̊
Therapist: That's just a little too much effort try again — very gently. . . .
Patient: p'ɑ̊ p'ɑ̊ p'ɑ̊
Therapist: Listen to that hollow sound. It's just like tapping the top of a bottle. It tells me that you are working a little too hard. . . . Try saying 'paper, paper'.
Patient: p'e̥ɪ p'ə̥, p'e̥ɪ p'ə̥
Therapist: Fine now try 'bubble, bubble'.
Patient: bʌb'Ω̥, b'ʌbΩ
Therapist: Did you hear that voice beginning to come on the second 'bubble'. Try it again. . . .

Visual Feedback. The therapist's main task when teaching injection is to monitor carefully the patient's attempts. If too much tension is evident then it is necessary to persuade the laryngectomee to employ less effort. Some individuals will initially exhibit insufficient effort and they need to be encouraged to build up oral air pressure step by step until they achieve a useful working pressure.

A simple water manometer will display the intraoral pressure achieved by the laryngectomee. This provides clear and immediate feedback to both patient and therapist. Air pressure meters are somewhat more convenient but are more difficult to sterilise. The water manometer is so inexpensive that it can be regarded as disposable. A low-cost pressure transducer connected to the analog input of a microcomputer will provide the advantage of hard copy records and more accurate measurement and analysis.

Control of Respiratory Outflow. Control of excessive air escape via the tracheostoma can be achieved by observing some critical rules:

(1) There is no necessity for an initial intake of breath prior to an utterance.
(2) A marked intake of breath via the tracheostoma will lead automatically to a rapid and noisy outflow.
(3) Injection requires only gentle breathing and is not directly dependent upon thoracic pressures.
(4) The production of syllables does not need to be accompanied by noisy outflow of air via the tracheostoma.

A number of simple techniques can assist those who produce noisy stoma emission and consist mainly of completely reducing the effortful approach of the patient towards the production of voice. If he is asked to whisper he may be able to comply, but quite frequently he does not know how to inhibit oesophageal voice and is likely to produce a low volume voice of fair quality.

An effective control technique consists of persuading the patient to count quietly 'without voice' and then gradually raise the volume without taking in any more than a gentle breath. If he begins to breathe in and out noisily he must be persuaded to return to quiet counting. Sophisticated air flow detection techniques can be used to monitor air flow and provide visual feedback but the simple device of asking the patient to hold his fingers about an inch in front of the stoma can be just as effective.

Effects of Extensive Surgery

The current approach to radiotherapy and surgery for laryngeal carcinoma in the United Kingdom means that an increasing number of patients are likely to have sustained more extensive removal of tissue than in the past. This can include partial glossectomy and excision of the oesophagus, as well as surrounding musculature, as the surgeon seeks to remove lymphatic tissues which have been invaded by the carcinoma (Ranger, 1983).

The reconstructive procedures undertaken at the present time are much less protracted than the original attempts to construct a new oesophagus from superficial tissues from the abdomen. The original process of raising skin flaps and progressively moving these in stages to provide the necessary tissues was dramatically successful in some cases, but many patients suffered the long wait from one stage to the other only to succumb to a recurrence before the final reconstruction of the oesophagus.

During the mid-1960s an opportunity was afforded to compare the effects on communicative skills of two different surgical procedures. At the Middlesex Hospital, Le Quesne and Ranger (1966) were attempting to achieve one type of solution. The excision of larynx, oesophagus and proximal affected tissues was immediately followed by drawing the patient's stomach up into the mediastinum and suturing a direct connection between pharynx and stomach.

At Guy's Hospital, London, other colleagues (Reading *et al.* 1966) were engaged in a different approach with similar cases. The ENT surgeon was responsible for the removal of the larynx and oesophagus, but another surgeon would remove a section of the colon at the same operation, and then transplant the tube as a connection between pharynx and stomach. Earlier attempts had been made to follow the course of the oesophagus, but Reading *et al.* preferred to establish a new route below the superficial tissues of the thorax, over the rib cage, entering the stomach just below the sternum. A prime advantage was that it was possible for the patient to move solids which lodged in the colon by means of digital massage.

A majority of patients at the Middlesex Hospital during the period in question achieved serviceable phonation, some with remarkably little aid from the speech therapist. Two women, for example, were admitted and had their operations while the speech therapist was away on holiday. Both had achieved fluent phonation by his return. Others, despite considerable efforts, were unable to obtain any useful phonatory output and were generally recommended to use an artificial larynx.

The principal reason for failure to achieve pseudophonation was a lack of appropriate contractility in the pharyngogastric segment. The method of instruction employed was injection, as the interference with respiratory function caused by the operation made insufflation virtually impossible. As in the case of patients who have undergone simple laryngectomy, the stomach pull-up patient must possess a means of trapping air. In his, usually her, case the reservoir consists of the extended portion of stomach tissue just below the pharyngogastric junction. The inability of a few patients to achieve excessive inhibitory contraction facilitates the transfer of air and can make them easier to teach than a more straightforward laryngectomee.

Experience with the colon transplant patients at Guy's indicated that the majority were not able to achieve a colonic voice. The problem was very similar to the difficulty experienced by stomach pull-up cases in that the pharyngocolonic segment rarely possessed contractile capability. The exposure of the mechanism above the rib cage was such that one could observe the whole process with the naked eye and in a few cases intervene to provide an improved system.

The method of choice was inevitably injection as the presence of the colon outside the thorax meant that it was not possible to induce air by insufflation. It is relatively simple to observe the whole process in such cases without the aid of cineradiography. When the patient attempts to produce a syllable commencing with a plosive one sees an immediate inflation of the transplanted colon. The air pressure reduces immediately when the plosive is released. In the majority of cases observed the junction is too large and too flaccid to operate as a useful sphincter. Logemann (1983) reports comparable findings and also suggests techniques similar to those which we employed at Guy's to assist these patients. We had a small number of patients who developed the art of digital pressure to virtuoso level.

One man who had demonstrated his excellent oesophageal voice to generations of medical students suffered a recurrence and underwent oesophagectomy with an extraothoracic colon transplant. At first he was only able to achieve communication with the aid of an artificial larynx, but subsequently learnt to operate his colon as if he were playing bagpipes. He would inflate the colon on the injection phase, trap the air with his fingers and then expel air with the palm of his hand, producing a quieter and less periodic output than his original oesophageal voice. As he once said 'It'll do when me batteries run down!'

We experimented with inflatable cuffs, on or near the surface of the pharyngocolonic segment, with only minimal success because of the slow response to the changing demands of pressure and relaxation. It is not impossible that a system activated by electromyographic input from the thoracic musculature and controlled by a microprocessor could achieve an improved performance.

The introduction of simple shunt techniques (Blom, Singer and Hamaker, 1982; Panje, 1981) can be dramatically effective with patients who have undergone standard laryngectomy, but is less likely to help the patient who has undergone pharyngolaryngo-oesophagectomy. The presence of a useful pharyngocolonic or pharyngogastric sphincter mechanism is as vital in such cases as it is in the standard laryngectomy (Perry, 1983; Logemann, 1983).

The electronic and prosthetic field has moved particularly slowly, although current Swedish and Dutch work on prostheses with variable intonation output is very encouraging. The size and innovative flexibility of the silicon chip would appear to be ideal to employ in such devices and interesting developments may be anticipated in the near future.

An account of the rehabilitation processes for communication by means of an artificial larynx or with the aid of specific surgical techniques have been ably reviewed and discussed by Salmon (1983) Edwards (1983) and Perry (1983). Similarly, the detailed discussions of management by Murrills (1983) and Perry (1983) offer the reader comprehensive accounts of current approaches and rationale.

Improvement of Voice Quality

A number of authorities emphasise the need to work directly on the improvement of voice quality with the oesophageal speaker. Personal experience has shown that it may be easier to achieve co-operation in the female patient who is likely to be more critical of the low frequency aperiodic phonation than male patients (see Gardner, 1971).

Techniques are very similar to those employed with a dysphonic patient who continues to have a larynx. The principal aim is to seek to encourage awareness and constructive criticism of voice quality in the individual, to teach him how to listen to his own voice and other voices.

Minimisation of excessive tension, and the establishment of a relaxed but effective pattern of respiration, are just as important for the laryngectomee as for any other dysphonic patient and the development of improved pitch and resonance can be achieved through very similar exercises (Shanks (1983), and Fawcus Chapter 10 of this volume).

References

Ardran, G. M and Kemp, F. H. 'The Mechanism of the Larynx, Part II: The Epiglottis and Closure of the Larynx,' *British Journal of Radiology*, 40, 372 (1967)

Berry, R. J. 'Radiotherapy and Chemotherapy', in Edels Y. (ed.) *Laryngectomy: Diagnosis to Rehabilitation* (Croom Helm, London, 1983)

Blom, E. D., Singer, M. I. and Hamaker, R. C. 'A Tracheostoma Valve for Post-laryngectomy Voice Rehabilitation', presented to the Annual Meeting of the American Broncho-Esophagological Association, Palm Beach, Florida, 3 May, 1982

Czermak, J. 'Uber die Sprache bei luftdichter Verschliessung des Kehlkopfs', *Wiener Akademie für Wissenshaften*, 35, 65 (1859)

Damsté P. H. *Oesophageal Speech* (Hoitsema, Groningen, 1958)

—— 'The Glosso-pharyngeal Press', *Speech Pathology and Therapy*, 2, 70 (1959)

Diedriech, W. M. and Youngstrom, K. A. *Alaryngeal Speech* (Charles C. Thomas, Springfield, Illinois, 1966)

Edels, Y. *Laryngectomy:Diagnosis to Rehabilitation* (Croom Helm, London, 1983)

Edwards, N. 'The Surgical Approach to Speech Rehabilitation', in Edels, Y. (ed.) *Laryngectomy: Diagnosis to Rehabilitation* (Croom Helm, London, 1983)

Gardner, W. H. *Laryngectomee Speech and Rehabilitation* (Charles C. Thomas, Springfield, Illinois, 1971, 1978)

Greene, M. C. L. *The Voice and its Disorders* (Pitman Medical, London, 1980)

Keith, R. L. and Darley, F. L. (eds) *Laryngectomee Rehabilitation* (College-Hill Press, San Diego, California, 1979)

Le Quesne, L. P. and Ranger, D. 'Pharyngo-laryngectomy with Immediate Pharyngo-gastric Anastomosis', *British Journal of Surgery*, 53, 105–9 (1966)
Logemann, J. A. 'Vocal Rehabilitation after Extensive Surgery for Post-cricoid Carcinoma', in Edels, Y. (ed.), *Laryngectomy: Diagnosis to Rehabilitation*. (Croom Helm, London, 1983)
Luchsinger, R. and Arnold, G. E. *Voice – Speech – Language. Clinical Communicology: Its Physiology and Pathology*. (Constable, London, 1965)
Moolenar-Bjil, A. 'The Importance of Certain Consonants in Esophageal Voice after Laryngectomy', *Annals of Otology (St Louis)*, 62, 979 (1952)
—— 'Connection between Consonant Articulation and the Intake of Air in Oesophageal Speech', *Folia Phoniatrica (Basel)*, 5, 212 (1953)
Murrills, G. (1983) 'Pre- and Early Post-operative Care of the Laryngectomee and Spouse', in Edels, Y. (ed.) *Laryngectomy: Diagnosis to Rehabilitation* (Croom Helm, London, 1983)
Negus, V. E. *The Comparative Anatomy and Physiology of the Larynx* (Heinemann, London, 1949)
Panje, W. R. 'Prosthetic Vocal Rehabilitation following Laryngectomy; the Voice Button', *Annals of Otology*, 90, 116–20 (1981)
Perry, A. 'The Speech Therapist's Role in Surgical and Prosthetic Approaches to Speech Rehabilitation, with Particular Reference to the Blomsinger and Panje Techniques', in Edels, Y. (ed.) *Laryngectomy* (Croom Helm, London, 1983)
Ranger, D. 'The Problems of Repair After Pharyngolaryngectomy', *Proceedings of the Royal Society of Medicine*, 57, 1099–103 (1964)
—— 'Extensive Surgery for Post-cricoid Carcinoma', in Edels, Y. (ed.) *Laryngectomy: Diagnosis to Rehabilitation* (Croom Helm, London, 1983)
Reading, P. V. and Brian, R. H. 'Colon Transplantation into the Pharynx and Cervical Oesophagus', *British Journal of Surgery*, 53, 933–42 (1966)
Salmon, S. J. 'Patients Talk Back', in Salmon, S. J. and Goldstein, L. P. (eds) *The Artificial Larynx Handbook* (Grune and Stratton, New York, 1979)
——, 'Artificial Larynx Speech: A Viable Means of Alaryngeal Communication', in Edels, Y. (ed.) *Laryngectomy: Diagnosis to Rehabilitation* (Croom Helm, London, 1983)
Schlosshauer, B. and Mockel, G. 'Röntgenkinematografische Darstellung der Pseudosprache nach Laryngektomie', *Archiv für Ohr, Nase und Kehlheilken* 165, 581, 638 (1954)
—— and Mockel, G. 'Evaluation of X-ray Tone Films in Laryngectomized Patients', *Folia Phoniatrica (Basel)*, 10, 154–66 (1958)
Shanks, J. C. 'Development of the Feminine Voice and Refinement of Esophageal Voice', in Keith, R. L. and Darley, F. L. *Laryngectomee Rehabilitation* (College-Hill Press, Houston, Texas, 1979)
Shanks, J. C. and Duguay, M. 'Voice Remediation and the Teaching of Alaryngeal Speech', in Dickson, S. (ed.) *Communication Disorders, Remedial Principles and Practices* (Scott, Foresman, Chicago, 1974)
Snidecor, J. C. *Speech Rehabilitation of the Laryngectomized* (Charles C. Thomas, Springfield, Illinois, 1962)

17 AN INTERDISCIPLINARY VOICE CLINIC

Tom Harris, Sara Collins and David D. Clarke

Introduction

In principle, there are two sources of therapeutic advancement in medicine and related fields. One is the invention of new elements of treatment, such as specific diagnostic procedures, therapeutic techniques or instruments, and the other a matter of bringing together existing elements of treatment into new and more effective combinations. It is often the first of these two which attracts more attention, but in some fields, of which the treatment of voice disorders is one, very striking advances can be made by adopting the second method.

The ingredients of a combined approach to the treatment of voice disorders mainly involve the disciplines of laryngology, speech therapy and experimental phonetics. On occasions clinical psychologists and psychiatrists may need to be involved, and the equipment and expertise of physiotherapists is also extremely valuable. In addition to the personnel, the technology that has been developed and adapted from other branches of science also plays an important part. In particular the use of stroboscopy, combined with the advances in laryngoscopy, laryngography, and air flow measurements now make laryngeal examination more accurate, informative, and easier (Williams, Farquharson and Anthony, 1975; Abberton and Fourcin, 1972; Berry *et al.*, 1982; Laver, Hiller and Hanson, 1982).

Interdisciplinary voice clinics have been established for a considerable time in Scandinavia, on the continent and in the United States. The concept has also been developing in the United Kingdom for some time, but despite the pioneering work of Simpson (1971) the effectiveness of the multidisciplinary approach has been little researched in this country until recently (Harris, Collins and Clarke; in press).

The Oxford Voice Clinic has been operating since 1982. It has developed considerably in the time it has been running, both in its aims and in its scope. It was originally set up in order to:

(1) Provide re-evaluation of voice patients who were not progressing with treatment as well as expected – the so-called problem cases.
(2) Provide additional diagnostic information in cases where there is no visible abnormality of the vocal folds but where the voice quality is abnormal.
(3) Identify other contributing medical factors among voice patients and to provide the appropriate treatment.

During the time the clinic has been running, however, other important aims have developed as we have acquired the necessary equipment and knowledge. These include:

(1) Earlier diagnosis of carcinoma or residual disease in patients previously irradiated for carcinoma of the larynx. This has become possible through the acquisition of a stroboscopic light source for laryngeal work and, as a result, more accurate guidelines are available for assessing which patients must be biopsied, and which are safe to review.
(2) A dramatic reduction in the number of patients requiring direct laryngoscopy simply because they were not possible to examine in an outpatient clinic.
(3) The opportunity to investigate the nature of voice disorders, their course of recovery, and the efficacy of the treatment provided.

The Oxford Voice Clinic employs a laryngologist and a speech therapist on a regular basis, and where possible uses the expertise and instrumentation of a phonetics department. This is either indirectly through analysis of tape recordings made of our patients, or directly through patient attendance at Oxford University Phonetics department. Here measurements can be taken of air flow and fundamental frequency for objective assessment, while a further potential advantage arises from the visual feedback of the patient's performance using a laryngograph which can be a useful adjunct to therapy.

The voice clinic is still for the most part a tertiary referral clinic for 'problem' cases. This means dysphonic patients attending outpatient clinics are not automatically seen in the voice clinic. Many are seen by an ENT surgeon and referred directly to the hospital speech therapist. She sees and assesses them, either providing treatment herself, or passing them on to their local therapist for treatment. As a result it has been possible to compare the performance of these two groups in order to evaluate the effectiveness of the multidisciplinary approach, determine the different characteristics of the two groups, and monitor patients' satisfaction with their treatment.

Method

Samples

Fifty patients from the voice clinic and 50 who had been assessed in the outpatient ENT clinic and referred to speech therapy were randomly selected and asked to complete a questionnaire. All the patients were seen between August 1982 and December 1984, and had completed therapy. Patients with psychiatric disorders were not included, nor were laryngectomees. From the outpatient group, 36 patients returned their questionnaire and 37 from the voice clinic group.

Questionnaire

The questionnaire contains three sections.

The first related to the characteristics of each group, and included the following information: the patient's age, sex, smoking habits, concomitant disorders, the nature of their work and voice use, the length of time before seeking help and seeing a specialist, whether or not the voice returned to normal; it also investigated the time this took, and the length of time off work or prevented from participating in various activities because of their voice disorder.

The second section deals with the course of the voice disorder. A nine-point rating scale (ranging from very dissatisfied (9), dissatisfied (8), fairly dissatisfied (7), slightly dissatisfied (6), neutral (5), slightly satisfied (4), fairly satisfied (3), satisfied (2), and very satisfied (1), was used to assess the following voice qualities:

(1) Voice quality.
(2) Pitch range.
(3) Volume.
(4) Comfort.
(5) Overall pitch.
(6) Vocal stamina.
(7) The comments of others.

Figure 17.1: Category Scheme for Diagnosis

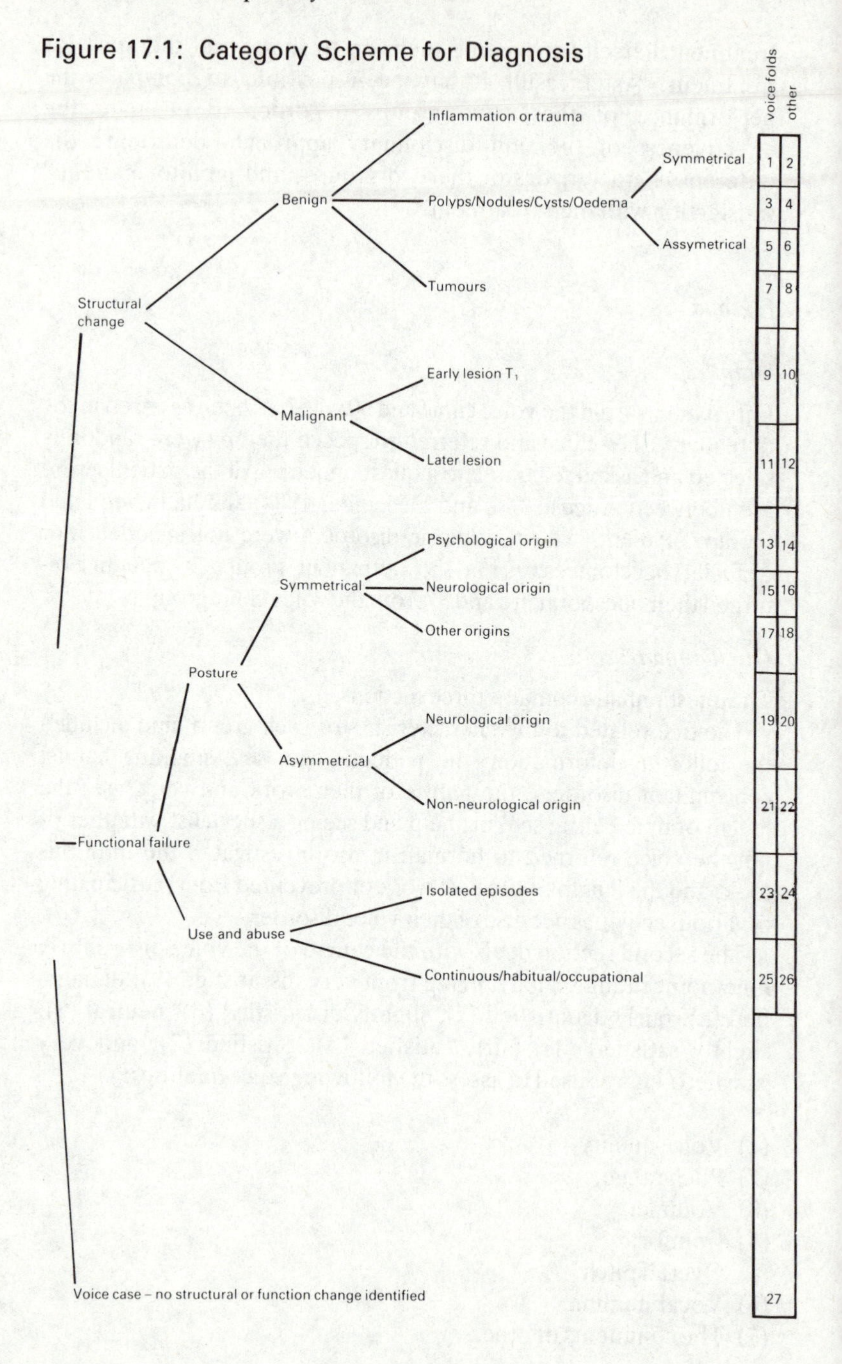

The patients completed these scales to rate their voice before the disorder, when at its worst, and following treatment.

The final section included questions to determine how many people were involved in the assessment and management of the voice disorder, and the patient's rating of how satisfied they were with this on the same nine-point scale described earlier. The following group of people were rated:

(1) The general practitioner,
(2) The local speech therapist,
(3) The hospital doctor,
(4) The hospital speech therapist,
(5) The voice clinic.

Screening of Case Notes

In addition to the questionnaire, the case notes for all the patients were reviewed and the main items of information transferred to a summary sheet. Diagnosis was recorded by assigning each case to one of 26 coding categories, or else category 27, 'NAD' (nil abnormal discovered) in the cases where no specific pathology had been found. The category scheme for diagnosis is summarised in Figure 17.1.

Results

The Characteristics of the Samples

As a separate matter from the criteria by which the two samples were originally selected, they were found in the course of analysing the results to have a number of other similarities and differences which are summarised in Table 14.1. This, of course, means that this was not a fully controlled trial on perfectly matched samples, but nevertheless gives a good preliminary indication of the kinds of people receiving the two sets of treatment and how they fared. Given the smallness of the samples collected, a number of the differences were not statistically significant, but nevertheless they provide an interesting summary of the information collected so far, and a guide to further research.

In order to assess the severity of the disorder of the two groups, the mean of ratings were calculated as given by the patients to the

Table 17.1: The Characteristics of the Two Samples

	Outpatient	Voice Clinic
Mean age	52.7	50.9
Per cent males	35.5	44.4
Per cent smokers	32.3	2.2
Per cent reporting neck problems	33.3	25.0
Per cent reporting reflux	22.6	25.7
Per cent reporting persistent sore throats	38.7	28.6
Per cent reporting tremor/ rigidity	6.7	6.1

Table 17.2: Voice Properties Before Disorder and at Worst Rated (1–9)

	Outpatients	Voice clinic
Before disorder		
sound quality	7.69	7.97
pitch range	7.50	7.73
power	7.58	7.87
comfort	7.52	7.53
pitch	7.58	7.90
stamina	7.28	7.56
opinion of others	7.38	7.59
When at worst		
sound quality	3.68	3.34
pitch range	3.38	3.48
power	3.32	3.37
comfort	3.29	2.88
pitch	3.74	3.83
stamina	3.24	2.48
opinion of others	3.43	4.36

sound, range, power, comfort, pitch, stamina and other's opinions of their voice before having a voice disorder, and when their voice was at its worst. These results are shown in Table 17.2

The voice clinic samples report rather worse disorder of the qualities of sound, comfort and stamina in particular.

The course of events was worked out for the voice clinic samples showing how each of the seven voice quality variables changed from before the disorder, to its height, and then to the time following treatment. This is shown in Table 17.3.

Table 17.3: Time – course of Treatment for Voice Clinic Sample – means on a Rating Scale of 1–9

	Before Disorder	At Worst	After Treatment
Sound quality	7.97	3.34	7.41
Pitch range	7.73	3.48	6.40
Power	7.87	3.36	6.81
Comfort	7.53	2.88	6.21
Pitch	7.90	3.83	7.00
Stamina	7.56	2.48	5.88
Opinion of others	7.59	4.36	7.30

Generally all the variables show a positive trend and recover well, but there are differences. Pitch range, comfort, and power are the properties that remain problematic even after treatment. Comfort and stamina fall to the lowest levels during the disorder and the opinions of others shows the least marked depression during the disorder.

A number of other methods reflect on the effectiveness of diagnosis and treatment in the two groups, and these are shown in Table 14.4.

These results suggest that patients in the voice clinic group are seen by a specialist sooner; are more likely to be viewable at indirect laryngoscopy; have less time away from work or hobbies because of their voice problem, and also feel that there is greater consistency in the people by whom they are seen in the clinic. Furthermore they rate the joint voice clinic as the most helpful agency seen by either group of patients, and most significantly (statistically significant at $p>0.01$) many more voice clinic patients

Table 17.4 Effectiveness of Diagnosis and Treatment

	Outpatient	Voice Clinic
Months before seeking help	11.0	6.6
Months before seeking ENT specialist	10.1	4.5
Per cent viewable at IDL	82.1	94.4
Months off work or other activities because of voice	8.7	5.6
Rated constancy of clinical personnel (1–5 scale)	3.71	4.37
Rated helpfulness of professional groups (1–9 scale):		
general practitioners	7.68	6.50
district speech therapists	8.39	7.89
hospital doctors	8.19	7.97
hospital speech therapists	8.54	8.44
joint voice clinic	—	8.61
Per cent NAD	46	6**

** $p \langle 0.01$ (test for the significance of the difference of two proportions, 2 = 3.71).

than outpatients have a specific pathology identified and recorded in their case notes.

Discussion

The main factors highlighted by this evaluation are that the patients seen in the voice clinic are generally worse at the height of their voice disorder than the outpatient group and yet achieve a comparable level of recovery. Also, significantly more voice clinic patients can be given a specific diagnosis, rather than fall in the 'NAD' (nil abnormal discovered) category. Looking in detail at the recovery of specific vocal attributes it is found that both comfort and stamina recover less well than such things as voice quality or volume. Since these are both attributes that cannot be objectively measured by doctors or therapists, they do not receive as much attention in treatment as the more easily measured attributes to which treatment is usually addressed. It is perhaps important to aim therapy more towards these problems, as it is likely these are some of the most distressing for the patients.

Secondary findings of the evaluation are that the voice clinic patient group were viewable at indirect laryngoscopy in the clinic more often, thus saving unnecessary hospital admission for direct laryngoscopy under anaesthetic. They were off work or inconvenienced by their voice disorder for less time than the outpatient group. Finally they received greater continuity of management in the voice clinic, which they seemed to prefer, as they gave it the highest rating. Their rating of the voice clinic was also higher than any of the forms of management received by the outpatient group, who of course had not been to the voice clinic and gave their highest rating to the hospital speech therapist.

Looking at working voices and trying to equate what we see with the sound we hear has always been somewhat 'hit and miss'. We hope that by evaluating our own performance as well as that of the patient, we may in the future be able to help improve the 'state of the art' into the 'state of the science' to the benefit of both the artists and the scientists concerned.

Acknowledgements

We would like to thank the ENT departments of the Radcliffe Infirmary, Oxford and the Royal Berkshire Hospital, Reading; also the Speech Therapy Department, Radcliffe Infirmary, Oxford.

References

Abberton, E. and Fourcin, A. J., 'Laryngographic Analysis and Intonation', *British Journal of Disorders of Communication*, 7(1), 24–30 (1972)

Berry, R. J., Epstein, R., Fourcin, A. J., Freeman, M., MacCurtain, F., and Noscoe, M. J. 'An Objective Analysis of Voice Disorder: Part 1 and 2', *British Journal of Disorders of Communication*, 17(1), 67–76, 84–90 (1982)

Harris, T. M., Collins, S. R. C. and Clarke, D. D. 'Multidisciplinary Voice Clinics: An Appraisal', Paper presented to symposium on *Recent Advances in Voice Conservation*, Royal Society of Medicine, London, 26 April 1985

——, Collins, S. R. C. and Clarke, D. D. 'The Oxford Voice Clinic: Preliminary Research Results', in Harris, T. M., Collins, S. R. C. and Clarke, D. D. (eds) *Developments in Voice Conservation* (Bruel and Kjaer, London, in press)

Laver, J., Hiller, S., and Hanson, R. 'Comparative Performance of Pitch Detection Algorithms on Dysphonic Voices', *Proceedings, IEEE International Conference on Acoustics, Speech and Signal Processing*, Paris, May 1982

Simpson, I. C. 'Dysphonia: The Organisation and Working of a Dysphonia Clinic', *British Journal of Disorders of Communication* 6(1), 70–85 (1971)
Williams, G. T., Farquharson, I. M. and Anthony, J. 'Fibreoptic Laryngoscopy in the Assessment of Laryngeal Disorders', *Journal of Laryngology*, 89(3), 299–310 (1975)

18 VOICE REFERRALS IN A GENERAL HOSPITAL

Eryl Evans

Introduction

This chapter describes the running of a voice clinic within the speech therapy department of a general hospital. The hospital itself is relatively small (400 beds) and deals mainly with acute problems, the inpatient population being largely transient. The ENT department, on the other hand, serves a large, rural catchment area and, therefore the proportion of ENT patients among the speech therapy caseload is high. Over a period of 12 months, just under half the patients referred to the department had some form of voice disorder, and this obviously influences the running of the department.

Apart from ENT referrals, other patients referred from within the hospital usually have acquired language disorders following cerebrovascular problems (excluding specific neurological and neurosurgical problems which are generally dealt with at a neighbouring hospital). The management of both sets of patients is vastly different, as the majority of ENT patients are referred as outpatients as opposed to inpatients, although there is a certain amount of involvement with the ENT ward. Most are seen following a consultation at the consultant clinics, and this obviously necessitates liaison with the outpatients' staff as well as the medical staff, and the close proximity of the ENT and speech therapy clinics can be both a blessing and a hindrance to the general smooth running of the department!

The information which follows is based on individual experience, in a specific situation, and the points discussed will not apply universally. The proportion of ENT patients referred and treated will vary from setting to setting, as well as depending on therapists' interest. However, some common issues can be raised, and some of these will be discussed.

What Sort of Person is Referred for Voice Therapy?

During a four-year period from April 1980, all patients referred for voice therapy have been classified, as far as possible, according to guidelines suggested by Simpson (1971) based on Luchsinger and Arnold (1965). A total of 360 were referred and classified as follows.

Dysplastic Dysphonia

No cases of congenital disorders of the larynx were referred. This is probably due to the paediatric department being situated at another local hospital.

Traumatic Dysphonia

Three cases were referred with dysphonia resulting from laryngeal injury. Two were as a result of direct blows to the laryngeal cartilages and one following damage to the strap muscles during surgery (this patient was transferred before therapy commenced). The laryngeal blows had caused immobilisation and swelling of the vocal cords, and swallowing and breathing were affected. However, there was no permanent nervous damage and both recovered without formal therapy other than advice. No functional problems occurred and vocal recovery was good.

Mechanical Dysphonia

This group of patients was the largest, with a total of 131 referred with dysphonia due to faulty voice production. They presented as either hyperfunctional or hypofunctional problems and were often long-standing and recurrent. Although the vocal problems were caused by laryngeal strain, the number of additional psychological problems described by some was sufficient for an additional 32 cases to be categorised under 'Mechanical dysphonia with strong functional overlay'. The distinction between these and cases of functional dysphonia is often difficult. The presenting symptoms of mechanical dysphonia included the following.

Reinke's Oedema. For this 23 cases were referred, with the severity of oedema varying from localised swelling to generalised laryngeal oedema. The majority made progress following therapy, but in eight cases vocal abuse persisted and surgical stripping of the vocal cords was necessary.

Vocal Nodules. For this 57 cases were referred where persistent vocal abuse had resulted in the formation of non-malignant nodes on the vocal cords. A proportion of these were seen post-surgery for the removal of the larger of two nodes, and others were referred so that voice therapy could attempt to reverse the disorder. Each group had its successes and failures, but generally the early diagnosis of nodules resulted in good therapeutic results. Post-surgery therapy, aimed at preventing reformation was also successful in most cases.

Contact Ulcer. Only one case was referred with a diagnosis of a contact ulcer. He presented with a well-established ulcer following prolonged, excessive voice use, and surgery was necessary. Following a period of complete voice rest, vocal recovery was good and therapy successfully carried out.

Tensor Weakness. For this 28 cases were referred with 'bowing of the cords', 'incomplete approximation' or similar diagnosis, where habitual vocal abuse had resulted in vocal cord weakness. There were no cases of permanent myopathy and all achieved a functional voice, although still weak under stress. There were often strong psychological factors which maintained the dysphonia beyond the point where the laryngeal condition had improved.

False Cord Phonation (Ventricular Dysphonia). For this 14 cases were referred where the ventricular folds were seen on laryngoscopy to approximate above the vocal cords during phonation. All but one achieved true vocal cord phonation following therapy, which was usually prolonged, due to the resistance to changing vocal habits. One lady totally failed to improve despite numerous approaches, but had complained of the disorder for 20 years!

Precancerous Lesions (Hyperkeratosis, Leukoplakia). Eight cases were included in this category. Although reported as being of 'obscure pathology' (Simpson, 1971) they are associated with chronic irritation or excessive vocal use, and regress under voice therapy. Two cases required stripping of the cords despite therapy, although there had been some reduction in severity.

Inflammatory Dysphonia

A diagnosis of 'chronic laryngitis' was made for 26 patients, where the irritation of the cords had been caused by factors other than mechanical ones. Ten had non-specific bacterial infections, secondary to respiratory infections and 16 were caused by irritation from fumes, dust or other environmental irritants. Despite therapy, six cases failed to improve due to the persisting irritant levels which could not be reduced.

Vasomotor Dysphonia

Four cases were referred with dysphonia due to unilateral monochorditis. The autonomic nerve supply to the larynx had been disturbed following allergic reactions, resulting in episodes of transient dysphonia. Three were teachers with additional pressures of voice use at work, who continued to have a predisposition to this condition, even when the dysphonia itself had improved.

Endocrine Dysphonia

A number of endocrine disorders may result in dysphonia, but only two categories were referred – two cases of puberphonia, and two of dysphonia due to thyroid imbalance. The young men with failure of vocal mutation at puberty were able to achieve a vocal quality and pitch more appropriate to their age and sex, and had no difficulty maintaining their 'new' voices. Two ladies reported frequent hoarseness following thyroid imbalance and on examination showed incomplete glottal closure. One failed to improve her voice due to excessive vocalis muscle atrophy, resulting in permanent bowing of the cords. The second lady was able to improve vocal quality following endrocrinological and voice therapy.

Functional Dysphonia

In this category 63 cases of dysphonia were referred, where the disorder is psychogenic in origin. (As mentioned previously, it is often difficult to differentiate this category from that of mechanical dysphonia with functional overlay.) The severity of the problems varied from long-standing aphonia to occasional weakness, and the majority of problems seemed to be triggered by anxiety. The variety of symptoms was surpassed only by the complicated and often tragic case history details. Only one patient refused any attempt at vocal rehabilitation, and recovery for the remainder varied from dramatic voice restoration to slow, gradual recovery requiring prolonged therapy. Frequent follow-up appointments were necessary to ensure maintenance of the voice. Ten cases were men, all with occupational pressures, although one had developed a functional dysphonia following treatment for laryngeal malignancy.

Paralytic Laryngeal Dysphonia

For this 33 cases were referred with paralysis of one or both cords. The interruption of the nerve supply was caused by a variety of disorders including a cerebral haemorrhage, pressure from a secondary tumour, surgical damage during thyroidectomy and one case where the cord palsy was the first symptom of motor neurone disease, although this was not diagnosed until later. Where a unilateral cord palsy was unresolved after six months of therapy, the ENT surgeons considered the injection of Teflon into the affected cord. This was most effective where a weak voice was possible, but tired easily.

Dysarthric Dysphonia

Five cases were referred where the dysphonia originated from disorders of the central nervous system, with laryngeal as well as resonatory and articulatory functions being disturbed. Three patients were suffering from multiple sclerosis, and had difficulty with phonation timing and vocal quality. During remission periods, all three found voice exercises helpful in controlling the voice. Two further patients were referred following reduction in vocal volume due to Parkinson's disease. Both benefited from work on breathing and the provision of pocket amplifiers, although long-term effects were minimal.

Myopathic Dysphonia

There were no referrals of dysphonia caused by a block at the neuromuscular junction, for example myasthenia gravis.

Arthritic Dysphonia

Two patients, with a history of polyarthritis, were referred with fixation of the vocal cords and acute inflammation of the larynx. Both reported difficult and painful phonation, and one improved as the arthritis subsided. Where the disease remained, the voice remained hoarse.

Neoplastic Dysphonia

Ten patients were referred following surgical removal of vocal cord polyps. Not all cases of polyps require voice therapy, and the voice usually recovers spontaneously. Where the hoarseness persisted after surgery, voice therapy was arranged, and in six cases there were obvious vocal abuse patterns which had contributed to the problem.

Alaryngeal Aphonia

For this 47 cases were referred for therapy following diagnosis of malignancy in the larynx which required laryngectomy. Due to the specialised management of this group, they are not included in the general information which follows.

Involvement with the ENT Department

An essential condition for the acceptance of a patient for voice therapy is a recent ENT report. Although 'the majority of voice disorders are the result of abuse and misuse of vocal mechanisms' (Boone 1977), the possibility of laryngeal pathology must be investigated before therapy is considered. When referrals are received from sources other than the ENT department, a request is made for the appropriate examination to be arranged, either by the referral agent or directly by the speech therapy department..

In an ideal situation, the speech therapist and ENT surgeon would interview dysphonic patients together, providing information required by both disciplines. Additionally, the interrelationship of the disciplines is emphasised for the patient. However, most speech therapists are pressurised by large caseloads and waiting lists and are unable to allocate time to attendance at ENT clinics, when not all patients are in need of therapy.

At present, we have a working relationship, which although not ideal, encompasses some of the requirements, and has obviously been developed for our specific situation. For example, due to clinical commitments, it is impossible for us to attend all the ENT ward rounds, but arrangements are made for attendance at the examination of specified patients. (Therapists experienced in ward rounds will appreciate that timing the arrival at patients is impossible, but a discreet telephone call from the ward staff is usually possible.) Our attendance at the ENT outpatient clinic is also restricted to specified periods, and where a patient cannot be seen during that time, arrangements are made for the speech therapist to be present for the laryngoscopy only. The opportunity to see the patient's larynx is invaluable as voice therapy can be more effective when based on experience of viewing laryngeal pathology.

It is also useful to meet the junior medical staff as they are appointed to the ENT department so that the speech therapist can introduce some concepts of her role in the management of their patients. There should then be carry over into the information received in referrals. Although it is difficult to insist on specific classifications, we can now expect information regarding presenting symptoms, condition of the larynx on indirect laryngoscopy and relevant medical investigations.

General Management of Voice Cases

The management of patients referred with voice problems depends a great deal on individual circumstances and facilities, but it cannot be too strongly emphasised that management must begin with the ENT examination. No patient is accepted for voice therapy, however mild the dysphonia, unless there has been a recent diagnosis by a laryngologist. This examination not only investigates the possibility of malignancy, but also provides essential information for the speech therapist regarding the condition and appearance of the vocal cords, larynx and related organs.

When the referral and all relevant information has been received, the initial interview is arranged. This may, or may not, be the first time that the patient has encountered the therapist and the latter often has to explain why the referral was made. (This situation is made much easier when the need for therapy is emphasised by the laryngologist.) Once the rationale for therapy has been explained, the case history and voice assessment is carried out. Details required during case history taking will vary according to the presenting problem, but adequate time is allocated for this first interview, and time allowed for treatment to commence at the end of the session.

From the information given in the laryngologist's report, the speech therapist is aware of the likely vocal symptoms and plan of treatment, and information obtained during the history will decide finer details. After taking the details and explaining and discussing the voice problem, the patient is given some immediate guidance on how to alleviate this. Advice is given regarding voice use so that it may be conserved for as long as possible. Specific situations are described so that the patient can relate the given information to his or her situation. The aim is to give this information and advice at a level which the patient can understand and, therefore, carry out effectively. Exercises are practised in the clinic and then written down for reference so that the likelihood of forgetting or misunderstanding is diminished. Greene (1972) advocates intensive daily therapy and this is obviously beneficial when attempting to instil new vocal habits. However, it is often impossible to offer such intensive therapy either due to clinical limitations, or employment difficulties for the patient. It is occasionally possible for a general practitioner to arrange sick leave for intensive voice therapy, but most can attend only once or twice weekly.

When the initial interview has been held, the laryngologist is informed of the outcome and the proposed plan of treatment outlined. A progress report is sent prior to the next ENT appointment along with a request for information regarding change in the laryngeal condition. As the speech therapy department is on the same site as the ENT clinic, it is possible to attend review appointments and receive the information firsthand. As treatment progresses review speech therapy appointments are coincided with ENT visits as it is important not to discharge the patient completely until progress can be maintained without supervision.

Facilities and Equipment Required

As for most therapists, the facilities and equipment desirable in dealing with voice cases are not those generally available. However, it is possible to run a successful voice clinic with basic equipment; Greene (1972) suggests the following essentials.

A Detailed Case History

This can be taken using a commercial form (such as Boone Voice Program for Adults, 1980), detailed headings as suggested by Luchsinger and Arnold (1965), or from the therapist's own guidelines. Our present format includes the categories:

(1) Present problem.
(2) Past history.
(3) General health.
(4) Occupation.
(5) Family and social history.
(6) Personality.

Each category contains subsections which might be relevant: for example, details of onset of voice problems, precipitating factors etc. Information required for specific voice disorders is included separately.

An Auditory Assessment of Dysphonia

While obtaining the history, the therapist will be listening and watching not merely to the information being given, but the way in which it is given, allowing insight into the person as a whole and not merely the symptoms presented. A tape recording of the dysphonic voice is essential, and although the quality of recording available to therapists is not always high, this is a useful tool, along with clinical observations of general tension, breathing, articulation and description of the voice itself.

Observation of Breathing

In addition to noting the method of breathing, whether clavicular, abdominal etc., the control of breathing for speech is noted and specific testing of phonation time and breath control carried out.

Observation of Oral and Laryngeal Movements

This is the way in which the patient uses his articulators for speech. Tension in this area can obviously relate to generalised tension of the laryngeal area. Laryngeal movements are observed by the ENT surgeon using either mirror laryngoscopy or fibreoptic laryngoscopy. In both cases, the speech therapist can view the larynx, either by means of a teaching attachment to the mirror or with an additional eyepiece on the fibrescope.

An ENT Report

This gives information regarding the appearance and health of the respiratory tract and the condition and movements of the cords.

Equipment Used in Therapy

This includes the following:

(1) A high quality tape recorder for assessment and recording progress as well as developing awareness in the patient.

(2) An amplifier to provide feedback for disorders where excess volume is used or amplification where insufficient vocal volume is produced.

(3) A pitch pipe which helps some patients achieve the optimum pitch for the voice.

(4) Videotaping facilities are becoming more commonly available and a visual as well as auditory record is informative for both patient and therapist alike.

(5) Printed exercise sheets — although many voice programmes have to be tailored to individual needs, we have a supply of printed exercises for the most common techniques of therapy. Relaxation and breathing exercises can be dealt with in this way, as can advice regarding vocal abuse for both inpatients and outpatients. However, these are always accompanied by explanation and discussion and do not replace therapy.

Some of the Problems

Therapists working with voice disorders could, no doubt, compile an extensive list of problems, which voice cases bring with them. Lack of co-operation from ENT surgeons can result in vague and sparse referrals. The patient is not made aware of the relevance of voice therapy and this leads to poor motivation to attend therapy (although this can also happen with the well-informed patient!). Feedback to and from the therapist is thus restricted and therapy becomes isolated. Patient motivation to carry out exercises may be poor once the absence of malignancy is confirmed. They may be reluctant to be absent from work 'just for my voice'. Where the patient is a professional voice user, employment pressures add to the tension already present.

Few therapists can boast ideal facilities and equipment, struggling instead in noisy, poorly equipped rooms where ingenuity is stretched in dealing with limited resources.

However, there continue to be many attractions to running a voice clinic in a general hospital, and these usually outweigh the problems, providing the therapist with a great deal of satisfaction.

References

Boone, D. R. *The Voice and Voice Therapy*, 2nd edn (Prentice-Hall Inc., Englewood Cliffs, New Jersey, 1977)

—— *The Boone Voice Program for Adults*. (CC Publications Inc., Oregon, Distributed by Taskmaster Ltd., 1980)

Greene, M. C. L. *The Voice and its Disorders*, 3rd edn (Pitman Medical, Tunbridge Wells, 1972)

Luchsinger, R. and Arnold, G. E. (1965) *Voice–Speech–Language, Clinical Communicology: Its Physiology and Pathology* (Constable, London, 1965)

Simpson, I. C. 'Dysphonia: The Organisation and Working of a Dysphonia Clinic', *British Journal of Disorders of Communication*, 6, 70 (1971)

AUTHOR INDEX

SUBJECT INDEX